THE SURVIVOR'S GUIDE TO SWINE FLU

THE COMPLEMENTARY MEDICAL APPROACH

JAYNEY GODDARD
FCMA, LIC.LCCH, DIP.ACH

PRESIDENT:
THE COMPLEMENTARY MEDICAL ASSOCIATION (THE CMA)

DISCLAIMER

The information in this book is in no way intended to replace the advice of your primary health practitioner – be this your doctor or your qualified complementary medical practitioner. If you wish to make any significant lifestyle changes you should do so under their guidance. We cannot claim to prevent or cure Swine Flu (H1N1) as none of the approaches that we recommend have yet been scientifically tested on the severe form of H1N1 that is currently circulating. This information has been produced in good faith and it is based upon scientific research and historical data. We present it to you so that you can take responsibility for making informed decisions about your own health care.

The Survivor's Guide to Swine Flu: The Complementary Medical Approach by Jayney Goddard

Copyright © 2009 Jayney Goddard-Hawkins. All rights reserved. Paperback edition is printed in the United Kingdom. E-Book edition created in the United Kingdom. No parts of the paperback or e-book edition may be reproduced or transmitted in any form or by any means, electronic or mechanical, including photocopying, recording, or by an information storage and retrieval system, without written permission from the publisher, CMA Publishing UK. For information contact CMA Publishing UK at Info@The-CMA.Org.UK

CMA Publishing UK is a division of The Complementary Medical Association (The CMA) and the logo is a registered trademark.

Designed by Dave Hawkins at Tzu Ltd.

Contact details; Results@Hawk-in.Co.UK

ISBN 978-0-9553457-1-5

Goddard, Jayney
The Survivor's Guide to Swine Flu:
The Complementary Medical Approach
– CMA Publishing UK
Includes bibliographical references.

AUTHOR BIOGRAPHY

Jayney Goddard FCMA, Lic.LCCH, Dip.ACH, is President of The Complementary Medical Association (The CMA), the world's largest professional membership organisation for qualified Complementary Medical practitioners and Complementary Medical training organisations.

A passionate and dynamic international speaker, writer, teacher and broadcaster, Jayney Goddard is considered to be one of the world's leading experts in the Complementary, Alternative and Integrated Medical fields. She consults for Governments world-wide to assist them in integrating Complementary Medicine into their healthcare systems and is committed to consistently raising levels of excellence within the Complementary Medical profession in general. Jayney is a Fellow of the Royal Society of Medicine and holds many official Advisory roles within high profile Complementary and Natural Healthcare organisations.

A prolific author, Jayney has written 4 encyclopædias (online) and is the Editor of the critically acclaimed "Complementary and Alternative Medicine: The Scientific Verdict on What Really Works" published by Collins. Jayney wrote "The Survivor's Guide to Bird Flu: The Complementary Medical Approach" in 2006, and has a number of other titles which are due to be published before the end of 2009. Jayney is the Editor of "With Our Complements" the Journal of The CMA and is a regular contributor to national newspapers and magazines in the UK and worldwide.

Jayney is a regular expert guest on a number of high profile television and radio shows in the UK and worldwide, she is also a popular Keynote Speaker at the various high level Complementary and Integrative Medical conferences around the world.

One of Jayney's most recent achievements was developing and hosting the "Scientific Research in Homeopathy" Conference held at the University of Westminster (London, UK). Jayney is also dedicated to helping practitioners develop both professionally and commercially and she facilitates regular workshops for practitioners. Jayney has a number of extremely high-profile public events planned for 2009 and beyond and you can keep abreast of these on The CMA website: The-CMA.Org.UK

ADVISORY NOTES

A NOTE TO PATIENTS WHO ARE TAKING CONVENTIONAL MEDICINE

We believe that it is very important for people to have as much information as they need – in order to make informed decisions about important matters such as their health and wellbeing. In this book we aim to help you do that by setting out for you the various options that you can consider. These will help you to improve your health and become less susceptible to a great range of illnesses, including viruses. The recommendations in this book have been scientifically proven to help people become healthier and it is possible that you may feel that you would like to reduce dosages of drugs or even stop taking certain forms of medication.

While it may, indeed, be possible for you to reduce dosages or even stop taking some kinds of medication, it is extremely important to point out that you must not do this without your doctor's consent and guidance.

This is vitally important as it can be very dangerous to alter your dosage or come off some forms of medication too rapidly and you will need your doctor's help to withdraw from certain prescribed drugs.

A NOTE TO DOCTORS

This book contains much sensible, thoroughly researched general health advice that is suited to the vast majority of people. Our recommendations are in no way intended to replace any advice that you may wish to give to your patients and we offer our recommendations to people on the basis that this will equip them to make informed decisions about their healthcare. Scientific evidence shows that should people follow the advice outlined in this book they will become generally healthier and fitter and be less predisposed to chronic degenerative disease.

However, please also be aware that research shows that in extremely unusual cases, one of the recommendations we make – eating garlic – may rarely, interact with anti-coagulant medication. In even more unusual situations, curcumin (derived from turmeric) may also act as an anti-thrombotic. If you are concerned about this, we suggest that you may wish to monitor patients' clotting factors. The Complementary Medical Association's website The-CMA.Org.UK has a full database of drug/herb/supplement interactions, if you wish to make sure that none of the drugs that your patients are taking interact with any of the nutritional or herbal recommendations in this book. In addition, should you have any questions or require clarification about any of the advice in this book please contact us at Info@TheCMA.Org.UK

A NOTE TO PRACTITIONERS OF COMPLEMENTARY MEDICINE

Throughout this book we stress that people must consult their practitioner in order to address any underlying health issues – in order for them to become as resilient as possible to viral infection and to benefit fully from the recommendations in this book. This book contains over 500 scientific references that support and verify many of the types of approaches that you may already take with your patients. We hope that this will be useful to you and will help to enhance your practice.

This book bridges the gap between complementary and conventional Medicine and we hope that you can use the information in this book to help your patients to understand that the advice that you are giving is supported by robust scientific data.

In addition, we believe that the information and research within this book will help to open dialogues with conventional medical doctors who will, no doubt, appreciate that hard science does, indeed, exist behind many complementary medical approaches. Ultimately, this will benefit the people who matter most of all – the patients.

The Complementary Medical Association will, in due course be holding a number of Swine Flu seminars aimed at medical professionals – both complementary and conventional and these will equip you with the information that you need in order to give your patients the very best information about Swine Flu and viral resilience. If you would like to know more please email The Complementary Medical Association at Info@The-CMA.Org.UK

If you are a fully qualified practitioner but you are not already a Member of The CMA we recommend you join. You can do this online at The-CMA.Org.UK

ANIMAL EXPERIMENTATION

This book bridges the gap between complementary and conventional Medicine and includes over 500 references to scientific experiments and some of these have involved animals. It is important to make clear that Jayney Goddard and The Complementary Medical Association do not support any animal testing that is either unnecessary, or for products that are not essential to human life.

Complementary medical approaches never advocate animal testing as the substances that we use e.g. vitamins, essential oils, herbs, homeopathic remedies etc. generally have a long history of use and a great deal is already known about them. Furthermore, animal physiology is vastly different to that of humans and this makes much animal experimentation redundant. We believe that it is wrong to inflict pain and that we are morally obliged to respect the lives of all creatures, while also considering that we do have a duty to promote human welfare and prevent human suffering.

ACKNOWLEDGEMENTS:

With love, respect and thanks to all who have made this book possible - you know who you are.

This book is dedicated to all who work tirelessly on behalf of The CMA: Hawkeye, Jill, Roberta, Ratna, Bruce, Tessa, Lesley, Bianca and to our ever-growing Membership body - people and organisations who examplify excellence across the entire field of complementary Medicine.

Reviews for "The Survivor's Guide to Bird Flu: The Complementary Medical Approach"

"An important and much needed overview on the subject of bird flu and more importantly, how to protect yourself from it." **Dr Mark Atkinson, Integrated Medical Doctor**

"When I was first asked to review this book by Jayney Goddard, I knew I was in for a good read. Goddard is the President of the Complementary Medical Association and an authority on several aspects of Complementary Medicine. . . . the book is a very good source of vital information that goes beyond 'Bird Flu', and I would recommend it for anyone who deals largely with the immune system as a specific area, and diseases that primarily affect it." **Dr Neil Slade BSc(Hons), PhD, LCH, CBiol., MIBiol.**

"As a former Army Officer turned therapist I am deeply aware of the historical effect of diseases on armies. Generally, armies have suffered more casualties as a result of disease than they have from enemy action. A lot of times these casualties could have been prevented by taking basic precautions and analysing the potential threats and putting in place the appropriate response. I find this book an excellent threat analysis with a belt and braces approach, both pro-active and reactive, to surviving the bird-flu." **Dan Kahn MSc, Bi-Aura Practitioner**

" . . . Jayney Goddard's brilliantly informative 'The Survivors Guide to Bird Flu: The Complementary Medical Approach' arrived in the Round Up offices this week and is an authoritative and indispensable handbook for anyone concerned about a possible pandemic.

Containing over 500 scientific references and historical evidence backing up the authors recommendations, the book bridges the gap between complementary and conventional Medicine and shows you what you can do, as an individual, to enhance your immune system and become as resistant to viral infection as possible." **Carl Munson, Journalist and Complementary Medicine Expert**

"The Book that everyone MUST buy!" **In the Know magazine - front page headline**

*"Jayney Goddard has produced an exceptionally readable and informative book. Technical terms and scientific research are clearly and simply explained throughout and the information is easily accessible to both the lay reader and those working in the health fields.
Although primarily aimed at how to survive bird flu this book can be widely used by all complementary health practitioners who want clear and concise information on promoting good health and well-being in their clients. It is also useful for the general reader who is keen to improve their general health.*

The author's extensive knowledge and practical advice combined with fascinating research into the history of pandemics and epidemics make this book compelling reading and as a practitioner in complementary therapies I am very glad that it has been written." **Lesley Lucas MSc, Massage Practitioner**

THE SURVIVORS GUIDE TO SWINE FLU: TABLE OF CONTENTS

GENERAL INTRODUCTION

Foreword by Dave Hawkins: Swine Flu raises a number of crucial issues for Complementary Medicine

CMA Members Survey: CMA Registered practitioners were surveyed (June 2009) on their approaches to - and opinions of how to treat Swine Flu.

Chapter 1: Introduction - Why should you consider a complementary medical approach to the prevention and treatment of Swine Flu?

Chapter 2: The History of Pandemics and Epidemics - From the first records to date - what can we learn from history?

Chapter 3: How Serious a Threat is Swine Flu? Where did it come from, what is its global spread and why is this strain so worrying?

Chapter 4: Potential Economic, Political and Social Effects - should this current H1N1 Swine Flu virus mutate to cause a seriously lethal pandemic.

Chapter 5: Swine Flu Time Line: To Date - How did this current pandemic start and a close look at its global spread and development.

Chapter 6: What is a Virus? - How do viruses spread? How does your body fight back? How does a virus get into your system? The pantropism of H1N1 Swine Flu - why this is of concern.

Chapter 7: What is Influenza? How does it affect your body? Viral pneumonia and secondary infections.

Chapter 8: Your Immune System & The Cytokine Storm - Why do some people die of flu? How does your immune system work? what is a cytokine storm and what can be done to prevent this phenomenon?

Chapter 9: Can We Treat Swine Flu with Conventional Medical Approaches? - An examination of the efficacy and safety of current Conventional Medical options - including Tamiflu, Relenza and vaccines.

Chapter 10: What is Complementary Medicine? What are the general principles of Complementary Medicine? How safe is it? Is there any research?

PREPAREDNESS

Chapter 11: Preparedness: Your Survival Unit - Who will be in your "Survival Unit" and what to consider in a survival situation.

Chapter 12: Preparedness: The Psychology of Survival - How to prepare yourself psychologically to maintain optimum chances of survival.

Chapter 13: Preparedness: Shelter - How to ensure that you have adequately prepared shelter.

Chapter 14: Preparedness: Water Supplies - How to find and maintain clean water supplies. How much water do you need to stockpile?

Chapter 15: Preparedness: Hydration & the Dangers of Dehydration - How to hydrate yourself correctly. Oral Rehydration Solution and how to make it. What to do to combat dehydration.

Chapter 16: Preparedness: Cleanliness and Sanitation - Correct handwashing procedures. The health ramifications of cleanliness. How to build a field toilet.

Chapter 17: Preparedness: Food Storage and Stockpiling - How to ensure that you have enough of the correct types of food and supplies.

Chapter 18: Preparedness: Exercise - How much is enough? How much compromises your immune system's response?

COMPLEMENTARY MEDICAL APPROACHES TO THE PREVENTION AND TREATMENT OF SWINE FLU

Chapter 19: Essential Oils - How to use essential oils to 'virus proof' your environment. Which oils are anti-viral and anti-bacterial.

Chapter 20: Herbs - Which herbs can modulate your immune system so that you are less predisposed to an overwhelming inflammatory response? Which herbs have anti-viral and anti-bacterial properties?

Chapter 21: Nutrition & Supplements - The Palæo-Mediterranean diet and how this modulates your immune system to be less predisposed to an acute overwhelming inflammatory response - as in a cytokine storm. Foods and supplements that will help you to be optimally healthy and less predisposed to chronic disease - including arthritis, Type 2 diabetes, heart disease, some cancers, stroke, Alzheimers disease, etc. How to harness the anti-ageing, energy boosting and mood enhancing effects of a correct nutritional approach.

Chapter 22: Homeopathy - The history of homeopathy. what homeopathy is and how it has performed thoughout history in epidemics and pandemics.

Chapter 23: Homeopathic Treatment of Swine Flu - The homeopathic Medicines that the author have identified as being useful for Swine Flu.

Chapter 24: Other Complementary Medical Approaches - A look at some other approaches that could prove useful in preventing and treating Swine Flu.

Chapter 25: Recommendations - A concise round up of all the recommendations in this book.

Appendix: The Six Phases of a Pandemic - The World Health Organisation's definitions.

Emergency Contact Forms - Two forms that you can use in case of emergency

FOREWORD - BY DAVE HAWKINS: HEALTHCARE WRITER

SWINE FLU RAISES A NUMBER OF CRUCIAL ISSUES FOR COMPLEMENTARY MEDICINE AND ITS PRACTITIONERS

Adapted from With Our Complements; The CMA Journal (Summer 2009 edition); Key Issues Raised by the Swine Flu Pandemic

KEY ISSUES RAISED

With the current spread of Swine Flu – officially a level 6 'pandemic' – which has killed hundreds of people in numerous countries, there are a number of issues for Complementary Medicine to face up to – and for all Complementary Medical and Natural Healthcare practitioners to consider.

ISSUE 1; LIARS, FAKES AND THIEVES?

In the US, the Food and Drug Administration (FDA) has started to *"identify and investigate individuals and businesses that wrongfully purport to promote products to prevent, or treat Swine Flu – and to take regulatory, or criminal action against them"*. (May 2009).

As a result of this a number of natural product and CAM sector associations in the States have gathered together to issue a warning to retailers not to stock or sell supplements that make these kind of claims (Natural Products magazine: May 2009).

This 'edict' covered dietary supplements – as this Group claimed they were *"unaware of any scientific data supporting their use to treat swine flu"*.

Now while all sensible people will applaud any efforts to prevent individuals and companies from selling 'unproven' treatments, or products to 'unwitting consumers', shouldn't we consider what this current 'stand' looks like to ordinary people and to governments and health care professionals around the world?

It looks as if all those so called 'con-men, fakes and Alternative health gurus' have been 'brought under control', doesn't it? It looks like a crackdown on Alternative Medical 'quacks' and their 'snake oil' salesmen. Essentially, the FDA's tactics infer that everyone in Complementary Medicine is suspect – they fail to differentiate between the vast numbers of highly qualified, ethical Complementary and Integrated Medical practitioners versus the tiny handful of potential profiteers – many of whom have no qualification in Complementary Medicine at all – and are simply 'bandwagon jumping'.

BUT IS THIS JUST ALL 'SMOKE AND MIRRORS' – AND PERHAPS A DIVERSIONARY TACTIC?

Perhaps the FDA is aware that the Conventional Medical options are not performing as planned: Tamiflu seems to be causing nasty side effects - and recommendations now are for it not to be prescribed to children. Reports in the British Medical Journal show Tamiflu and Relenza rarely prevent complications in children with seasonal flu, yet carry side effects. The BMJ states: *"For most children aged between 1 and 12, the risks associated with taking the drugs may well outweigh any benefits."*

As we know, a vaccine is being rushed into production and many scientists question whether it has been sufficiently tested - and also whether the proposed additives are safe. In the US, vaccine manufacturers are proposing to incorporate the controversial Thimerosal (mercury derived) preservative which has been linked to autism by some researchers and manufacturers also propose to add adjuvents to vaccines to 'make them go further'; proposed substances include aluminium- linked to Alzheimers disease and squalene - linked to auto-immune disease.

During this time of dire crisis, when people are actually dying from a pandemic flu, is there a valid role for qualified Complementary Medical practitioners to play?

Shouldn't someone be speaking up for the Complementary Medical and Natural Healthcare professionals at this time of acute healthcare 'crisis', rather than standing back and watching what's going on, from the sidelines? Bad things happen when good people simply keep silent and watch.

(It's worth noting that amongst the products targeted by the FDA as being a 'scam' lies a range of UV light devices - these have been identified as one of the products being sold that are 'patently fake'. All this is despite years of scientific research on the well established efficacy of UV light (especially from Eastern Europe) in killing viruses and other pathogens. It appears that the FDA can simply make defamatory statements like these above to support its crackdown on these supposed 'snake oil' salesmen.)

Also of concern is which other Complementary Medical therapies and natural healthcare treatments the FDA may lump into its 'Anti-Scam' campaign? Especially when they appear to be patently ignoring much historical and scientific evidence that suggests certain interventions they have targeted are efficacious and valid.

ISSUE 2; "THIS IS SERIOUS – BEST LEAVE IT TO DOCTORS WHO KNOW WHAT THEY'RE DOING"

Let's Play "Devil's Advocate" for a moment:
Since the outbreak of Swine Flu all of the public commentary and news has concentrated on the reactions of Conventional Healthcare and the distribution of 'essential drugs' to combat the threat of Swine Flu. What has happened to the voice of Complementary Medicine and Natural Healthcare?

From the outside it would appear that many practitioners are taking the view that this is no time for 'amateurs like us' to get involved. This is a serious health threat – so now's the time for us to take a back seat – and leave it to doctors – who know what they're doing. Sit back and wait until the promised new vaccine emerges later in the year, even though it will be rushed through with limited testing. Even though governments worldwide are seriously considering compulsory vaccination for the whole population (and visitors?).

Surely it is time for Complementary Medicine and Natural HealthCare and all of its Practitioners, to stand up and be counted? Does your Complementary therapy work? Or is it really time to 'hand over to the professionals'?

No-one in the field of Complementary Medicine would expect all Complementary Medical therapies, or Natural Healthcare approaches to work in the treatment, or prevention of Swine Flu, but what do fully qualified, professional Complementary Medical practitioners really think?(see CMA Practitioner Survey on next page)

ISSUE 3; "I'M NOT STAYING AROUND FOR ALL THIS!"

And what will happen in the UK, if doctors follow up with their threat and refuse to work through a pandemic – from fear of being sued?

This threat was brought to light by the British Medical Association (BMA) on behalf of their GP members. Whilst doctors who work in NHS hospitals are covered by NHS Indemnity insurance, doctors who operate local surgeries are not – and they are concerned that their insurance cover might not protect them against any legal claims made against them during a pandemic for "death–in–service".

One of the BMA's negotiators on Flu Planning said; *"Doctors will be putting their lives on the line and it is only right they can feel assured they are properly covered if anything goes wrong. We don't want to be going into it [a severe pandemic] with GPs feeling unsure where they stand. Doctors are only human and some will not want to go on the front line."*

http://www.hc2d.co.uk/content.php?contentId=11759

But where does that leave individual Complementary Medical and Natural Healthcare Practitioners? Should they deliberately decide NOT to treat patients who come to them with Swine Flu, for risk of being sued? Or should they "boldly go" where GP's may refuse to tread?

WHAT ABOUT THE CREDIBLE COMPLEMENTARY MEDICAL AND NATURAL HEALTHCARE PREVENTION REGIMES AND POTENTIAL EFFECTIVE TREATMENTS FOR SWINE FLU?

Having reviewed 'The Survivor's Guide to Swine Flu; The Complementary Medical Approach', I am convinced that there is sufficient scientific evidence to support a range of Complementary Medical approaches to help prevent the spread of Swine Flu – and to treat it successfully.

As the analyses in the book were mainly based on the H1N1 outbreak of 1918–1919 (The Spanish Flu), the findings still hold true today. I personally believe that one of the most successful treatments for H1N1 then, as it should remain today, is homeopathy. And the role of Herbal treatments, Essential Oils and the correct approach to Nutrition and Hydration remain as crucial as ever.

This book represents an informed view from Jayney Goddard, a professional practitioner, and world renowned expert who does believe that there is only one viable Medical approach – that of a sensible Integrated approach – not a conventional vs 'Alternative' war that only harms the people in need of the best healthcare they can get. She is brave enough to stand up and inform people of what their realistic health choices are in a crisis like this.

THE CMA POLLED ITS MEMBERS ON THIS ISSUE:

THE CMA MEMBERS' SURVEY: JUNE 2009

QUESTION
Do you believe that Complementary Medical Practitioners and Natural Healthcare Practitioners should openly discuss how to treat Swine Flu with their therapies, or should they leave it to Conventional Medical Practitioners to sort out?

A: Should discuss it openly	86%
B: Leave it to Conventional Medicine	7%; includes some responses from of our practitioners who are also conventional doctors.
C: Don't know	7%; worries re: having infectious patients in their practice rooms

A SELECTION OF COMMENTS:

"If I am asked if I can help, I will. If I am asked about conventional treatment, i.e. Tamiflu, vaccination, etc, I refer them to a suitable website and allow them to make up their own minds."

"By all means discuss remedies that actually work: The public have a right to know, for instance, that homeopathy has very good supporting stats from 1918 and is arguably more effective than Tamiflu."

"If we don't help strengthen peoples' constitutions, then what good are we?"

"While a number of complementary therapies could ease the symptoms, e.g. nutrition, herbs, acupuncture, allowing a swine flu patient into the treatment room wouldn't be good as there would be likely contamination to other patients (and self)."

"We should discuss it openly but I do however strongly advocate to work as closely with Conventional Medical Practitioners as possible. Together we hold all the pieces of the jigsaw."

"I personally feel that if a practitioner has any evidence that certain types of therapies are effective in treating swine flu they should discuss openly. In the event of a patient having a diagnosis of Notifiable Infectious Disease, the practitioner should ensure that it is safe to treat that patient and that she/ he has advised the patient not to view CAM as a substitute for any treatment that a doctor has prescribed."

"(A)...but also contact GP? Health authority."

"Having bought Jayney's book on Avian Flu, I certainly mention it and talk about the homeopathic and natural remedies that have been used to treat various types of flu in the past and that perhaps these can be used with current variants."

CHAPTER 1

INTRODUCTION

WHY SHOULD YOU CONSIDER A COMPLEMENTARY MEDICAL APPROACH TO SWINE FLU?

The World Health Organisation (WHO) has described Swine Flu as "unstoppable":

Dr Margaret Chan, Director-General of the WHO said (3rd July, 2009)

> *"As we see today, with well over 100 countries reporting cases, once a fully fit pandemic virus emerges, its further international spread is unstoppable,"*

She did go on to emphasise that the vast majority of patients, to date, had experienced only 'mild' symptoms and most had made a full recovery within a week, without any formal medical treatment.

This latest pandemic flu virus (H1N1) has shown that it can spread rapidly from person to person and from country to country and the WHO, and almost every single country who already have Pandemic Influenza Preparedness Plans in place (having been preparing themselves to face the potential threat of the global spread of the lethal Bird Flu virus (H5N1) over the last few years), have put these into practice swiftly and effectively.

HOWEVER IT IS THE ASSUMPTIONS UNDERLYING THESE PLANS – AND THEIR POTENTIAL INADEQUACIES - THAT MAY BE A CAUSE FOR CONCERN

Given the threat of a sudden, even more severe spread of Flu, these International and National Pandemic Preparedness Plans rely upon a standard, Conventional Medical approach, to keep you and your family safe.

At the heart of this programme is the reliance on the use of the anti-viral drugs Tamiflu and Relenza, and the development of swiftly produced new vaccines. There is also a reliance on the existing health systems in individual countries and a hope that they will be able to cope with an

Introduction

increased demand for care – and deliver an effective response.

The evidence to support this particular well-planned approach as the best way forward should the Swine Flu pandemic progress to an even more severe epidemic, is not necessarily compelling.

THE POTENTIAL STRAIN ON EXISTING HEALTH SYSTEMS?

Whilst the response from the health care authorities in most countries during the rapid spread of the virus in July, appears to have worked well, this might not be the case if the pandemic increases in its severity.

The 'mildness' of the symptoms, for most people and the advice to call a Helpline rather than visiting your local doctor in the UK, appears to have been successful and despite the massive surge in the number of people infected, the health system has managed to handle the outbreak effectively - so far.

A Report from The House of Lords (28th July) was hyper-critical of the UK Government's handling of the crisis over the previous 3 months, citing a confused and perhaps inadequate approach.

THE RELIANCE ON TAMIFLU?

One of the main concerns many experts have, is that there is a heavy reliance on Tamiflu in these Preparedness Plans. This reliance has been questioned by those who are concerned about the effectiveness of Tamiflu (see later).

Even for the people who can get hold of it from their country's, or the world's, supplies and stockpiles, what is the evidence, to date, that it has worked? And, given that some of these stockpiles have been around for a few years, are the supplies still within their 'use-by' date?

There is added concern that some of the people who have managed to get hold of Tamiflu may already be using it as a precautionary measure, even if they haven't caught Swine Flu yet. This has added to the debate about the possible extent of Tamiflu resistance.

Another concern is whether supplies of Tamiflu being sold over the internet are what they claim to be.

THE RELIANCE ON THE DEVELOPMENT OF AN EFFECTIVE, SAFE, VACCINE?

Many experts are also questioning the wisdom of rushing a vaccine out into the marketplace. Concerns about the potential effectiveness of this vaccine may be answered by testing on people who already have Swine Flu (rather than simply testing it on healthy volunteers) but worries about the potential safety hazards might not be so easy to answer.

Given the 'rush' to produce an 'effective' vaccine and the willingness of medical authorities and Governments to approve any and all of those developed, there is no way that anyone will be able to assess the medium-term, let alone the long-term, side effects that these new vaccines may produce.

On top of that, amongst those who have their doubts about the safety and the effectiveness of these new vaccines, there is a dread that Governments - as in the UK - are even considering the implementation of a compulsory vaccination programme.

"WHAT ARE MY OTHER OPTIONS?"

This book has been written with the sole intention of helping YOU examine the options you have when it comes to taking control of your health in the face of a potentially devastating viral infection like Swine Flu.

Our advice is; Don't Panic. But do take time to review the facts about Swine Flu and examine the range of medical options you have.

As you've started to read this book, we assume you are seriously interested in looking at the Complementary - as well as the Conventional Medical options open to you. In the following pages you will discover exactly which options you have and you'll be able to decide which approach you want to take.

TAKE THE NATURAL APPROACH TO BEAT SWINE FLU

We believe that it is entirely possible for you, as an individual, to prepare yourself to be optimally resistant to this H1N1 flu virus - and any other virulent viral infection - by taking a well thought-through Complementary Medical and Natural Healthcare approach.

In addition, should you be unfortunate enough to catch Swine Flu, you'll be equipped to understand how to take a Complementary Medical approach which could give you the ability to survive the illness.

The approach to tackling Swine Flu outlined in this book, is based on historical evidence and robust scientific research and will provide you with all the information you need to make better-informed decisions about what you need to do now, to safeguard your wellbeing. We'll show you how to implement simple lifestyle changes that will improve your general health and make you less likely to catch viral infections like H1N1 - and help you recover from viral attacks on

Introduction

your system.

This Complementary Medical approach does not rely on vaccination, or drugs, to help you cope with severe viral infections like Swine Flu, but uses natural herbs and a range of natural supplements, which, when linked to the development of good habits and a positive mental approach, will help you to prepare yourself so that you are as resistant to viral infection as you can be.

MODULATE YOUR IMMUNE SYSTEM

One of the key themes you'll find with this Complementary Medical approach to making yourself 'healthier' is that of 'modulation'. This is a way of making your immune system work more efficiently when faced with Swine Flu.

In contrast to the approach that many other books and natural healthcare experts have taken towards this topic in recent years, we do not encourage you to 'boost' your immune system when under attack from Swine Flu.

We don't believe that 'immune-boosting' is the correct approach to use against this particular virus - as you'll see later - because of the specific symptoms it causes. In fact, we strongly recommend that the last thing you should do, if you catch Swine Flu, is boost your immune system.

WE'LL EXPLAIN HOW A RANGE OF COMPLEMENTARY MEDICAL APPROACHES CAN HELP IN THE FIGHT AGAINST SWINE FLU

As mentioned above, there are a number of ways you can use Complementary Medical therapies and approaches against the threat of Swine Flu. These include the use of a numer of **immune modulating and anti-viral herbal medicines, immune modulating nutritients and supplementation, anti-viral essential oils (aromatherapy)** and **homeopathy**.

WHY WE EMPHASISE THE ROLE OF HOMEOPATHY

The historical evidence on how homeopathy has been successfully used to treat Swine Flu (H1N1) in the past, is quite compelling. Because of this, you will find an emphasis on homeopathy when it comes to treatment options.

You can read for yourself, the extensive, reliable doctors' reports that demonstrate the effectiveness of homeopathy in the US during the horrendous 1918-19 'Spanish Flu' pandemic. These reports explain the differences in the approaches taken by homeopaths, compared with conventional doctors, at the time, that produced mortality rates of less than 1% for those treated homeopathically (almost everyone survived), compared with the general mortality rates, for those who were infected and treated conventionally, of around 25 – 30%.

The current mortality rates for Swine Flu are very low at around 0.5% (of those reporting to their doctors with the virus and then undergoing treatment). The underlying concern for most health authorities is how they can cope effectively with the infections caused by this Swine Flu virus (H1N1), should it mutate into a more deadly version later in the year.

There is no evidence that this virus is mutating, or getting more virulent at this point in time (in terms of mortality) and laboratory testing around the world indicates the H1N1 virus appears to be behaving the way that it was when reports first started circulating in April 2009.

We do believe that a Complementary and Natural Healthcare approach will work effectively, but all we are doing in this book is helping you to make your own informed choice.

We're going to take you through the facts, then let you decide how you feel YOU can best survive Swine Flu.

THE 'COMPLEMENTARY' APPROACH TO TREATMENT

This approach is NOT an 'alternative' medical approach. It is a 'complementary' one and, as such, draws upon the latest medical research from the fields of virology, immunology and microbiology as well from scientific research into the specific lifestyle changes, herbal medicines and nutrients that we suggest in order to inform our recommendations for action.

CHAPTER 2

THE HISTORY OF PANDEMICS AND EPIDEMICS: FIRST RECORDS TO DATE

THE PELOPONNESIAN PLAGUE

Probably the earliest records of a major "plague" came from reports of the Peloponnesian war (430 B.C.E.). During this great war, between the Athenians and the Spartans, a terrible plague broke out and, in fact the Athenians lost over one third of their army. Until recently it was unknown what caused this disease but in January, 2006 researchers at the University of Athens discovered a mass grave underneath the city. They were able to isolate the bacteria that causes typhoid, from the teeth of people buried there.

What is also known about this disease is its extremely violent onset and the severity of its symptoms. The reason we have a report of this illness at all is because the Greek historian Thucydides actually contracted the disease but survived and was able to report it as follows:

"People in good health were all of a sudden attacked by violent heats in the head, and redness and inflammation in the eyes, the inward parts, such as the throat or tongue, becoming bloody and emitting an unnatural and fetid breath."

Thucydides then went on to describe other violent symptoms including vomiting, diarrhoea, sneezing, coughing and intense spasms. The skin of the victims was reddened and covered in pustules and patients were desperately thirsty.

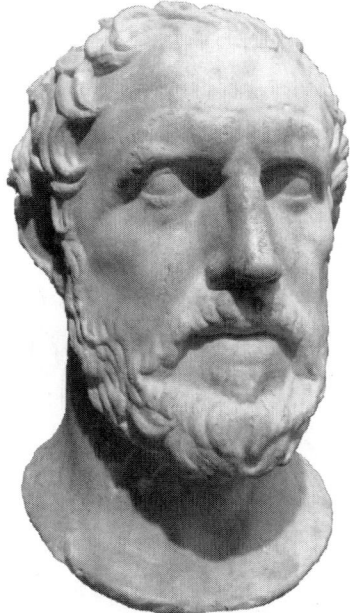

ΘΟΥΚΥΔΙΔΗΣ (THUCYDIDES)

Most victims died after about a week, sooner if the disease affected the bowels, as severe ulceration and the diarrhoea that this caused, proved to be fatally exhausting and dehydrating. The repercussions of this plague were terrible for the survivors too, as they had a legacy of extreme disfigurement to contend with and fingers and toes, even genitals, were lost and many survivors went blind. In addition to this – many people completely lost their memories and Thucydides reported they *"did not know either themselves or their friends"*.

According to Thucydides, this plague began in Ethiopia, and spread through Egypt and Libya, then into the Greek world. It eventually killed a third of the Athenian population, including the great Athenian leader and mastermind of ancient Greek glory – Pericles. The Peloponnesian Plague was self-limiting, as the infectious agent concerned was so virulent that it killed off its hosts at a rate faster than they could spread it.

The term "Pandemic" actually comes from the Greek – *"pan"* meaning "all" and *"demos"* meaning "people".

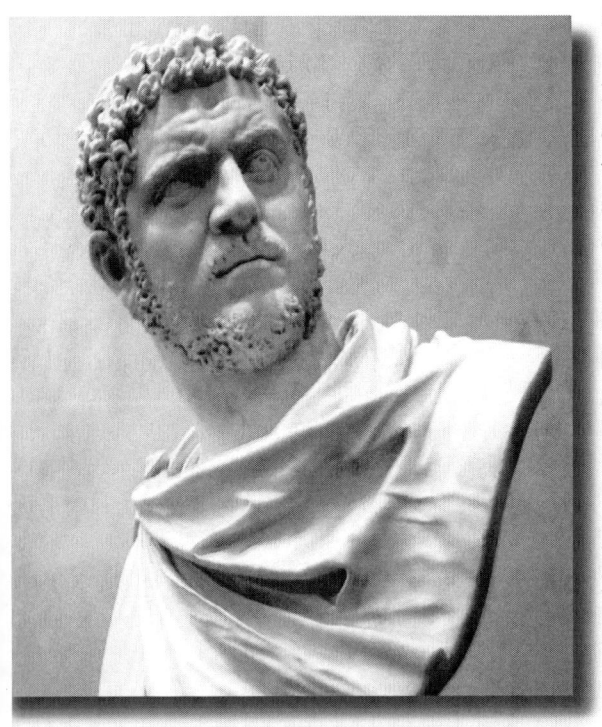

MARCUS AURELIUS ANTONIUS

ROME

In AD 165, troops returning from the battles at Constantinople and beyond, brought back with them not only the 'Victors Spoils', but also a deadly disease that was to wreak havoc on the Roman Empire, killing an estimated 5 million people. This plague had very high lethality, as a quarter of those who caught it died.

Two Roman emperors died from this plague, one of whom was Marcus Aurelius Antonius and thus the plague became known as the Antonine Plague. In AD 166, the Greek physician and writer Galen recorded some of the disease's symptoms in his writings "Methodus Medendi":

"A "nine-day illness" – fever, diarrhoea, inflammation of the pharynx and throat and eruptions on the skin, both dry and wet."

This description has since led scholars to believe that Galen was describing smallpox. Following the Antonine Plague, Rome was devastated by a second plague in AD 251 to 266, and, at its height, there were reports of over 5,000 people dying every day.

CONSTANTINOPLE

Although the Antonine Plague and the illnesses that followed were devastating – their death tolls were minimal compared to the devastation that occurred in the 6th century AD in the city of Constantinople.

Although details are sketchy, it is thought that the disease began in Ethiopia, or Egypt and spread northwards, and seemed to be linked to the routes taken by shipping which

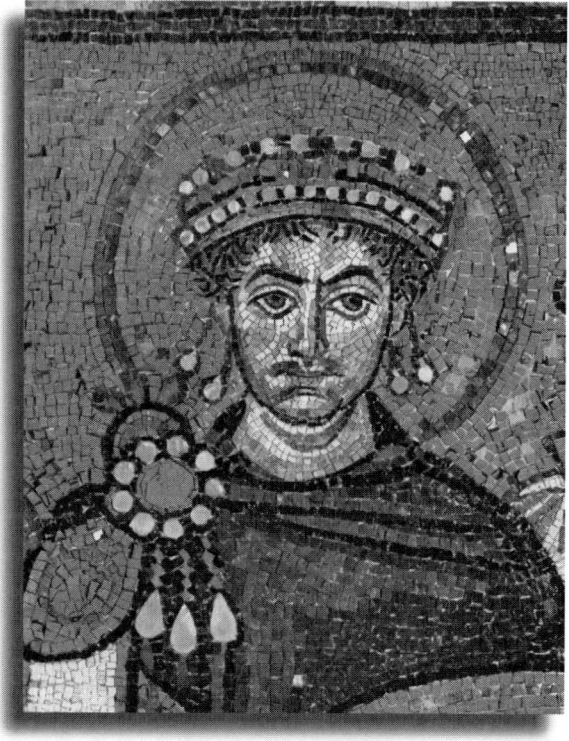

EMPEROR JUSTINIAN

supplied enormous quantities of grain to the city's vast public granaries. It is believed that rats on the ships carried fleas that bore the disease. However, this is disputed among researchers and there is evidence that supports the idea that the great plagues may have been water-borne.

The Justinian Plague (named after Justinian – the ruler of the time) was in fact the first great pandemic of the Bubonic Plague.

The Byzantine historian Procopius wrote that between AD 541 and 542, the disease was killing over 10,000 people each day in the city of Constantinople.

Overall, he estimated that it killed off 40%, or more, of the total population. The plague moved further out across the eastern Mediterranean, eventually wiping out a quarter of the region's population.

After a period of minor activity, the plague became virulent again and another major outbreak occurred and spread to the region that is now modern day France and eventually the death toll was around 25 million.

When one considers that the total population of the world in AD 500 was around the 200 million mark, this 25 million death toll is enormous. Proportionately, in terms of today's population which is just over 6.5 billion, this would equate to over 813 million deaths, globally.

A RESPITE, UNTIL THE BLACK DEATH

Europe did not have any major plagues for the next 800 years, until the 14th Century. From 1357 to 1350, the Plague of Justinian again travelled from the East and reared its very ugly head but this time presenting with another very marked symptom – that of blackened skin, due to the haemorrhaging underneath the skin.

This was the "Black Death". People fled in its path but this only served to spread the disease further.

In Europe alone, 25 million people died and there were reports that the Black Death also broke out in Asia and the Middle East too – it was a true global pandemic.

Bubonic Plague outbreaks occurred repeatedly in Europe, and reports show that it became more virulent as it passed from one generation to the next, until the 1700s by which time the death toll had reached an estimated 137 million.

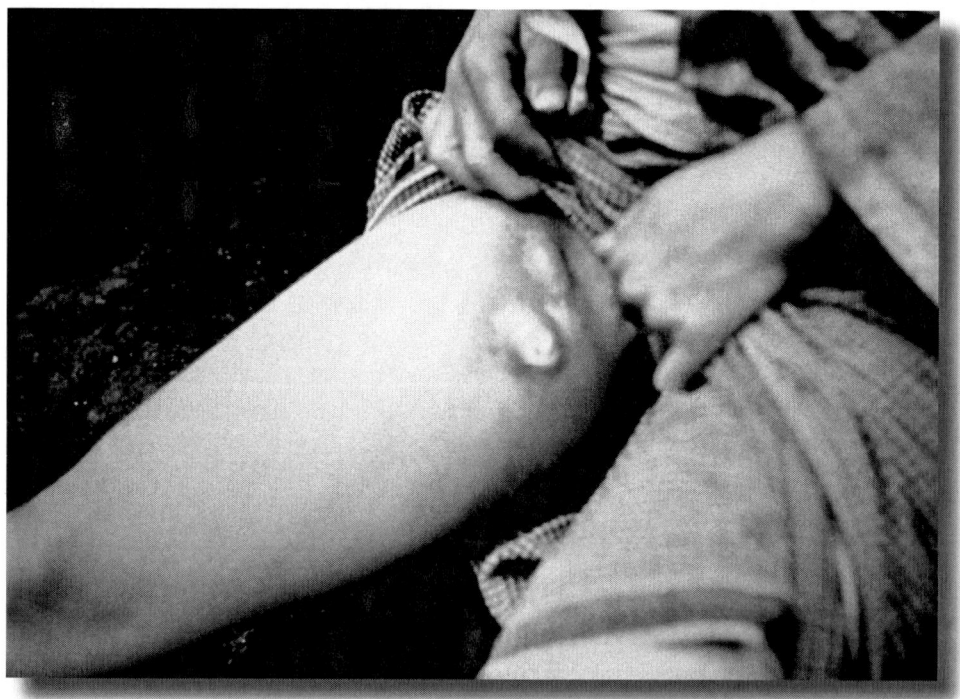

This plague patient is displaying a swollen, ruptured inguinal lymph node, or buboe. After the incubation period of 2-6 days, symptoms of the plague appear including severe malaise, headache, shaking chills, fever, and pain and swelling, or adenopathy, in the affected regional lymph nodes, also known as buboes. Source: Centers for Disease Control and Prevention's Public Health Image Library 1993

THE GREAT PLAGUE

One of the major outbreaks that we are very familiar with was the Bubonic Plague (Yersinia Pestis) of 1665. Symptoms included:

- Fever, headaches and chills
- Exhaustion and delirium
- Swollen, painful, and sometimes hot-to-the-touch lymph nodes called 'buboes', (hence the name 'Bubonic Plague')
- Septicaemic blood infection
- Coughing blood
- Lung infection, usually causing death in one to three days

There was a 50% death rate among those who contracted the disease – more or less similar to the current lethality of Bird Flu. The death toll was 500,000 people – half the population of London at the time – today this would equate to a death toll of over 3.5 million – just in London.

There is much speculation as to why the disease eventually faded away – possibly it was to do with the fact that in 1666 the Great Fire of London occurred – thus driving away rats (and their infective fleas) if indeed rats were to blame. However, it is more likely that improved sanitation measures contributed to the greater overall well-being of London's inhabitants as the City was largely re-built after The Great Fire and sewerage systems were improved.

CHOLERA

The next great pandemic was definitely worse in crowded cities – where poor sanitation provided a perfect breeding ground for bacteria and the spread of infection. Cholera had been described as early as 500 B.C.E. in Sanskrit writings and again later the 16th Century by Portuguese physician, Garcia de Orta.

However, in 1816 the disease suddenly accelerated, became enormously virulent and spread like wild-fire across the world. It is a disease that still kills, in significant numbers, today.

- 1849 10% of the population in St Louis in the USA died
- 1832: 500,000 New York city residents died
- 1847: 53,000 Londoners died
- 1865: 30,000 Pilgrims undertaking the Hajj in Mecca died.
- 1885: Chicago, USA – 80,000 people died.
- 1892: 8,605 residents of Hamburg in Germany died
- Globally in 2000, over 5,000 people died

Already endemic to India and the subcontinent, from the early 1800's the disease spread along trade routes into Russia and Eastern Europe, before shifting to Western Europe and even North America. The only continent untouched by cholera was Antarctica.

The most recent large cholera outbreak occurred in 1961, starting in Indonesia, and though modern sanitation has curbed the disease's power, it is still a killer today and is associated with unsanitary conditions.

INFLUENZA PANDEMICS

The best data that we have for various influenza pandemics are relatively recent although more sketchy records do stretch back 300 years: The most detailed information that we currently have is as follows:

1889-1890: THE ASIATIC FLU

This was first reported in May, 1889 in Bukhara, Russia. By October, it had spread to Tomsk and the Caucasus. After this it moved quickly to infect people in Western Europe and finally reached North America in December 1889, South American countries in February–April, 1890, India in February–March, 1890 and finally, Australia in March–April, 1890.

Scientists believe that it was caused by the H2N8 type of flu virus and we do know that it had very high virulence and lethality levels, with approximately 50% of those who contracted the disease dying. This was the most lethal pandemic of the 19th Century.

1918-1919: THE SPANISH FLU

The "Spanish Flu", 1918–1919. Known at the time as Swine Flu, was first formally identified in early March 1918, in American troops training at Fort Riley, Kansas. There are, however, some reports that the first wave of this flu actually began in the major staging post for the Allied forces in Étaples in France in 1916.

By October, 1918, it had spread to become a world-wide pandemic on all continents. It was unusually lethal and virulent, and came in three distinct "waves", ultimately 'vanishing completely' within 18 months.

In the first six months, 25 million were dead; and it is unknown how many died globally but various estimates put the total of those killed worldwide at between 40 to 100 million. In India it is thought that around 17 million died, 500,000 in the United States and 200,000 in the UK.

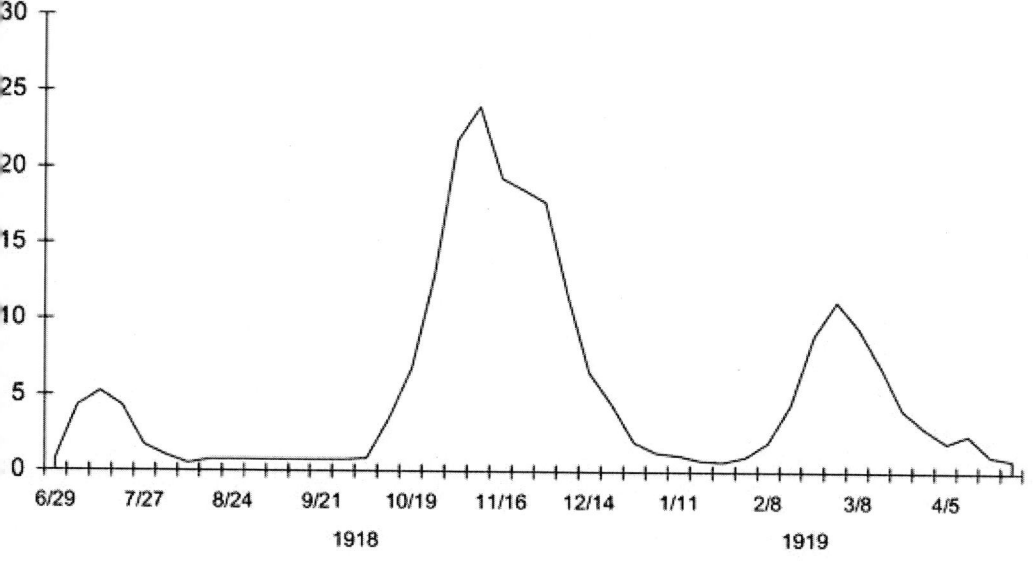

Three pandemic waves: weekly combined influenza and pneumonia mortality, United Kingdom, 29th June 1918 – end May 1919[1]

Scientists have managed to recover traces of the virus responsible from the Alaskan permafrost where bodies of people who died from the flu were well preserved. The USA's Centre for Disease Control (CDC) scientists have identified it as a type of H1N1 Influenza virus.

One of the "unusual" factors about this influenza pandemic was that the type of people who succumbed to it were different from the kinds of people who are usually vulnerable to influenza, which normally affects the very young and the elderly, who have weaker immune systems.

In 1918, the group most badly affected were those who were "young and fit". However, it is very important to remember that ,"The War to End All Wars", had been raging and it is as well to consider whether this was in fact, a concomitant issue.

For example, the men at Fort Riley were under enormous strain as they were seeing people in terrible condition, returning (or not!) from the Western Front and indeed, were anticipating their own transfer over to the trenches. This would have taken an enormous toll on their supposedly "fit" immune systems.

In 1918, the influenza pandemic broke out on the Western Front when World War 1 was drawing to its climax. The pandemic had no real impact upon the outcome of the war as both sides were affected to equal degrees. However, from the personal perspective, this pandemic was a disaster, and dwarfed all the other casualty lists of the war.

An shocking statistic and food for thought, from Dr David Payne in an article on the excellent website; www.westernfront.co.uk

> "To give this pandemic some perspective, if the graves of the 750,000 Western Front Commonwealth dead and missing were concentrated into a single location, they would occupy an area of about 3 square kilometres or 1.2 square miles. If all the dead of the 1918–1919 flu pandemic – 40,000,000 – were similarly concentrated, their graves would cover an area of around 160 square kilometres or 62 square miles."

1957-1958: ASIAN FLU

The "Asian Flu", 1957–58. Another Avian Influenza, H2N2, was responsible for about 70,000 deaths in the United States and figures vary for the global death toll. H2N2 was initially identified in China in late February, 1957 and the Asian Flu spread to the United States by June, 1957.

1968-1969: HONG KONG FLU

The "Hong Kong Flu", 1968–69. Caused by the virus H3N2, the Hong Kong Flu caused about 1 million deaths around the world. This virus was first detected in Hong Kong in early 1968 hence its name. Influenza A (H3N2) viruses still circulate today and still cause deaths.

BIRD FLU: H5N1

Bird Flu, or Avian Influenza (H5N1) – has killed millions of birds and has only shown minor signs of a mutation that would make it easily transmissible between humans. One of the reasons for the great concern about Bird Flu, is its lethality among people who have contracted it. The figures are alarming, to say the least, and currently stand at around 60%. This is more lethal than any previous flu pandemic throughout history.

References:

1 Jordan E. Epidemic influenza: a survey. Chicago: American Medical Association, 1927 at http://www.cdc.gov/ncidod/eid/vol12no01/05-0979.htm#21

CHAPTER 3

HOW SERIOUS A THREAT IS SWINE FLU?

Swine Flu is caused by the Influenza A virus H1N1, which can affect 'swine' (pigs, etc), birds, humans and probably, like recent cases of Bird Flu (H5N1), a variety of other mammals.

So, despite the fact that almost every country in the world is thought to have been affected, this bout of Swine Flu has been described as 'mild', although for the relatives and friends of those who have been infected and not survived, this may appear to be an insensitive description.

It is estimated that 'normal "seasonal flu"' kills around 250,000 – 500,000 people worldwide every year. The number of deaths varies, depending on the virulence of specific seasonal flu viruses. The estimate for mortality from seasonal flu in the USA, for example, is that around 36,000 people die from it every year.

This is only an estimate in the US (as it is in most countries), as influenza only gets listed as a 'cause of death' in less than a thousand cases every year (849 in 2006) – as only the 'secondary infection' or the 'final cause of death', are actually recorded.

In estimating the potential mortality rates from Swine Flu in the UK, Sir Liam Donaldson , (Chief Medical Officer), has quoted a range of between 3,000 and 65,000 potential deaths this year, saying that the lower number is in line with normal estimates for deaths from seasonal flu in the UK.

A WORLDWIDE PANDEMIC

Swine Flu is a serious threat to the health of everyone on the planet. The world's official health agency, the World Health Organisation (WHO) declared it an official pandemic on June 11th 2009 and by early July, 2009 reported that, as far as records showed, it had infected a large and growing number of people (6th July, reported 94,512 confirmed cases and 429 deaths).

How Serious a Threat is Swine Flu?

After this date the WHO stopped producing detailed worldwide statistics on its spread and more up-to-date estimates were released by the European Centre for Disease Prevention and Control (ECDC). Just under 2 weeks later, by the 19th July, the ECDC reported 137,215 confirmed cases and a rise in the number of deaths to 779. By the end of July they reported that there had been just over 1,000 deaths.

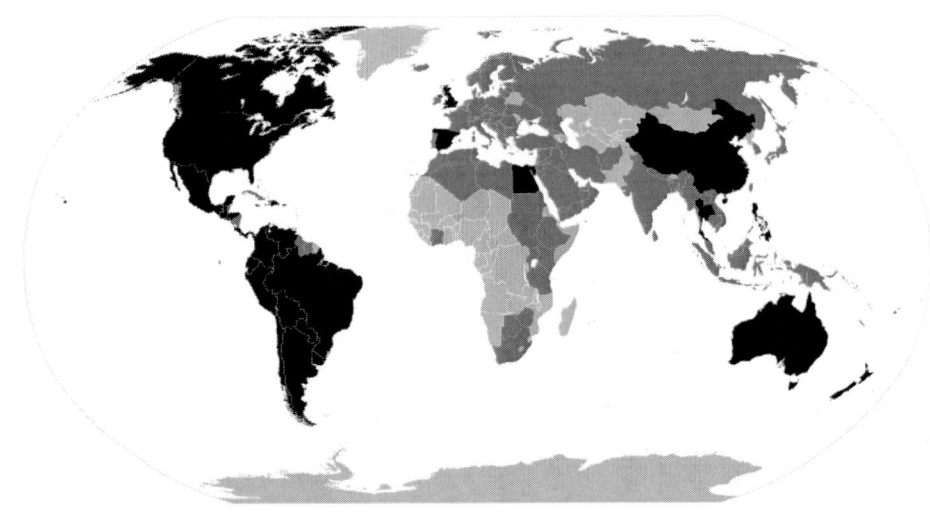

Deaths   Confirmed cases   Unconfirmed or suspected cases

Spread of Swine Flu; latest news on the WHO and BBC websites:
http://gamapserver.who.int/h1n1/atlas.html?select=ZZZ&filter=filter4,confirmed
http://news.bbc.co.uk/1/hi/uk/8083179.stm

The number of deaths in the UK started to rise dramatically in July 2009, rising to 29 by mid-July and ended the month at 30. Despite the fact that it had by then affected almost every country on the planet (130 according to the WHO by the end of July), including tiny ones like Vanuatu, the concerns over the spread of this Swine Flu virus were felt in different ways in different countries.

ECDC figures released by the end of July 2009, showed that, apart from the UK (with unofficial reports of 100,000 plus, people affected), the only other countries in Europe to report any deaths were Spain, with 6 deaths and Hungary (1 death).

In countries including Germany (834 reported; 19th July), France (475), Greece (323), Italy (258), there had been few reported cases across most of Europe - let alone any deaths. The approach taken to this outbreak by most European countries, whilst being cautious, did not appear to be the same as in countries, like the UK and the USA, where there had been a number of deaths.

E.g. Italy put a warning in place about travel to the UK; France 'invented' a pandemic level '5A', rather than going to the WHO's highest, level 6.

Countries with confirmed cases of pandemic (H1N1) 2009 in the European Region (44): Albania, Andorra, Austria, Belgium, Bosnia and Herzegovina, Bulgaria, Croatia, Cyprus, Czech Republic, Denmark, Estonia, Finland, France, Georgia, Germany, Greece, Hungary, Iceland, Ireland, Israel, Italy, Kazakhstan, Latvia, Lithuania, Luxembourg, Malta, Monaco, Montenegro, Netherlands, Norway, Poland, Portugal, Romania, Russian Federation, Serbia, Slovakia, Slovenia, Spain, Sweden, Switzerland, The former Yugoslav Republic of Macedonia, Turkey, Ukraine and United Kingdom.

http://www.euro.who.int/influenza/ah1n1 27th July)

Africa has been hardly affected according to reported cases and deaths (1 in Egypt by the end of July) and Asia has not seen many cases, or deaths (July 19th: only 30 deaths in the whole of Asia - and 24 of these came from Thailand alone: Phillipines (3): China (1); Singapore (1); Brunei (1).

By the end of July just over half of all deaths had been reported from Latin American countries from Mexico through to Central America and down through South America.

The worst affected countries, in terms of mortality were:

USA	263
Argentina	137
Mexico	125
Canada	45
Chile	40
Australia	31

In the UK the number of reported cases had risen to around 100,000 in the week of 20th July, 2009 and a new series on NHS health lines and websites were inundated as soon as they were opened, as people searched for information on the virus - and on how to get hold of the recommended anti-viral drug, Tamiflu. The new NHS website received over 9,000,000 hits in its first two hours of going live.

How Serious a Threat is Swine Flu?

The 'estimates' given out by various authorities of the numbers of people who have been infected are exactly that, just estimates. Medical experts have explained that these are only 'reported numbers' – and the reality is that many more people have been infected and have not reported to their doctors, or health care specialists, for treatment.

SWINE FLU DEATH RATE ESTIMATES 'FLAWED': JULY 15TH 2009:

According to UK Researchers, the current estimates of the proportion of people who would die, if they contracted Swine Flu, are flawed, because no-one knows how many people have been infected in the first place (e.g. people who stay at home and recover without ever calling their doctor), that not all deaths from Swine Flu are being attributed to it (many deaths from Swine Flu may be being seen as deaths from other causes, e.g. heart attacks, pneumonia) and because no-one, currently, has any idea of the time lags between catching the virus and onset of symptoms and mortality. (http://www.newscientist.com/article/dn17466-swine-flu-death-rate-estimates-flawed.html?DCMP=OTC-rss&nsref=online-news)

"WHAT IS SO UNUSUAL ABOUT SWINE FLU?"

What is so different about this particular wave of Swine Flu, is that it is spreading so quickly in the Northern hemisphere outside of 'flu season'. It is also affecting people from groups who are normally considered to be at low risk (e.g. 25–40 year olds), rather than those people who are traditionally considered to be the most vulnerable e.g. the over 70's.

Given the probability that Swine Flu might spread again in the Northern Hemisphere this winter, in the real flu season, medical experts are studying the spread of this version of Swine Flu in Australia and New Zealand (10) – their 'winter' flu season - with intense interest. (As we have seen, it has also been extremely virulent in the May – July period in Argentina and Chile).

"WHO IS MOST AT RISK?"

A paper published in the New England Journal of Medicine at the end of June, 2009, contained a study of the ages of all cases of severe pneumonia reported in Mexico between March 24th and April 29th 2009, which were then compared with those of 2005–2006, 2006–2007 and 2007–2008. (The data covered 2,155 cases; 821 hospitalisations: and 100 deaths).[1]

It showed relative spikes in the death rates for the age groups 20–44 (with less noted spikes for teenagers and then children; and for 45 – 54 year olds) and a surprisingly low relative level of mortality amongst anyone over the age of 60.

They concluded:

> "These data show a sudden increase in the rate of severe pneumonia and a shift in the age distribution of patients with such illnesses, which were concurrent with person-to-person circulation of (the Swine Flu) infection in Mexico……which was reminiscent of past pandemics and suggested relative protection for persons who were exposed to H1N1 strains during childhood, before the 1957 pandemic. If resources or vaccine supplies are limited, these findings suggest a rationale for focusing prevention efforts on younger populations."

In the UK in mid-July the concerns were about the effect it was having on children under–5 and babies (with 134 serious cases and 4 dead; 20th July 2009) and on pregnant women.

On 24th July the WHO reported that in most countries the majority of 2009 cases were still occurring in younger people, with the median age reported to be 12 to 17 years (based on data from Canada, Chile, Japan, UK and the United States of America). Some reports suggest that persons requiring hospitalisation and patients with fatal illness may be slightly older.[2]

By the end of July an advisory panel to the Centres for Disease Control (CDC) in the US recommended that pregnant women should be among the first to get the swine flu vaccine. They also recommended that high priority should also be given to caregivers of infants; health-care workers; children and adults under 24. They then said vaccinination should be considered for people with underlying medical conditions such as diabetes or chronic heart disease.[3]

LOW MORTALITY RATE:

Unlike the potential threat of Bird Flu (H5N1) that global health authorities have been preparing for, Swine Flu (H1N1) has already demonstrated the ability for human-to-human transmission but has not exhibited such high potential mortality rates. (As we have seen, Bird Flu has shown mortality rates of around 60%, while the current outbreak of Swine Flu has an estimated mortality rate of around 0.5%).

"WHERE DID IT COME FROM?"

Although the H1N1 virus has been known about since 1918–19 (having been identified initially – at the time - not as 'Spanish Flu', but as 'Swine Flu') and has been traced in many outbreaks all around the world over recent years, its latest source appears to be in Mexico.

Some people have identified the starting 'source' of this particular outbreak as an industrial pig farm in the rural town of La Gloria in Mexico, but this has not been confirmed. [4]

How Serious a Threat is Swine Flu?

Reports of serious complications from this strain started to emerge in April 2009, although some reports suggest it was circulating in Mexico as early as January 2009. The origins of this particular version of H1N1 have been circulating in pigs for around 10 years:

"We found that the common ancestor of the (new H1N1) outbreak and the closest related swine flu viruses existed between 9.2 and 17.2 years ago, depending on the genomic segment...." [5].

"WHICH ANIMALS CARRY THE SWINE FLU VIRUS?"

The current Swine Flu outbreak has been ascribed to an infection in pigs in Mexico. However it has been known for some time that H1N1 has been 'living', in a latent form in the livers, gut and respiratory tracts of some birds for the last 90 years.

There has yet to be any evidence that it has affected any significant numbers of pigs in Mexico, or elsewhere (certainly not to the point where they need to cull any herds of pigs). But it certainly has developed a mutation that enables it to be transmitted directly from human–to–human. This strain of Swine Flu (H1N1) is far more virulent than recent ones and is now considered to be a 'Highly Pathogenic Influenza' or 'HPI' for short.

The other HPI flu virus that has been the focus of attention in recent years - Bird Flu (H5N1) - was first seen spreading in South East Asia in 1997, becoming deadly to himans at the end of 2003 (although it was first reported in Scotland in 1959). It has since spread to a number of countries and has recently caused deaths in Egypt. (421 reported cases, worldwide, as at July 2009,with 257 deaths). It is difficult to find exact figures to ascertain how many poultry have either died from this flu or have had to be culled. Certainly some countries are not forthcoming with their data and have internal policies to suppress information. Some estimates say that 200 million domestic poultry have died so far, but this is likely to be on the low side.

So, just like Bird Flu, the Swine Flu virus will exist in wild birds such as ducks, geese and swans as well as shore birds such as gulls. All this time the H1N1 virus has been asymptomatic in many birds, which means that they have the virus and can spread it but it doesn't make them ill.

"WILL SWINE FLU AFFECT PETS?"

Bird Flu has been known to have been responsible for killing animals and birds in around 40 different species. These include a range of wild birds, including geese, storks, egrets, herons, and falcons, and some mammals, including a number of tigers that caught the disease from infected poultry at a tiger breeding zoo in Thailand.

There was evidence that the tigers initially caught the H5N1 virus from chickens that they were fed and that there was then a subsequent transfer of the virus between tigers. All in all, 147 tigers died or had to be euthanized.

Domestic cats have also been seen to be vulnerable to the Bird Flu virus and so far no-one has estimated the effect this latest outbreak of Swine Flu might have on cats and domestic pets. There are no reports of any domestic animal fatalities as a result of H1N1 yet, although of course, all viruses can mutate to affect different species.

"HOW DOES SWINE FLU SPREAD?"

Swine Flu (H1N1) is currently being transmitted from human carrier to human carrier. Visitors returning from trips to Mexico appear initially to have carried the disease.

It would appear that the virus has been transmitted between people who were in close contact and also between people in the vicinity of each other.

To see the spread of Swine Flu on a day-by-day basis visit the BBC website (http://news.bbc.co.uk/1/hi/uk/8083179.stm).

"WHY IS THIS STRAIN SO WORRYING?"

H1N1 has already demonstrated an ability to infect people, cause severe disease and kill. And this has occurred even amongst 'healthy' sections of the population. So, as this new strain of H1N1 spreads through the population, few people, if any, would have a natural immunity to it and an even more severe pandemic may occur.

Having said this, as pointed out earlier, a research study in the US has shown that the virulence of Swine Flu is particularly low amongst the over 60's. They attribute this to the fact that many of these people would have been exposed to the virus the last time it was highly virulent – during the 1957 Asian Flu epidemic. The theory is that anyone over 52 years of age would have been exposed to it then – and probably still carries a natural immunity to it now.

However the 1957 Asian Flu wasn't an H1N1 strain, it was an H2N2 strain.

"CAN A MORE SERIOUS PANDEMIC BE AVERTED?"

As you know, the WHO made the latest Swine Flu outbreak an official 'Pandemic' in June 2009 based on its observed spread between humans at such rapid rates.

When these programmes were originally put in place it was probably expected that a worldwide infection such as Swine Flu might have been more deadly. But the current pandemic is certainly a worldwide phenomenon with over 137,000 notified cases, probably millions more – and over 1,000 deaths.

The concern is two-fold:

Either, that this wave of infection – or a following one – may be more deadly and have a higher mortality rate, closer to that of the recent Bird Flu infection (around 60%).

Or, if it infects more people, that the number of deaths would be significant. For example, if the population of the US (300m) all caught it – and 50% had it badly enough to report it/seek treatment, and the death rate was (as it currently stands) 0.5%, it would kill around 750,000 people. In the UK – on the same assumptions – it would kill around 150,000.

If, as appears more likely the current Swine Flu pandemic affects millions of people, but only a small proportion catch it severely enough to need treatment – 5%, rather than 50% - the mortality figures for the US would be around 75,000 and the UK 15,000.

If current Government pandemic preparations are followed, it is unlikely that a severe pandemic could be averted. Even if the anti-viral drugs that they have stockpiled were effective – they simply do not have sufficient stocks to treat enough people to stop the virus in its tracks.

Even if an effective vaccine is developed in time to treat people, looking at the historical precedent - whether the vaccine is actually safe may only be discovered years after it has been used.

References:
1 http://content.nejm.org/cgi/content/full/NEJMoa0904023
2 http://www.who.int/csr/disease/swineflu/notes/h1n1_situation_20090724/en/index.html
3 http://www.suntimes.com/lifestyles/health/1692502,CST-NWS-swine30.article
4 http://content.nejm.org/cgi/content/full/NEJMp0904012
5 http://www.nature.com/nature/journal/vnfv/ncurrent/pdf/nature08182.pdf?__xsl=/mobil/cms-common.xsl

CHAPTER 4

POTENTIAL ECONOMIC, POLITICAL AND SOCIAL EFFECTS

Aside from the enormous health ramifications, the impact of a virus like Swine Flu, could lead to severe economic, political and social crises.

THE ECONOMIC COSTS?

In November, 2005, a senior World Bank economist estimated the bill, if Bird Flu were to spread around the globe, at up to $800bn a year, which would knock around 2% off global gross domestic product (GDP). Another 'think tank' (the Lowey Institute: Australia), estimated that the loss from a world flu pandemic would be around $4.4 trillion – the size of Japan's total economy, with 142 million deaths globally (2006).

And that was before the Credit Crunch took such a slice out of world GDP figures.

More recent estimates of the economic effects of the current pandemic point to a fall in GDP worldwide of 5% (The Oxford Group), and to a fall of 7.5% in the UK. (This estimate assumes that UK GDP will fall by 4.5% this year anyway, and that a severe outbreak of Swine Flu would take another 3% off this: (20th July ,2009: Ernst & Young ITEM Club). [1]

It is very difficult to know how accurate any of these figures are. Much depends up on the actual virulence of the virus – if it increases its mortality, and its impact upon society and as yet, scientists have no way of predicting this.

Apart from its effect on business in general, this H1N1 pandemic could be devastating for the farming (pig–rearing) industry and everyone in it, if, despite the absence of any evidence to implicate the consumption of pork with the spread of Swine Flu, people start to panic and stop eating pork – even from unaffected areas. (Various countries reacted to the latest Swine Flu outbreak by banning the import of pork products from Mexico and other affected countries).

The recommendations from the UK Government state:

> *"Swine influenza viruses are not transmitted by food. You can not get H1N1 (swine) influenza from eating pork, or pork products. Eating properly handled and cooked pork and pork products is safe. Cooking pork to an internal temperature of 160^0F kills the H1N1 (swine) flu virus as it does other bacteria and viruses."*

While the economic effects of a major, virulent, pandemic could be serious, it could be ruinous for farmers. What has yet to be seen in any Pandemic Preparedness Plans are any proposals for how Governments will support farmers whose livelihoods could be decimated overnight.

We believe that Governments in every country – rather than waiting for more cases to occur - as they have tended to do with other farming-related disasters (e.g. the BSE and the Foot and Mouth outbreaks in the UK) – should take steps right now – to assist farmers to make realistic Preparedness Plans, based on existing ones for Bird Flu, and have support plans ready from day one in order to avert the economic disaster that could happen in this sector.

It is easy to concentrate upon the potential negative economic impact this current bout of Swine Flu might cause, however, it is worth noting that for the 2,000 new recruits needed to man the NHS phone lines in July, 2009, it has brought positive benefits.

Also, with companies that manufacture and supply various drugs and vaccines looking at a massive increase in demand, there will be profits to be made during this pandemic. (E.g. the reports (23rd July), on Biota Holdings' (Australia), massive rise in royalties on the sale of Relenza, which may soar even higher, as they were planning on a tripling of production. Biota's payments from GSK, rose from around A $400,000 in April - June, 2008, to A $8,900,000 for its Relenza sales in the three months ending June, 2009).

Baxter, one of the first pharmaceutical companies to produce a Swine Flu vaccine (having taken out patents on an H1N1 vaccine in August, 2007) had to announce (16th July, 2009) that they couldn't take any more orders for their vaccine.[2]

And the man who was head of the research team that invented Tamiflu for Gilead Sciences in the

1990's. Dr Norbert Bischofburger, is sitting on a large number of share options in the company, as well as earning around £450,000 a year and taking several million pounds in bonuses.[3]

THE POLITICAL COSTS?

A survey produced for the World Economic Forum in April 2006 found that a human flu pandemic now ranked alongside terrorism as the risk most concerning global businesses and political leaders.

Early suspicions amongst some commentators are that the latest outbreak of Swine Flu may be a 'human–developed' event. (See reports on "The Gibbs Article" on the internet. The paper by highly respected scientist Adrian Gibbs was submitted to the WHO and claimed that the current H1N1 virus developed from a lab experiment - the WHO have publicly refuted this - although they did point out that they had welcomed the paper, given the status and credibility of Adrian Gibbs - furthermore, they welcome other such papers as it is helpful for as many scientists to give their attention to the development and spread of H1N1 as possible.)

According to a leaked confidential Home Office Report on the potential Bird Flu pandemic, reported on by the Sunday Times in 2006, the UK Government were predicting that up to 320,000 people could die as a result.

They considered the use of mass graves, as a worst-case scenario, in the case that a severe flu pandemic were to strike. They admitted that this level of mortality would overwhelm the country's burial services, leading to delays in burial and cremation of up to four months. A cabinet committee gave the Great Plague burial pits (as used during the seventeenth century), as an example of a solution.

The report claimed that it would take Local Authorities in Great Britain about three months to bury and cremate about 48,000 people who died of flu. Therefore a 320,000 death toll would push back burial and cremation schedules by around 17 weeks. A pandemic death rate of 2.5% would overwhelm burial and cremation services, said the report.

Following various political upheavals in the UK in 2009, with all the reports of sleeze in politics, increasing death tolls from Iraq and Afganistan and the likelihood of a Conservative win at the next General Election, some commentators consider that firm handling of the Swine Flu crisis by the Prime Minister might help improve the chances of the Labour Party winning the election.

In the US, President Obama should have all the political clout he needs to ensure an effective governmental response to any outbreaks.

THE SOCIAL EFFECTS?

Governments already have measures in place to cope with any potential civil unrest that a severe pandemic like Swine Flu may cause.

The UK Government has already made plans for hospitals, doctors and pharmacies to be guarded by the police and the army should it be necessary. They have also made plans for mass burial sites and fast-track death certification by doctors, to cope with the anticipated numbers of fatalities, should the virus mutate and cause high mortality rates.

As we have seen, the estimates put forward by the Chief Medical Officer in the UK (July, 2009) are for between 3,000 and 65,000 deaths from Swine Flu.

HOW WILL KEY SECTORS COPE WITH A MORE LETHAL PANDEMIC?

BUSINESSES
Various businesses and companies will also have preparations in place to work out how their operations will carry on, in the event of a severe pandemic. One of the key opportunities will be to establish how they can operate with most of their staff, where possible, working from home.

THE POLICE AND THE ARMY
In the UK and the USA, police forces have detailed plans for responding to a major and serious flu pandemic like this. They have already completed simulation exercises as part of their preparedness planning.

Police tasks will include guarding GP's surgeries and hospitals, where antiviral medications are stocked. They will keep order and prevent civil unrest and will be co-opted into helping mortuary staff. Large gatherings such as football matches would be cancelled to curb the spread of infection. If mass graves are required for corpse disposal – as has been suggested by the British Government, it is likely that the police and the army will be required to dig and supervise the use of these.

SCHOOLS
At present, it is down to each Local Education Authority to decide for itself whether to keep their schools open. Children are one of the main sources for the spread of any infectious disease, however, given the potential virulence of Swine Flu, this may not be the case.

HOSPITALS
All elective surgery (routine surgical procedures that are planned as a matter of choice e.g.

cataract surgery - as opposed to life saving surgery) would be cancelled as all hospital beds would be required for people who have serious flu symptoms, such as Acute Respiratory Distress Syndrome (ARDS) and Viral Pneumonia. There is already a countrywide shortage of respirators in the UK, which would be crucial for keeping patients alive. Doctors are planning for a pandemic but without the equipment they need there is not much that they can do.

Hospitals will have to put triage systems into place so that patients are given treatment according to the perceived severity and relevance of the treatment i.e. *"is there any point in treating a particular patient – what are his or her chances of recovery"* etc. This puts enormous strains on doctors, nurses and hospitals both in terms of work load and ethically.

SHOPS

It will be difficult to maintain the "Just in Time" supply chain for getting food and other vital provisions into shops. It is likely that supermarkets are setting up some form of preparedness plan but when interviewed they are reluctant to share the details of this. Hauliers are likely to run into problems as they may well have many people off sick and also may not have any supplies to deliver. There might have to be rationing which would limit how much each family could buy – if any stocks are available.

TRANSPORT

There is little evidence to suggest that public transport organisations have planned for a pandemic. Should Swine Flu cause a severe pandemic it is likely that train and bus drivers would be unwell, so transport companies would only run restricted services. The British Government has requested detailed plans to ensure that commuters could still travel to work.

The most important thing to take from all of this very worrying information is that it is essential to Plan Carefully and not Panic!

Remember, even though we are in a Phase 6 Pandemic - this current adaptation of the H1N1 virus may not develop to be as virulent as in 1918 – but if it is – once you have read this book, you will know how to prepare properly for it.

REFERENCES

1. http://www.telegraph.co.uk/finance/5865495/Swine-flu-threatens-deflation-slump-Ernst-and-Young-ITEM-Club-report-warns.html
2. http://www.reuters.com/article/rbssHealtheareNews/idUSN1646263220090716
3. http://www.dailymail.co.uk/news/worldnews/article-1202298/The-clever-inventor-profiting-swine-flu-pandemic.html

CHAPTER 5

SWINE FLU: TO DATE

TIMELINE FOR THE 2009 SWINE FLU OUTBREAK; FACTS AND NEWS REPORTS:

MARCH 18TH: Mexican authorities begin picking up cases of what the World Health Organization calls an "Influenza-like-illness"(ILI).

MARCH 18TH – APRIL 11TH: Media in Mexico start to report on an increase in 'flu-like' illnesses across the country.

APRIL 12TH: A 39-year old woman suffering from an acute respiratory illness undergoes treatment for five days in a hospital in the state of Oaxaca, Mexico, and subsequently dies.

Mexican health authorities trace people who have been in contact with the woman and find some are displaying mild symptoms of pneumonia.

The authorities point out that over 5,000 cases of pneumonia occur annually in Oaxaca state and that they consider the woman's death to be an isolated incident.

APRIL 16TH: Mexican health officials get in contact with the Pan-American Health Organisation, about the illness.

APRIL 18TH: Mexican health officials visit 21 hospitals around the country and confirm an increase in this type of case across the country.

APRIL 21ST: The Health Department in Oaxaca state confirms a second death from this 'atypical pneumonia'. Having been prepared to face a potential 'Bird Flu' outbreak over the previous few years, the hospital establishes a quarantine area in its emergency room.

Swine Flu: To Date

APRIL 22ND: The Mexican health ministry issues a nationwide alert about a potential avian flu outbreak and samples are sent to Canada for testing.

APRIL 23RD: Mexico reports these first cases of H1N1 to the World Health Organisation (WHO). In the US, public health officials announce that seven people in California and Texas have been diagnosed with a flu virus known as H1N1, but all seven have recovered.

Mexican officials send out case definitions and ask for any records of this kind of case since March 1st. The reports showed that during the March 1st – April 30th period (2 months), a total of 1,918 suspected cases had been reported, including 286 probable and 97 confirmed cases.
A total of 84 deaths were reported. A majority of case-reports were for hospitalised patients, reflecting the concentration of surveillance efforts within hospitals. However, the Mexican Ministry of Health also received reports from sites conducting routine seasonal Influenza surveillance of patients with Influenza – like illnesses (ILI). Of 1,069 patients with suspected and probable cases for whom information was available, 755 were hospitalised, and the remaining 314 were examined in outpatient settings or emergency departments. Suspected or probable cases were reported from all 31 states and from the Federal District of Mexico. The four areas with the most cases were Federal District (213 cases), Guanajuato (141), Aguas Calientes (93), and Durango (77).

APRIL 24TH: Health authorities around the world go on alert as the World Health Organisation announces that several hundred cases of Swine Flu in humans have been suspected over the past weeks in Mexico. They include what is eventually identified as around 15 fatalities, although many more are initially blamed on the virus, while there are nearly a dozen cases in the United States.

Mexican authorities speak for the first time of an "epidemic." More than 1,000 people in the country are placed under observation.

Schools, universities, theatres and museums are closed down in Mexico City to prevent the spread of the disease.

Neighbouring Latin American countries declare health alerts or announce preventative measures.

APRIL 25TH: The WHO Director-General, Dr Margaret Chan, convenes an Emergency Committee meeting in Geneva under International Health Regulations (2005). This is the first such meeting called to advise the Director-General on a public health emergency. It recommends that a Public Health Emergency of International Concern (PHEIC) be declared. The WHO warns of the "pandemic potential" of the new Swine Flu virus, which can be transmitted from human to human.

The Survivor's Guide to Swine Flu

More cases are found in the United States.

Mexico toughens measures against the disease and orders people who are sick or showing symptoms of the disease to be isolated.

The South-East Asia Regional Office's Strategic Health Operation Centre activated.

APRIL 26TH: The United States declares a health emergency after the confirmation of a total of 20 cases in the country, including eight students in New York.

Canada announces its first cases of Swine Flu.

Countries around the world step up vigilance and precautionary measures as WHO warns that the virus can mutate at any time and become much more dangerous. Public meetings are suspended in Mexico.

APRIL 27TH: The first confirmed cases in Europe, in Spain and Scotland, in people who have returned from Mexico.

The WHO raises its alert level from 3 to 4 on a scale of 6, signaling a "significant increase in risk of a pandemic." It warns that no region in the world is safe from the virus.

Communicable Diseases Surveillance and Response Unit presents the first Influenza A (H1N1) update at Monday morning meeting in the Regional Office for South-East Asia with specifics on the number of cases and areas affected. Mexican virus is confirmed as the H1N1 "Swine Flu" virus.

APRIL 28TH: The epidemic continues to progress, affecting all five continents in the world.

A state of emergency is declared in California.

Several countries suspend their pork imports from infected regions, despite reassurances that this is a human – to – human transmissible virus and that there is no evidence of transmission to humans from 'infected' pork, or pork products.

Joint South-East Asia Regional Office IHR Task Force and Crisis Management Team meeting held with the Regional Director.

APRIL 29TH: The first confirmed death in the United States for H1N1 is a 23-month old Mexican child.

Swine Flu: To Date

The virus spreads in Europe, where first cases are confirmed in Germany and Austria. New cases are declared in Spain, of which one person had not been to Mexico.

The WHO raises its pandemic alert to level five, calling on countries to prepare for an "imminent" pandemic.

The WHO officially refers to this disease as New Influenza A (H1N1).

At a 'Daily International Health Regulations' (IHR) taskforce discussion the WHO forms four core working groups to cover Surveillance/Monitoring & Laboratory, Logistics and Management, Communication and Health Education and Medical & Health Systems.

APRIL 30TH: The European Union rules out a French idea to suspend flights to Mexico. The WHO does not recommend limiting travel but Britain, Canada, France, Italy and the Netherlands advise people against travelling to Mexico.

The WHO, the Food and Agriculture Organisation and the World Organisation for Animal Health (OIE) issue a joint statement stating that pork and pork products "will not be a source of infection" if handled in accordance with good hygienic practices.

MAY 1ST: Mexico begins a five-day shutdown at the start of May Day weekend to try to contain a flu epidemic which the government now says appeared to be "not so aggressive" as initially feared.

The first confirmed case of Swine Flu in Asia is recorded in Hong Kong after a Mexican man who arrived via Shanghai tested positive. Guests and staff at the hotel where he had stayed are placed under quarantine for a week.

The WHO says it has "no doubt" that a successful vaccine against the Swine Flu virus could be developed within the next six months.

MAY 2ND: Mexican authorities say the flu epidemic appears to be "in a stabilisation phase", but the toll in the country rises to 19 dead and 454 confirmed infections.

The WHO says 16 countries have officially reported 658 confirmed cases of Influenza A(H1N1), but that there is no indication that it has begun to spread in a sustained manner anywhere outside of North America.

Canada reports the identification of the A(H1N1) virus in a swine herd in Alberta. It is highly probable that the pigs were exposed to the virus from a Canadian farm worker recently returned from Mexico, who had exhibited flu-like symptoms and had contact with the pigs.

Three new countries (Costa Rica, France and Republic of Korea) have reported cases.

MAY 3RD: The WHO says 18 countries have officially reported 898 cases of Influenza A(H1N1) infection.

The WHO decides to deploy Tamiflu (Oseltamivir) to 72 least developed countries.

MAY 4TH: The WHO says 21countries have officially reported 1,085 cases of Influenza A (H1N1) infection, with 26 deaths.

Three new countries (Colombia, El Salvador, and Italy) have reported cases.

The WHO Director-General addresses the UN General Assembly: she stresses the uncertainty about the current pandemic, discusses the various lessons that can be learned from past pandemics, the fact that there are limited amounts of antivirals and vaccines, and the need for solidarity.

MAY 5TH: The WHO reports 1,490 cases from 21 countries and 30 deaths.

The WHO dispatches 2.4 million courses of antivirals to 72 countries most in need, including Mexico.

The WHO Scientific Committee meets to discuss a range of issues including the development of the Influenza A (H1N1) virus and issues around the virus' severity.

MAY 6TH: The WHO reports 1,893 cases from 23 countries and 31 deaths. Two new countries (Guatemala and Sweden) report cases.

The WHO's South East Asia regional office distributes about 60,000 doses of Tamiflu (Oseltamivir) and Personal Protection Equipment to its Member States.

MAY 7TH: The WHO reports 2,371 cases from 24 countries with 44 deaths.

One new country (Poland) confirms one case of A/H1N1.

Dr Keiji Fukuda, Assistant Director-General briefs the Association of Southeast Asian Nations on the WHO's pandemic response and the implications of moving from phase 5 to phase 6.

MAY 8TH: The WHO reports 2,500 cases from 25 countries and 46 deaths.

One new country (Brazil) confirms four cases of A/H1N1.

Swine Flu: To Date

MAY 9TH: The WHO reports 3,453 cases from 29 countries and 48 deaths.

Four new countries (Argentina, Australia, Japan and Panama) confirm cases of A/H1N1.

MAY 10TH: The WHO reports 4,393 cases from 30 countries 42 deaths.

One new country (Norway) confirms two cases.

The WHO reviews the latest information on vaccines with the International Federation of Pharmaceutical Manufacturers and Associations (IFPMA), the Developing Countries Vaccine Manufacturers' Network, and other Influenza vaccine manufacturers.

MAY 11TH: The WHO reports 4,789 cases from 30 countries and 53 deaths.

MAY 12TH: The WHO reports 5,269 cases from 30 countries and 61 deaths.

Thailand confirms its first two cases of H1N1, two teenagers who had recently returned from Mexico. Eighteen passengers on the same flight who sat close to the two teenagers were contacted and given Tamiflu (Oseltamivir).

MAY 13TH: The WHO reports 6,302 cases from 33 countries.

Two new countries Cuba, and Finland confirm cases.

The "Gibbs article" comes out. Written by one of the scientists who helped develop Tamiflu, it hypothesizes that the origin of this new H1N1 virus might have grown in eggs and released in an accident.

MAY 14TH: The WHO reports 7,457 cases from 34 countries, and 65 deaths.

One new country (Belgium) confirms one case.

Indian Drug manufacturer, Cipla, receives pre-qualification by WHO for production of Tamiflu (Oseltamivir).

A vaccine advisory group meeting held by WHO to ascertain whether enough evidence exists to recommend large-scale A(H1N1) vaccine production.

MAY 15TH: Seven new cases of Swine Flu confirmed in Britain while the Foreign Office lifts its travel restrictions into Mexico. Four children in London and three people in Greenock, Scotland have the virus. Total UK cases at 85.

The WHO comments on 'The Gibbs Article' and says that it does not believe that the Swine Flu virus resulted from a laboratory accident.

US health officials say there are 100,000 infected in the country, whilst also easing the warning on travel to Mexico.

Texas health officials report that a man from Corpus Christi died on Friday, raising the number of U.S. deaths to five.

The CDC also reports 4,714 confirmed and likely cases.

GlaxoSmithKline announces plans to begin production of a Swine Flu vaccine once it receives a seed sample of the latest H1N1 virus.

MAY 16TH: India's first confirmed case of H1N1 reported.

MAY 17TH: 39 countries have officially reported 8,480 cases of Influenza A(H1N1) infection and 72 deaths to WHO.

Japan reports 21new confirmed cases from students at three high schools in Kobe and nine students at a High School in Osaka. All the new cases appear to have acquired the virus independently and have not travelled recently to countries affected by Influenza A(H1N1).

MAY 18TH: Japan reports 118 new cases over the last 24 hours.

All 72 countries receive their consignments of Tamiflu (Oseltamivir) antiviral courses that the WHO started sending on 5th May. The WHO sent out 3 million courses of the drug.

MAY 19TH: UN Secretary General Ban Ki-moon and WHO Director General Dr Margaret Chan meet with around 30 pharmaceutical manufacturers and discuss the need for equity and fairness in access to vaccines for developing countries.

MAY 22ND: 62nd World Heath Assembly concludes with the Director General emphasizing that *"the decision to declare an Influenza pandemic is a responsibility, and a duty, that she takes seriously"*.

Weekly Epidemiological Record focuses on Clinical observations on H1N1 patients.

JUNE 1ST: The WHO carries out consultations with over 30 experts from 23 countries to consider countries' needs and concerns and the steps WHO needs to take when considering when and if to go to Phase 6.

Swine Flu: To Date

JUNE 10TH: An article published online in Nature, suggests that transmission to humans occurred several months before recognition of the existing outbreak.

JUNE 11TH: The WHO Director General declares that *"the world is now at the start of the 2009 Influenza pandemic"*.

The WHO officially raises its infectious diseases alert to Phase 6, its highest level, in recognition of the fact that the virus is now undergoing communitywide transmission in Australia as well as in North America.

The announcement makes this the first global Influenza epidemic in 41 years. The last one in 1968 ("Hong Kong flu") killed an estimated 1 million people worldwide.

The figures for this epidemic, to date are announced at 27,737 laboratory-confirmed cases and 141 deaths, although health officials believe many times that number have been infected but have not been tested because their disease was mild.

JUNE 12TH: A further 67 patients in England are confirmed with Swine Flu, pushing the UK total to over 1,000.

Egypt reports three new cases of Swine Flu as two children and a Colombian visitor test positive for the A(H1N1) virus.

An elderly New York woman infected with the swine-flu virus dies in Las Vegas.

JUNE 13TH: A second, dedicated, Swine Flu clinic has to be opened in a Canberra hospital in Australia in order to cope with demand.

JUNE 14TH: US Health Secretary says production of a vaccine for Swine Flu is being set up in case a vaccine programme is recommended.

Korea's confirmed cases of Swine Flu rise to 61.

The number of confirmed Swine Flu cases in Missouri is 51, with one death.

Thailand's prime minister urges public calm as Swine Flu cases triple over the previous three days

17 Swine Flu cases in India

The Survivor's Guide to Swine Flu

JUNE 15TH: A person with Swine Flu dies in Scotland and becomes the first known death of a Swine Flu patient outside of the Americas.

JUNE 16TH: The premature baby son of Britain's first Swine Flu victim dies — just 24 hours after his mother - but not from Swine Flu.

The FDA in the US demands that dozens of internet sites remove any claims relating to Swine Flu.

A 9-year-old boy in Miami-Dade County died from Swine Flu, making him the first death in Florida.

Salt Lake Valley Health officials confirm a fifth Utahn infected with the H1N1 Swine Flu virus has died.

Connecticut reports its third Swine Flu death.

JUNE 17TH: The number of UK Swine Flu cases reaches 1,582 in the UK, after 110 more people in England test positive for the virus.

The Swiss pharmaceuticals company Novartis AG, announces it has produced the first batch of Swine Flu vaccine which will be sent off for testing – and which "is being considered for clinical trials." (This batch was made in Germany; they are building a new plant in North Carolina: the US Government had already placed an order with them for $289m of vaccine, in May).

A Spanish tour operator says that two Caribbean countries have turned away a cruise ship because of fears of Swine Flu among crew members

JUNE 18TH: Three people die in Illinois, bringing the total of deaths in the US to eight.

A 47-year-old woman in Utah whose mother contracted Swine Flu while living with her - was denied the antiviral Tamiflu twice by doctors, then went on to die from the flu herself.

JUNE 19TH: The number of Swine Flu cases rise to 21,449 in the US and the number of deaths to 87.

Dedicated testing facilities for Swine Flu set up across Glasgow using existing NHS accommodation to house nine testing facilities including health centres and clinics.
Seven new cases of the H1N1 virus confirmed taking the total number of cases in Scotland to 537.

Swine Flu: To Date

Three adults and four children test positive for Swine Flu, bringing the total for Saudi Arabia to 29.

An Australian man suffering from Swine Flu dies.

519 confirmed cases in China

JUNE 20TH: China continues to wield some of the toughest controls to combat the spread of the so-called Swine Flu.

Fourth Swine Flu death reported in New Jersey.

Maryland health officials say they've confirmed 334 cases of Swine Flu.

Swine Flu forces cancellation of Caribbean Games.

Total number of people affected with Swine Flu in India is 50.

JUNE 21ST: An eighth-grader at Buffalo's Harvey Austin School 97 stricken with Swine Flu and other ailments dies.

Indian cases up to 59.

Fiji in the middle of the pacific confirms its very first case of Swine Flu.

The Chief Medical Officer in the UK writes to health authorities urging hospitals to test all patients who show signs of flu-like symptoms. He wrote: *"Transmission from person to person in this country is increasingly common. There is evidence that sporadic cases are arising with no apparent link either to cases elsewhere in the UK or to travel abroad."* The letter followed an earlier warning from him that millions of Britons could fall victim to Swine Flu in the coming months.

JUNE 22ND: AVI Biopharma a developer of RNA-based drugs announces it has signed a contract with the US Defense Threat Reduction Agency to develop Swine Flu drugs.

Delta Air Lines says the H1N1 virus has sapped travel demand, resulting in a $250 million hit on the carrier's second-quarter revenue.

A 49-year-old woman with Swine Flu dies in the Philippines in the country's first death related to the virus.

The Survivor's Guide to Swine Flu

The seventh case of H1N1 (swine) flu is reported in the Czech Republic.

JUNE 23RD: Another 149 cases of Swine Flu are confirmed in the UK, bringing the total to more than 2,900.

California's ninth death from Swine Flu.

Australia reports its second Swine Flu-related death.

JUNE 24TH: The WHO says there have been 52,160 cases of Swine Flu confirmed - in about 100 nations.

Argentine health officials say seven more people have died from Swine Flu, bringing the number of deaths to 17.

The Texas Department of State Health Services reports that as of June 17, there were 2,354 confirmed cases of Swine Flu and 10 deaths.

The Palestinian Ministry of Health reports that a Palestinian woman from Ramallah has been diagnosed with Swine Flu.

Reports out today reveal that the Canadian government delayed sending alcohol-based hand sanitizer to Native American reservations battling the H1N1 flu virus out of fears people would drink it.

JUNE 25TH: The number of people infected with Swine Flu crosses the 3,000-mark in Australia.

A 30-year-old woman with Swine Flu dies, making her Florida's second Swine Flu fatality.

JUNE 26TH: The US accounts for half of the reported number of cases, with nearly 28,000 laboratory-confirmed cases of the virus, with 56,000 cases globally reported to the World Health Organization.

On top of this at least 1 million Americans have contracted the H1N1 Influenza, according to mathematical models. The data shows that the virus is continuing to spread in the US, even though the normal flu season was over and that an increasing proportion of victims were being hospitalised.

The CDC said that although 1 million infected appears to be a high number, between 15 million and 60 million Americans are infected by the Influenza virus during a normal flu season.

Swine Flu: To Date

At least 3,065 in the US had been hospitalised and 127 have died.

The very young are most likely to be infected, the CDC said, but older patients seem to suffer more. The average age of Swine Flu victims is 12, the average age of hospitalised patients is 20 and the average age of those who have died is 37, she said. The spread was highest in New England and the Northeast.

In the Southern Hemisphere, which was one month into its flu season, several countries have been badly affected.

Chile has had more than 4,000 laboratory-confirmed cases and seven deaths,

Argentina more than 1,200 cases and 17 deaths.

Australia 3,200 cases and four deaths.

French pharmaceutical company Sanofi-Aventis announces it has begun large-scale production of a vaccine.

Swine Flu claims the lives of two Michigan residents, putting the state's death toll up to seven.

Organisers at the Glastonbury Festival go on alert after it emerges that an infected man was planning to attend.

Bangladesh confirms its first ever case of Swine Flu.

The WHO issues reassurances that Swine Flu remains stable and shows no signs of mixing with other Influenza viruses.

JUNE 27TH: Once a hotbed for infections, Tennessee reports the number of cases is dropping.

A teenager in Arizona dies, bringing the death toll statewide to nine.

A 26-year-old Perth woman becomes the fifth Australian to die.

JUNE 28TH: India reports four fresh cases of Swine Flu, taking he total number of people infected with the virus to 93.

The number of confirmed Swine Flu cases in Nebraska is 111.

Two deaths confirmed in Thailand. Plus 1,209 confirmed cases (1,100 recovered).

The Survivor's Guide to Swine Flu

South Korean - six more people infected, bringing to country's total to 202

A 9-year-old Buffalo girl dies of Swine Flu -- the second Buffalo School District student to die of the disease in a week.

JUNE 29TH: Roche Holding says that a patient in Denmark has developed resistance to Tamiflu, but that the drug is still effective in the circulating H1N1 Swine Flu virus.

The total number of Swine Flu cases in Scotland has tops 1,000.

Nepal reports its first 3 cases of Swine Flu.

JUNE 30TH: Nine more cases of Swine Flu confirmed in Wales, taking the total to 26.

A Connecticut man dies, the state's sixth death linked to the H1N1 virus.

New Jersey reports its 6th Swine Flu death.

JULY 1ST: Officials in the US officially warn people off holding 'Swine Flu parties'.

28 staff sent home from the Wimbledon Championships with suspected Swine Flu.

The official figure for the number of people who've contracted Swine Flu in the UK is 6,538.

The mayor of Buenos Aires, declares a state of emergency to help control the spread of Swine Flu.

JULY 2ND: Britain faces a projected 100,000 new Swine Flu cases a day by the end of August, the nation's health minister said yesterday. Britain has officially reported 7,447 Swine Flu cases and three deaths, but officials acknowledge the real number of cases is far higher, since many have not been tested. Britain is the hardest-hit nation in Europe amid the global Swine Flu epidemic. Many flu experts believe numbers could jump exponentially now that the virus is entrenched. Few people have natural immunity, allowing it to spread rapidly.

Health officials say the number of Swine Flu cases in Illinois has risen to more than 3,100, with 13 deaths.

Argentina overtakes Canada as the country with the third highest number of Swine Flu deaths as it reports 17 more H1N1 flu deaths, bringing the total to 43 to 44. (US top with 127 deaths, followed by Mexico, 116).

Swine Flu: To Date

Hong Kong's retail sales fall more sharply in May than in the previous month, mainly because of a sharp drop in tourist arrivals stemming from fears about the spread of Swine Flu.

JULY 3RD: Dr Margaret Chan the WHO Director-General opens a Swine Flu forum in Mexico by saying that the spread of the virus worldwide is now unstoppable.

The number of Swine Flu cases in Argentina rises dramatically, with the new health minister reporting an estimated 100,000 cases.

Japan and Hong Kong report they have each found a patient with the type of Swine Flu that has proven resistant to Tamiflu.

First Swine Flu death in India.

Reports that the virus is showing signs of rebounding in Mexico.

The WHO reports that at least 337 people have died from Swine Flu, which has also sickened 80000 others in 121 countries.

JULY 4TH: First Swine Flu death in London.

Three people die in New Zealand, the country's first fatalities from the H1N1 virus.

JULY 5TH: Swine Flu total in Wales hits 50; there are also 28 "clinically presumed" cases of Swine Flu.

Australia reports its 11th death linked to Swine Flu. The number of cases totals 5,298.

Syria reports its first confirmed case.

JULY 6TH: New Zealand orders 300,000 doses of Swine Flu vaccine

UN Secretary-General Ban Ki-moon says the world body may need over $1 billion to fight the Swine Flu pandemic for the rest of this year

Philippines seeks extra $390 m for anti-flu drive.

Australia reports 12th Swine Flu Fatality

JULY 7TH: Reports that Tamiflu has surpassed Viagra as the most commonly spammed drug on the internet.

The Survivor's Guide to Swine Flu

Thailand reports the deaths of two more people afflicted with Swine Flu, bringing the country's total to nine.

Argentina moves towards popular unrest as people start to question the government's handling of the H1N1 flu outbreak that has killed 60.

JULY 8TH: Fourteen cases of Swine Flu detected among US soldiers stationed at the biggest military base in Afghanistan.

A San Francisco teenager diagnosed with a Tamiflu resistant strain of Swine Flu.

San Quentin State Prison says it will stop accepting inmates from 19 Northern California counties Wednesday because of fears over the Swine Flu.

Australia Reports 18th Swine Flu Death.

The WHO announces that it is stopping counting and tracking the number of cases – as it is too high.

JULY 9TH: Fourteen patients are now thought to have died in the UK after contracting Swine Flu.

US plans for autumn Swine Flu vaccination campaign.

Nearly 100 new cases of Swine Flu diagnosed in Wales in the space of one day. There are now 279 cases of flu in Wales – up from 183 earlier in the week.

JULY 10TH: Vietnam reports three more Swine Flu cases

JULY 11TH: A vaccine against Swine Flu is not likely to be ready before the first wave of an expected pandemic hits, an expert has said.

Second death in Hawaii linked to Swine Flu.

California to receive more than $30 million in federal grants to help prepare for an expected resurgence of Swine Flu in the coming Influenza season.

First Georgia (US) Swine Flu death reported.

First Nunavut death reported, with 32 more cases of H1N1, bringing the total number of cases in the territory to 372.

Swine Flu: To Date

JULY 12TH: Reports say that a Swine Flu vaccine will be rushed through saftey checks to be ready to use in the UK.

The US announces another $1 billion order for Swine Flu vaccine.

Britain records 15th Swine Flu death.

The Air Force Academy in Colorado Springs, Colorado is dealing with the state's largest outbreak of Swine Flu.

Illinois health officials report one more death and a hundred more cases of the Swine Flu this week. That brings the statewide death toll up to 14, with more than 3,200 confirmed cases. Over half the cases are reported in young people from ages five to 24.

JULY 13TH: Study published that shows that 1918 flu survivors seem immune to Swine Flu; and that this may apply to those who lived through the 1957 Flu pandemic.

The number of people diagnosed with Swine Flu in New Brunswick jumps by more than 50 per cent in three days, with 33 confirmed cases.

JULY 14TH: Swine Flu calls to GPs 'jump 50%' in the UK. Figures for England and Wales show that those aged five to 14 had the highest infection rate, at 159.57 per 100,000.

Hawaii's second Swine Flu-related death confirmed.

US Swine Flu vaccinations could begin in October with children at schools among the first in line.

Health authorities estimated up to 6,000 Australians could die from Swine Flu in a "worst case scenario" during the current Southern Hemisphere winter.

JULY 15TH: Worries that the Swine Flu pandemic may affect the annual Hajj to Mecca despite low rates of infection in the Middle East, standing at just over 1100 cases, with no reported deaths. Iin Saudi Arabia the total number of reported infections is just 114.

JULY 16TH: Britain's Chief Medical Officer says that up to 65,000 deaths could occur if the pandemic worsens, with a minimum of 3,100 deaths expected, with the official death toll at 29.

The French government orders 28 million doses of Swine Flu vaccine from Sanofi Pasteur.

The Survivor's Guide to Swine Flu

Swine Flu starts to spread even faster across much of Britain, with 55,000 new cases in England in the last week.

JULY 17TH: US Swine Flu cases surpasses 40,000 and deaths rise to 263.

Four more people in London die after contracting Swine Flu.

For the latest World News Updates on Swine Flu and Complementary Medicine go to The CMA website (The-CMA.Org.UK).

Figures are also available at:

http://www.searo.who.int/LinkFiles/Influenza_A(H1N1)_Chronology_of_Influenza_A(H1N1).pdf
http://www.wpro.who.int/NR/rdonlyres/5D3B17F6-8F19-4269-A547-C5F61C1AC8E2/0/MMWRswineoriginfluMexico_mm58d0430a2.pdf
http://news.bbc.co.uk/1/hi/health

CHAPTER 6

WHAT IS A VIRUS?

The disease 'influenza' is caused by a virus (as opposed to parasites, bacteria or fungi). A virus is an infectious agent composed of a nucleic acid, DNA or RNA, which is surrounded and enclosed in a coat of protein.

PROTEINS?

A protein is any one of a group of complex large organic molecules that contain carbon, hydrogen, oxygen, nitrogen and usually sulphur. They are composed of one or more chains of amino acids.

Proteins are fundamental components of all living cells. This includes animal cells, bacteria and even viruses – which are somewhere between living and non-living matter.

Proteins are found in many substances, such as enzymes and hormones, all of which are necessary for the proper functioning of an organism. Animals and humans need protein in their diet for the growth and repair of tissue and this can be obtained from foods such as meat, fish, eggs, milk, and legumes.

VIRUSES ARE TINY

Unlike bacteria, viruses have no cell walls and are so tiny that they can pass through ultrafine filters that manage to hold back bacteria. This helps them to enter our cells. (In fact, viruses were originally called "filterables" by scientists, as they were able to pass through the very finest filters that could hold back bacteria and other minute organisms.)

What is a Virus?

They have the ability to move from cell to cell and in fact "have to do so", as viruses are what are known as "obligate parasites", organisms that cannot live independently from their host.

HOW THEY REPRODUCE?

They do not reproduce by themselves and have to "steal" genetic material from other cells, as they lack the cellular machinery for self reproduction. While other organisms such as bacteria, parasites and fungi are clearly alive as we would understand the term, viruses, confusingly, exist in a twilight zone, somewhere between death and life as mentioned above – as at no stage in their existence cycle do they reproduce on their own.

So, a virus' existence is entirely dependent upon its ability to commandeer the machinery (DNA or RNA depending on the type of virus) of one of your living host cells and this renders the cell incapable of doing all the things that it is supposed to do – normally – to keep us alive and well.

All a virus does is reproduce – inside its host's cells – making enormous numbers of copies of itself – and then spread itself.

HOW THEY SPREAD?

Viruses are constantly trying to find ways of spreading themselves. They do this by infecting a host – in the case of Swine Flu the usual hosts are pigs but other species, including humans are being infected, as we know.

The host is of no importance to the virus – it is just simply "a ride" - a way for the virus to replicate.

The illness that the virus induces causes symptoms – and these symptoms can include sneezing and coughing, which is an excellent way for the virus to get out of your body and into other peoples' bodies – where it can then begin to hijack a series of cells from the new host.

So, 'making you ill' is usually beneficial to a virus. But if it makes you too ill - so that you can't socialise - or in extreme cases - if the virus kills its victim this will interfere with its ability to 'hitch a new ride' and subsequently reproduce. So the virus may then mutate into a less aggressive form.

HOW YOUR BODY 'FIGHTS BACK'?

Of course the host – your body – isn't going to stand for being ill for weeks on end, coughing and sneezing and shedding virus left, right and centre, so it too, responds.

Your immune system learns to recognise the virus and will make anti-bodies which begin to fight this specific virus.

Most of the time we do get better after a viral infection but, the virus will continue it's mission to spread among other people so, although we personally may have won the battle, we have not won the war.

The virus can then 'mutate' over time – in other people – and may (theoretically) come back to infect you again at a later date – in a slightly different form.

THE POTENTIALLY DEADLIER INFLUENZA VIRUS

The family of viruses that influenza belongs to are called orthomyxoviridae (from "myxa" meaning "mucus" in Greek) which has three members, types A, B and C.

Types A, B and C all infect people, but only Type A is capable of causing pandemic influenza.

As we have seen, all viruses are small and the Influenza A is considered to be a medium-sized virus. The average diameter of a human hair is about 80,000 nm. (nm is a nanometre – one billionth of a metre.) In its spherical form, Influenza A is about 120nm, so its size is somewhere between a cold virus (rhinovirus) at a very tiny 20nm and a comparatively gigantic, 200nm Ebola virus. The Influenza A virus is more than 100 times smaller than a human red blood cell and much smaller than bacteria.

ONE OF THE SIMPLEST MICRO-ORGANISMS AROUND

Compared to almost any other micro-organism, viruses are simple in structure, consisting of little else than genetic material (DNA or RNA) that decrees how the virus is built and gives it any other particular features that will help it to trick a host cell to gain entry and begin to make new copies of itself from this blueprint. So, as we have seen all the Influenza A virus wants to do is get into your cells and turn these 'host cells', into a photocopier machine to produce more influenza viruses.

INFECTION

Hijacking your cells for this purpose is called infection.

One of two things can then happen. First of all, the host cell may just be used to make copies of the virus and this can be of very little consequence to the host cell. Alternatively, the consequences of infection can be disastrous and the host cell dies and viral copies are let loose and go on to infect and kill more cells.

What is a Virus?

Our immune system tries to defend us in the face of a viral attack, but viruses are prepared for this and have developed their own set of counter-attacks, which are built into the virus' structure.

THE CONFIGURATION OF THE H1N1 VIRUS

The genetic blueprint for the virus' composition is contained at its core and this is surrounded with a protective covering of protein called a capsid.

As you know, in human cells there is a double helix configuration of DNA (deoxyribonucleic acid). This is in contrast to H1N1 viruses, which have only a single strand of ribonucleic acid (ssRNA).

THE HIJACK APPROACH

A good analogy to describe how a virus hijacks a cell and uses the cell's internal 'machinery' to make copies of itself is as follows:

> Imagine a factory manufacturing cars. This factory is your cell. Now imagine that someone (the virus) turns up and says; "Right – here's the plan (viral genetic blueprint), I want you to stop making cars but I want you to use your tools to make tricycles instead. And, I'm not going to pay you and in fact I might even make you all redundant and close the factory down, or if I am in a really bad mood I will blow the factory up".

It's an unlikely scenario of course. After all, how would someone like this be able to get into the factory in the first place? They would have to use trickery and subterfuge.

And this is exactly what a virus does.

GETTING INTO YOUR SYSTEM

When an influenza virus arrives in your respiratory tract it is still technically on the outside of your body, it has not yet been able to gain entry to your cells. So, in order to achieve this, it has some very special characteristics that make it able to penetrate the cell walls that line your respiratory tract.

Influenza A is an 'enveloped virus', which means that it is enveloped in an additional covering of sugars and fats on its surface, called a phospholipid bilayer (also called 'lipid bilayer' or 'lipid-protein bilayer'), which is what it uses to enable it to gain entry.

The Survivor's Guide to Swine Flu

The hard, shell-like, capsid – made of the virus' own protein - is covered with this phospholipid bilayer. This lipid-protein bilayer, also contains material that has been stolen from the virus' previous home, as it exploded out of the last cell it was in.

Crucially, this viral envelope also has viral protein spikes, with sugars (carbohydrates) attached that stick through it, giving it a typical 'sputnik' look.

The protein-sugar combination in the lipid bilayer is called a glycoprotein.

There are three glycoproteins that poke through the surface of the virus. Our own immune system can "recognise" them, if your body has previously been exposed to a particular virus, and will make anti-bodies against them, providing it has time to do so.

Some viruses are so lethal that they kill the "host" before the immune system has time to "recognise" a virus and make the antibodies to it.

A REPRESENTATION OF THE H1N1 VIRUS[1]

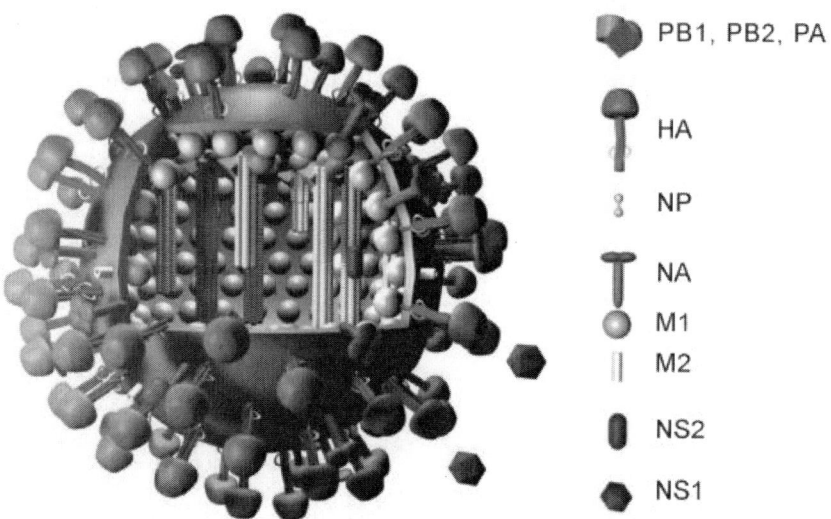

The three glycoproteins on a virus are called;

- Hemagglutinin (HA)
- Neuraminidase (NA)
- M2

What is a Virus?

There are 16 broad immune classes, or types of HA glycoprotein and 9 different immune classes of NA glycoprotein. (In fact, while we know that antibodies to M2 do exist, very little is known at this time about their role in immunity.)

The different HA immune classes are designated (named) H1 to H16.

The NA immune classes are designated N1 to N9.

So, for example the influenza subtype that is currently causing grave concern in Swine Flu is "Influenza A" H1N1. So we can infer from this that this particular Swine Flu has **glycoprotein spikes** of the classes **Hemagglutinin (H), 1 and Neuraminidase (N), 1.**

That's why we refer to is as **H1N1**, for short.

HOW WE FIGHT OFF THIS FLU INFECTATION

One of the problems for humans facing an influenza as powerfully infectious as H1N1 appears to be, is that the immune classes (the H1 or the N1) will also vary slightly from time to time and this affects how well our antibodies can recognise them.

These differences give rise to the different strains of the virus that arise from time to time, but these differences are not as large as the differences between the major classes (e.g. H1 vs H5).

TO USE A MENTAL EXERCISE TO CLARIFY THIS IMPORTANT POINT:

> Imagine a world where you have only ever seen three types of flower; roses, hollyhocks and orchids. You know that they are flowers and they are all very different from each other.
>
> They don't look alike at all.
>
> These are the equivalent of H5, H6 etc. and N1, N2 etc.
>
> Naturally, flowers come in different colours – so these various colours in a particular type of flower could be considered to be subtypes.
>
> So if you have only ever seen roses, hollyhocks and orchids in your entire life and then you suddenly come across a tiny daisy, you may not recognise it to be a flower at all.

This is the equivalent for your immune system of coming across a new strain of virus. Of course you will eventually work out that it has a stem, petals etc, so it must in fact be a flower, although it bears no resemblance to any that you have ever seen before. This all takes time.

So, to relate this to flu; your immune system may be slow and even possibly unsuccessful in recognising different strains of the same 'viral subtype', in normal flu.

However, most human immune systems have no experience of the current H1 subtype of Swine Flu at all, so they cannot recognise it. This is why we are at such great risk from this virus. The only way that our immune systems will ever be in a position to 'learn' about this viral subtype is by being infected.

As mentioned previously - some authorities are saying that anyone who lived through the Asian Flu outbreak of 1957 could have this kind of immunity to the current H1N1 virus – although the 1957 virus was H2N2.

One of the main concerns about H1N1 is that your immune system needs time to recognise the virus and to make antibodies to it and as discussed above, this may be a luxury that we can ill afford. Although the current Swine Flu virus is classified as 'mild' in most people, the concern is that should the H1N1 virus mutate to be similar to the H1N1 virus of 1918, it could cause enormous damage – before your immune system has time to make the much needed antibodies. So they may not even be made at all if a person falls ill and dies rapidly, as it can take about a week – or sometimes longer to make antibodies. (Back in 1918, people were developing symptoms in the morning and were dead by dusk.)

NOW WE KNOW ABOUT HA AND NA, WHAT DOES THE M2 PROTEIN DO?

Although little is known about the M2 protein, scientists call it an ion channel and it is relevant and important in the 'uncoating' process as discussed above. It is known that the M1 protein is a matrix protein and the M2 protein is a membrane protein and recent research suggests the M gene may be involved in determining host tropism. [1] (More about tropism and pantropism later in this chapter.)

Pharmaceutical companies are attempting to target this protein with the use of antiviral drugs such as amantadine and rimantadine. These M2 blockers are the "older" type of drug used to combat influenza.

WHAT HAPPENS TO THE SWINE FLU VIRUS ONCE IT ATTACHES TO ONE OF YOUR CELLS

As we have explained, in simple terms, viruses use trickery; the spikey HA and NA glycoproteins act as a key, which, when successful, allows them to attach to your cell in the right place and 'match' other parts on the outside of your cells. Your cell thinks this is just a normal part of your

What is a Virus?

bodies' system coming to deliver nutrients and allows it in.

Once the virus latches on to one of your cells, it begins to cause the cell wall to develop a pit – into which the virus begins to sink. Eventually this pit deepens and deepens, until it totally engulfs the virus.

To explain in a bit more detail, there are special regions on the HA glycoprotein of the virus, called 'receptor binding sites' and these can attach to a host cell if the host cell has a specific receptor molecule.

Imagine a special key fitting a special lock:

Like the influenza virus, the host cells in the respiratory tract also have lipid bilayers and these too are studded with glycoproteins – which they use, in the normal course of events to let the 'good things' the cell needs – to enter the cell.

A host cell glycoprotein (sugary-protein) sits on the 'receptor molecule' for the Influenza A virus and this host cell glycoprotein is tipped with a particular kind of sugar called sialic acid.

Human cells have a particular type of sialic acid called N-acetylneuraminic acid (NeuAc) and when this is attached to the cell's glycoprotein, by yet another sugar called galactose, it creates a 'potential' receptor for the Influenza A virus to attach itself, via the HA protein spike.

It is 'potential' because there is one additional subtlety here: it depends upon the precise way in which the NeuAc, sialic acid is attached to the galactose (Gal). There are several possible linkages, of which two, the α-(2,3) and the α-(2,6) linkages, are necessary for influenza virus recognition. The numbers and the Greek letter "alpha" describe which atoms are connected to which on the sialic acid and the galactose.

It has been recognised for a long time that, pigs as well as humans have both types of linkages and so can be infected by Avian Influenza, Swine Influenza or Human Influenza and sometimes all three at the same time. In fact, the current H1N1 virus is a combination of human, bird and pig strains.

For a while, when Bird Flu was under the microscope, it was believed that bird respiratory and intestinal tract cells had "NeuAc-α-(2,3)-Gal" linkages while human respiratory tract cells had "NeuAc-a-(2,6)-Gal" linkages. However, scientists now believe that human respiratory tracts have both. Research also indicates that human viruses "prefer" the NeuAc-α -(2,6)-Gal linkages and that bird viruses "prefer" NeuAc-α-(2,3)-Gal linkages. (Also see our 'Further Reading' section at the end of this chapter)

This is crucial information in the fight against Swine Flu (and Bird Flu), as Conventional and Complementary Medical scientists are working hard to figure out ways that viruses can be prevented from attaching themselves to host cells – thus stopping them from entering and wreaking havoc.

This is why pigs are often implicated in viral change – as the virus can mix with other similar viruses inside a pig's body and create a whole new strain. This is called genetic "reassortment" and "recombination".

The 1918 pandemic flu was known as "Spanish Flu" because media reports of if its existence first came from Spain because there was a media blackout in many other countries due to the war. But before that it was also called "Swine Fever", as it was thought to have originated from pigs.

ONCE INSIDE YOUR CELLS

The virus is now inside a little bubble (called a vesicle) that is totally enclosed and this is now inside the cell. Once inside the vesicle, the internal environment of the cell, which is quite acidic, causes the viral covering to fuse with the vesicle's wall and this releases the genetic material of the virus into the your host cell.

This ultimately allows it to gain access to the 'duplicating' equipment it needs to make new

MORE CAUSE FOR CONCERN: WILL SWINE FLU BE AS POTENTIALLY LETHAL AS BIRD FLU COULD BE?

It appears that Bird Flu viruses of the H5 and H7 subtypes have mutations that insert extra amino acids (the building blocks of proteins) at the 'cleavage site' and that this expands it, so that a wider variety of tissue proteases can perform the cleavage operation. In order to do their work, these proteases need a variety of particular amino acids and these are the ones with basic groups on their side chains. These include the amino acids, lysine, arginine and histidine.

The kind of H5 influenza that is not too serious – "Low Pathogenic Avian Influenza" (LPAI) H5s have only one basic amino acid at the cleavage site. However, if there are 'polybasic amino acids' at the cleavage site, this is characteristic of the deadly form of H5 "Highly Pathogenic Avian Influenza" (HPAI) viruses and these are the ones that have killed millions of birds and humdreds of humans, over the last few years.

Whether the same will be true of the current Swine Flu virus we have yet to discover.

copies of itself. The process of fusing with the vesicle is called 'uncoating' and requires 'cleavage' of Hemagglutinase to happen.

At some point (exactly when and where isn't completely clear to scientists yet), in order to be infective, the hemagglutinase glycoprotein has to be cut ('cleaved') into two pieces. This is done by a special kind of enzyme called a protease. The site on hemagglutinase where this must occur (the cleavage site) is quite tiny. Therefore, the types of proteases that can trigger infectiveness are limited to only a few types of tissues.

In humans, these are found predominantly in the respiratory tissues and in birds they are located in the intestinal tract tissues.

Because in humans, these proteases are found mainly in our respiratory tract, H1N1 predominantly affects our respiratory organs and this is why people who have contracted H1N1 can show such severe signs of respiratory distress, although – alarmingly – patients have also presented with gastro-intestinal symptoms too. This fact is worrying because it infers that the current H1N1 virus is able to affect the cells other than those in the upper respiratory tract, making it potentially more lethal.

REASSORTMENT AND RECOMBINATION

The worry has always been that a strain of flu, e.g. Swine Flu could mutate in this way, to make it even easier for human–to–human transmission and if the virus becomes more virulent this could lead to a deadly pandemic on the scale of that in 1918. A change occurring in the HA binding site via a mutation as outlined above would allow the virus to efficiently bind to a human receptor cell, and start to create copies of its new mutated self – which then infects people. This could allow a virus that previously only affected pigs, or birds, to be transmitted from person to person.

There is much scientific controversy over viral mutations like these, as to whether random mutations, i.e. picking up errors along the way – due to the sheer numbers of viruses that exist and the numbers of replicants that each virus is able to produce - will cause the H1N1 virus to increase it's human to human infectivity.

However, there is another theory called 'recombination' and this may also be the driving force behind the viral changes that occur. The theory that leading scientists in this field are currently considering – that of 'cleavage' – is supported by scientists, Mark and Adrian Gibbs in Australia and Henry Niman in the US.

They propose that the driving force in genetic variation is not the error-prone, or seemingly random duplication of genetic material that picks up errors along the way that lead to mutations.

They believe that the driving force behind this change is the process of "recombination", where pieces of genetic material from different genes in the virus, or from similar genes of two different viruses, swap pieces between themselves and recombine to produce a new set of hybrid genes.

So, there is evidence from research on material from the Spanish Influenza epidemic that the HA glycoprotein of the 1918 virus is derived from both Pig Influenza virus and Human Influenza viral sources. This evidence demonstrates that the beginning and the ends of the virus' RNA are from the human version of the flu virus, but the middle section is from a virus that was circulating in pigs at the time. But the pathogenicity and virulence of influenza viruses is almost certainly multigenic, i.e. it requires cooperating changes in more than one gene.

Therefore, we can't predict a virus' virulence at this time, although there are many tantalising clues as to what might be going on and further exploration of Niman and Gibbs ideas may well be helpful.

It is also unknown if there are relative contributions of mutation and recombination as additional sources of genetic variation. It is known, however, that if we can predict a virus' potential virulence then we may well be able to develop strategies to deal with that particular virus ahead of time, rather than being in the situation of having to react to a new, virulent form of flu, 'instantly' which, of course, means delays in the production of drugs and vaccines to combat it.

Now that scientists can start to understand how the Swine Flu virus mutates, they can start to understand how to manufacture appropriate drugs which will, hopefully, combat it. With a potentially dangerous virus – like Swine Flu – the time it takes to react could cost lives.

MORE ABOUT REASSORTMENT AND RECOMBINATION

Viral material – RNA – is a single strand of genetic material, formed of eight separate pieces, called segments. These are a bit like our chromosomes. In Influenza A, six of these segments have a protein each, while two segments have two proteins each.

For a virus to 'be a virus', it needs all eight pieces, but these can come from different viruses.

So, if a host, such as a pig, or a human is infected by both a bird virus and a human, or pig, virus at the same time, the segments are in a common pool within the host cell.

These can get mixed up (reassorted) and can end up producing viral strands that have some

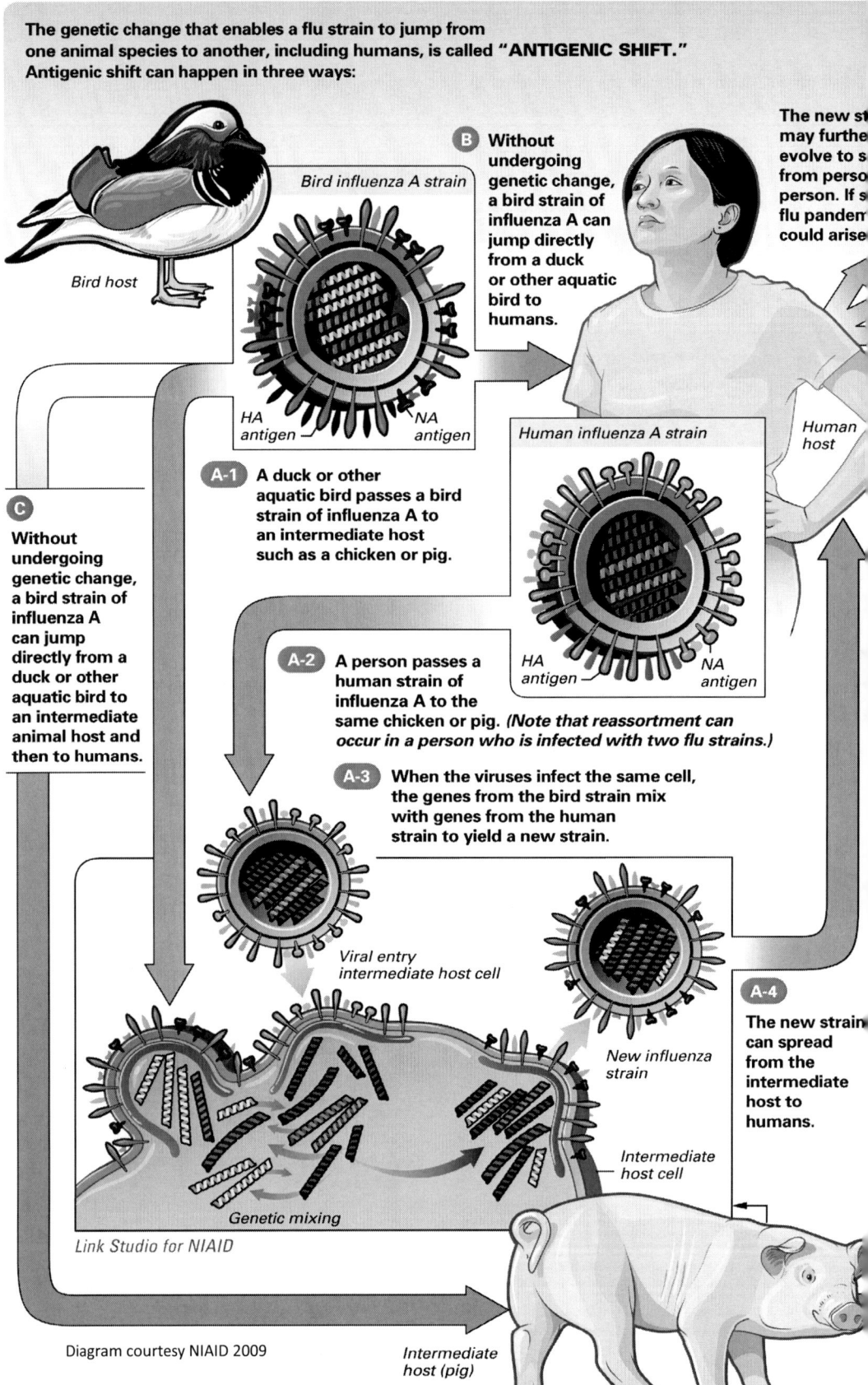

segments coming from one virus and some from another. This can produce a crossbreed or hybrid of Swine, Avian and Human Influenza viruses.

Since eight segments from two different viruses can make 256 different combinations, i.e. 16 segments in total can combine in 16 different ways, many scientists believe that reassortment is likely to have a big role in developing any serious pandemic strain of influenza.

It is also believed that there is also some requirement for random mutation, or recombination that might affect the "binding site" of HA. We do know that reassortment can produce major changes in an influenza virus, which together with other mechanisms, can produce the kinds of hybrid bird and mammal viruses involved in pandemics.

These mutations are not the only, or even necessary, factors that determine the level of pathogenicity (the ability to cause disease) or virulence (severity) of a virus like Swine Flu. Recent analysis of the 1918 pandemic influenza suggests that subtle variations in the configuration of the cleavage site and the presence or absence of sugar sidechains at various places may also relate to and play a major part in producing the virulence and pathogenicity of a virus.

HOW DOES A NEW SWINE FLU VIRUS GET OUT OF A HOST CELL AND INTO NEW CELLS?

Once the Swine Flu virus has made enough copies of itself, these copies group together just inside the host cell's outer wall. Next, they then begin to 'bud' through the surface stealing some of the host cell's membrane and taking it with them so that they can make a new viral lipoprotein envelope. This procedure is fraught with difficulty and actually a very "wasteful" process. Sometimes, it is possible for the wrong eight viral segments to get packaged together or it is even possible for more than eight segments to incorporate and these viruses are then no longer effective. It is estimated that this happens around 90% of the time. However, there are just such vast numbers of viruses made that this inefficiency becomes almost irrelevant.

Last of all the virus has a couple of hurdles to deal with. The first of these is that on exiting the host cell, the virus can "grab" onto the glycoprotein spike of the host cell and this leads the new virus to try to re-infect the host cell. Secondly, the viral particles that have sialic acid stuck to their HA from passing through the cell membrane can clump together and become immobilised. The virus has a solution for this problem though – the other viral glycoprotein spike (NA) is an enzyme that can clean sialic acid from the cell surface and also from the HA spike and this allows the release of the newly produced virus.

PANTROPISM

If, as appears to be happening with the current outbreak of Swine Flu, other body systems aside from the Upper Respiratory Tract (URT), are being infected, there is cause for concern, as mentioned previously. The problem happens when the polybasic amino acids at the cleavage site render the virus 'pantropic', meaning that the virus can affect a wide variety of tissue types, such as the nervous system, kidney, heart etc.

There is evidence that the H1N1 1918 influenza was pantropic in nature and that many organ systems were affected, not just the respiratory tract as is the case with a "normal" Influenza A.

REFERENCES & SOURCES:

1 Bildbeschreibung: 3D Modell Influenzavirus Quelle: Eigene Herstellung Zeichner: M. Eickmann Datum: 01.10.2005
Antigenic shift diagram courtesy of the National Institute of Allergy and Infectious Diseases

FURTHER READING:

To learn more about the way that they influenza A virus binds to cell-surface receptors, the following article may be of use:

Binding of the influenza A virus to cell-surface receptors: structures of five hemagglutinin-sialyloligosaccharide complexes determined by X-ray crystallography.
by: M. B. Eisen, S. Sabesan, J. J. Skehel, D. C. Wiley Virology, Vol. 232, No. 1. (26 May 1997), pp. 19-31.

Abstract:
The structures of five complexes of the X-31 influenza A (H3N2) virus hemagglutinin with sialyloligosaccharide receptor analogs have been determined from 2.5 to 2.8 A resolution by X-ray crystallography. There is well-defined electron density for three to five saccharides in all five complexes and a striking conformational difference between two linear pentasaccharides with the same composition but different linkage [alpha(2-->6) or alpha(2-->3)] at the terminal sialic acid. The bound position of the terminal sialic acid (NeuAc) is the same in all five complexes and is identical to that reported previously from the study of mono - and trisaccharides. The two oligosaccharides with NeuAc alpha(2-->6)Gal linkages and GlcNAc at the third position have a folded conformation with the GlcNAc doubled back to contact the sialic acid. The pentasaccharide with a terminal NeuAc alpha(2-->3)Gal linkage and GlcNAc at the third position has an extended (not folded) conformation and exits from the opposite side of the binding site than the alpha(2-->6)-linked molecule of the same composition. The difference between the conformation of the pentasaccharide with a 2,6 linkage and the trisaccharide 2,6-sialyllactose suggests that 2,6-sialyllactose is not, as previously believed, an appropriate analog of natural influenza A virus receptors. The oligosaccharides studied are NeuAc alpha(2-->3)Gal beta(1-->4)Glc, NeuAc alpha(2-->6)Gal beta(1-->4)Glc, NeuAc alpha(2-->3)Gal beta(1-->3)GlcNAc beta(1-->3)Gal beta(1-->4)Glc, NeuAc alpha(2-->6) Gal beta(1-->4)GlcNAc beta(1-->3)Gal beta(1-->4)Glc, and [NeuAc alpha(2-->6)Gal beta(1-->4)GlcNAc]2 beta(1-->3/6)Gal-beta-O-(CH2)5-COOCH3. http://www.citeulike.org/user/oceanwind/article/4301590

CHAPTER 7

WHAT IS INFLUENZA?

AND HOW DOES MY BODY COPE WITH IT?

Influenza, or 'flu' for short, is the name given to a collection of a particular group of symptoms and signs that most of us are quite familiar with.

These include sudden fever, feeling chilly, headache, feeling "ill", body aches and pains and loss of appetite.

Generally, the fever may last a few days and may also be combined with swollen glands, sore throat, cough, painful eye movements and a runny nose. Sometimes, once the main onslaught of the flu is over, you may begin to feel better but you can suddenly become ill again as your body succumbs to a "secondary" infection.

SECONDARY INFECTIONS

This secondary infection is sometimes known as an "opportunistic" infection and is suggestive of the idea that bacteria (usually) will pounce upon a person in a weakened state and disease will take hold.

Even if you manage to avoid the secondary illness, you can be laid low after a bout of flu and this can last for weeks. In fact, in some people this debilitation can last for years and it is thought that certain illnesses like Chronic Fatigue Syndrome may have their aetiology (medical origin) in an influenza infection. Sometimes people talk of having a gastric or tummy flu and this is not actually influenza at all – and bad colds can often be confused with flu but they are a totally different type of virus.

"HOW DO I KNOW IF I HAVE FLU?"

Although many diseases may start off with the same types of symptoms, until your immune system recognises the nature of the invader, your body sounds a 'general alarm', which results in you getting a typical fever, with muscle aches and pains and a general feeling of being "ill".

All these sensations are very important as they are due to the release of substances called cytokines – which your body automatically releases as its 'first' response to fighting an "invader".

Some other diseases start off in the same way as flu and may actually feel the same as flu – in their initial stages. These include a wide range of infections such as smallpox, anthrax and of course, other respiratory viruses. The diseases that present in a similar manner to flu are called Influenza-Like Illnesses or ILIs.

In the early days of this Swine Flu outbreak it was difficult to definitely say whether people had caught a late form of seasonal flu – or whether they had Swine Flu, as the symptoms start off the same.

In fact with Swine Flu's 'cousin', Bird Flu, in recent years, one of the big problems seen in people who had actually caught Bird Flu was that the disease presents in different ways – most people show symptoms of respiratory distress, however some patients have presented initially with severe diarrhoea and then went on to develop Acute Respiratory Distress Syndrome (ARDS). Doctors call a disease that has many different presentations, or changes its symptoms, "Protean". Protean is derived from "Proteus", an ancient Greek god who had the ability to change his shape at will.

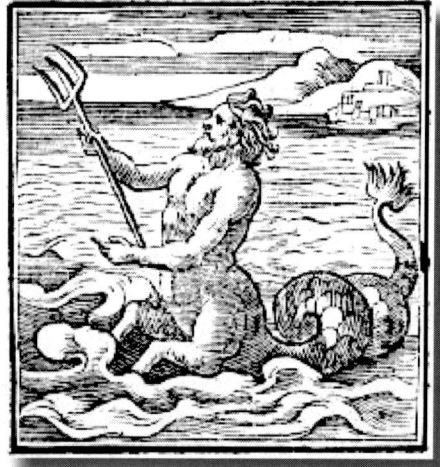

Proteus - woodcut by Jörg Breu displayed in the Book of Emblems by Andrea Alciato (1531)

The body's response in all these cases has been to send out its equivalent of a general 'SOS' alarm. It can be hard for doctors to recognise and differentiate between diseases in these early stages as they will often 'present' in a similar manner as outlined above, so the doctor has to make a 'differential diagnosis' to decide what the problem actually is.

The Survivor's Guide to Swine Flu

There is a standing joke among medical staff about the how to make this differential diagnosis in this early stage of an infection – an easy way to decide whether the patient has real influenza or merely a bad cold:

> *"Put a £50 note in the middle of a field. If the patient can crawl and get it he has a cold. If he can't be bothered – he has flu".*

"DO THESE VIRUSES CAUSE DISEASE?"

At this stage it is as well to explain that influenza viruses and other pathogens – (disease causing agents) are, in themselves, not able to 'cause' disease (pathogenicity) nor are they responsible for the severity of the disease (virulence).

Both these factors are brought about as a result of 'the relationship' between the virus and its 'host'. In the case of Swine Flu for example, it is the relationship between the host and the H1N1 virus that determines the severity of the disease.

So, a large part of this book will look into ways that we can modify this relationship between the virus and YOU (the host), so that you can become more resistant to the H1N1 virus and limit the damage that this virus can cause to you if you do contract it.

There are a number of excellent 'preparedness strategies' that you can put into place that will help you to accomplish this. These are all based upon sound Complementary Medical principles, that are backed up and underpinned by extensive scientific research.

"THE 'TERRAIN' IS EVERYTHING"

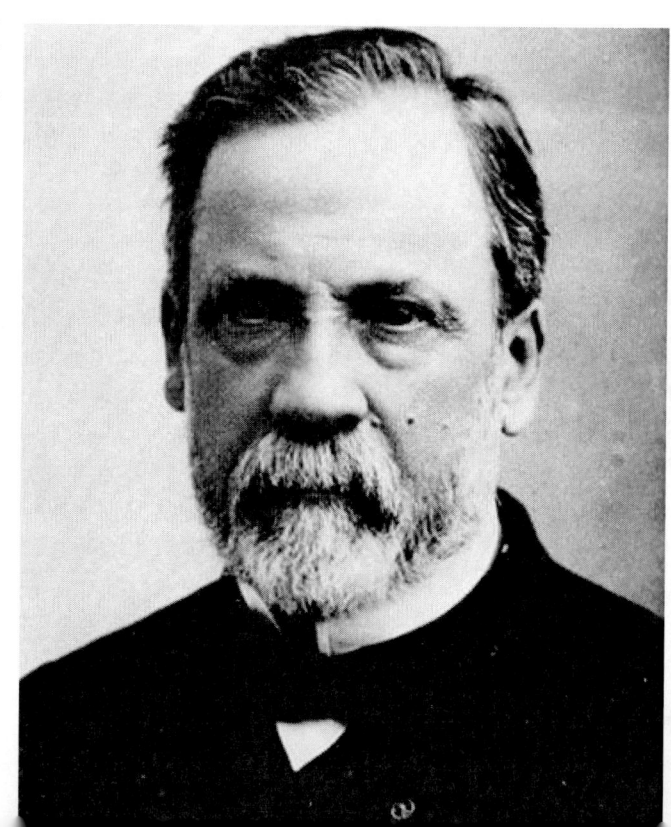

Louis Pasteur (pictured) – "the Father of Germ Theory" – and one of the great medical theorists and practitioners, originally proposed that infectious agents (germs) are all around us and that they are "lying in wait for us" in order to infect us.

Essentially in Pasteur's original picture, the host (you) were a 'sitting duck' and had nothing to do with whether or not you were infected. It just happened – pretty much as the luck of the draw.

However, later on in his career, Pasteur had a re-think. He was a brilliant man and after many long years of dedicated work, he came to the conclusion that, in fact, the host has a lot more to do with whether an infection would occur than previously thought. An apocryphal tale tells of him recanting his beliefs about infection on his deathbed and saying "I got it wrong, the terrain is everything".

By this he meant that the "internal ecology" and well-being of the individual have much more relevance than he at first thought. In general, the healthier you are, the less likely most viruses, etc. would be to establish a hold in your body. The less healthy you are, the more likely certain viruses and diseases would be to infect you.

Today, the importance of the state of the 'terrain' is absolutely accepted as a crucial factor in whether one person gets ill and another doesn't – and has been proven by scientific research. However – just over a hundred years ago, people stuck rigidly to Pasteur's original ideas and his later work was ignored. Co-incidentally, this was when vaccination began and so there may well have been a good reason for vaccine manufacturers to promulgate Pasteur's original theories.

WE LIVE WITH VIRUSES AND BACTERIA EVERY DAY

Regardless of the type of environment that we inhabit – from the desert to the sea shore, from the highest mountains to the deepest valleys, we are surrounded by bacteria, viruses, fungi and an assortment of other microscopic organisms. Most of the time these live on us, in us and around us and we are never even aware of them, we certainly can't see them. In fact, we actually depend upon some bacteria for our well-being – such as the 'good bacteria' found in our gut that have numerous functions, including helping us to make vitamins from food that we eat.

Sometimes, these organisms can be parasitic and just tagging along on and inside us for a free ride. These don't actually do us any harm but they are not beneficial either. And finally, a harmless micro-organism can enter that wouldn't normally cause many problems at all, save for the fact that if it gets into the wrong person at the wrong time, the results can be disastrous. An example of this is in a person who is infected with HIV which severely affects the immune system. They may be feeling completely well but because their immune system is compromised (depleted), and they are more susceptible to infections that affect them badly and any new bacterium or virus can be potentially very dangerous.

A more specific example of this is the overgrowth of candida (a yeast). Candida is usually just a mild annoyance in some people. In most people it is usually not noticed at all but it is usually present somewhere within us. However, if a person with HIV succumbs to a candida infection it can run riot and can be life-threatening.

So, an infectious organism (and the virulence or strength with which it infects) is therefore not solely a function of the invading organism. It is 'the relationship' between host and organism that defines the outcome of any infectious situation.

INFLAMMATION IN VIRAL INFECTIONS E.G. SWINE FLU

The typical symptoms of viral respiratory infections are caused by inflammation of the upper and lower "respiratory tract" (your mouth, throat and lungs). Inflammation is the reaction of local tissue to some harm or injury (e.g. an infection).

Inflammation is such an important factor in Swine Flu that it is useful to spend some time defining in broad terms what it actually is: Inflammation is a dynamic process and is not a specific condition. It is a cascade of intricate reactions that take place inside the body and this is usually in response to a particular stimulus such as an injury or pathogen (an organism that has the ability to cause disease).

Inflammation is part of your body's defensive reaction and is essentially protective in nature as it is designed to shorten the harm that an injury or a pathogen might cause and to promote healing. One of the problems that we face particularly in Swine Flu is that the inflammation itself becomes harmful if our body's response is too vigorous. This is the "Cytokine Storm" that overwhelms the body and causes enormous problems, sometimes leading to death. We cover the Cytokine Storm in more depth in the next chapter.

RESPIRATORY INFECTIONS

Biology teachers tell us that our respiratory tract (RT) is a bit like an upside down tree with the roots at the top and the leaves at the bottom. It's a good analogy – it incorporates the mouth, nose, throat, as the inverted roots and the 'wind pipe' as the tree trunk. Further down in your chest are the lungs and these divide into smaller and smaller sections right down to the 'alveolar sacs' which are a little like tiny leaves on an enormous tree. These come into intimate contact with tiny blood vessels (capillaries) that allow a gas exchange, so that oxygen passes into the blood from your lungs and waste gases – i.e. carbon dioxide – is returned from your blood into your lungs and eventually exhaled.

Coughing, choking and sputum production (phlegm production) are all ways that the body has of protecting the alveoli and keeping them clear of obstruction.

However, viruses like Swine Flu can affect cells in any part of your respiratory tract from the mouth and nose right down through your throat and into the lower respiratory tract where your

Current medical thinking is that the Bird Flu virus (H5N1) has not easily passed easily between humans – yet – because it seems to "favour" and latch onto the cells in the lower part of the lungs where it is not easily coughed or sneezed out. It may be that the latest version of Swine Flu does latch onto the cells in the upper respiratory tract, but we have yet to be sure of this. (See the section on Pantropism in Chapter 6).

trachea, bronchi and alveoli can be affected.

One of the problems in influenza is that there is a tendency for a condition called tracheobronchitis to develop and this is inflammation of the lower respiratory tract. Infections such as this, by 'primary lung pathogens', such as viruses are major causes of illness and death. In medicine, a suffix "itis", is used to describe an inflammatory situation, as in laryngitis (inflammation of the larynx), bronchitis (inflammation of the bronchi), or sore throat – pharyngitis (inflammation of the pharynx or back of the throat).

ANTIBIOTICS?

Even though we know that viruses are not susceptible to antibiotics, patients with acute respiratory viral infections (e.g. even for a mild cold) are nearly always prescribed antibiotics in order to prophylactically treat potential secondary infections – and this is one of the major reasons for inappropriate antibiotic prescribing in industrialised countries.

It is this inappropriate prescription of antibiotics that is believed to be one of the main underlying reasons why antibiotics – the old 'wonder drugs' – are becoming less effective in treating various diseases and for the emergence of "Super Bugs" such as MRSA.

WE SURVIVE MOST ORDINARY INFECTIONS

Most "upper respiratory tract infections" (URTIs) are usually sudden in onset and recovery is usually spontaneous (i.e. you recover without special treatment or medical intervention). The influenza virus, as opposed to most other virally caused URTIs (e.g. a cold caused by the rhinovirus), is also characterised by high fever, severity and a long, drawn-out recovery.

People with ordinary influenza infections suffer to varying degrees, but even the sickest will usually recover. (As we have seen, the average number of deaths in the US from 'normal' flu is currently put at around 36,000 deaths a year – in a population of just over 300m people [around 0.01%]).

Some people can carry the virus and don't even know they are infected or have only minor, virtually unnoticeable symptoms. We do not have any idea of what this proportion is for people who have Swine Flu (i.e. how many people are carriers – but have no symptoms).

However, even though the percentage of really serious illness and death is quite small overall, the fact remains that in epidemic and pandemic situations, infection is so widespread that (even if the percentage of people who die is small), it can add up to tens of thousands of people in an ordinary year and in a major pandemic it would likely be in the millions, tens of millions and even hundreds of millions globally. The truth is that nobody knows for certain. It is worth noting though that influenza virus strains that cause pandemics also tend to be more virulent, so the mortality rate is higher than is seen in ordinary Influenza A infections.

PRIMARY VIRAL PNEUMONIA

Among the most serious potential consequences of any influenza infection is a 'Primary Viral Pneumonia'. Pneumonias are inflammations of the lung tissue caused by infections and this can also be called pneumonitis.

Primary Viral Pneumonia can cause an accumulation of fluids and dead cell debris in the tissues and spaces of the respiratory tract. On an X-ray these show up as shadows or 'infiltrates' on the normally clear lung. Sometimes pneumonia may not be too severe and the person can keep on with their day to day life – there is a term for this; 'walking pneumonia', but in normal flu seasons about 2% of the pneumonia cases are serious, and during pandemics this figure may reach 20% or more. Currently, the majority of people who have contracted Bird Flu (H5N1) have also had severe lung involvement and it appears that this also applies to the severe Swine Flu cases.

Primary Viral Pneumonia will tend to start much like a typical flu, however after a short time – usually a few days – it turns into wheezing, with a shortness of breath and pain on inhaling. In very severe cases the patient may cough up blood, or blood-tinged sputum and there is high mortality. This is Acute Respiratory Distress Syndrome. Patients with this syndrome will very often need to be put onto a respirator in order to facilitate breathing. There is an acute shortage of respirators in every area of the world and these are used at full capacity at all times – even when there is no serious epidemic of respiratory disease. In a severe pandemic situation, this lack of access to respirators will present enormous problems. This is just one of the many reasons why it is so imperative that you take steps to prepare yourself and your loved ones in case H1N1 should mutate.

If Swine Flu continues to spread and is as virulent as it was in 1918, lots of things that we currently take for granted will not be available. The USA's White House Report on Pandemic

Preparedness released in May 2006 warned of serious anticipated disruptions to medical services:

"In the event of multiple simultaneous outbreaks, there may be insufficient medical resources or personnel to augment local capabilities".

Furthermore, State, Local and Tribal Governments should:

"......anticipate that all sources of external aid may be compromised during a pandemic"

MORE ABOUT OPPORTUNISTIC OR SECONDARY INFECTIONS

As discussed briefly earlier in this chapter, in viral influenza, secondary complications can also arise as a result of opportunistic bacterial infection. This was a major factor in the extremely high mortality levels in 1918. If the bacteria can be identified; and if these bacterial infections can be treated with an appropriate antibiotic; safely, without side effects – we should use that antibiotic.

In the field of Complementary Medicine, there are many anti-bacterial and anti-viral options, including herbs and some essential oils that have been demonstrated to be very efficacious. However, in a life or death situation it is entirely sensible to use the best – and most appropriate medicine available – and this may well be an antibiotic drug which can safely be used alongside a Complementary Medicine. This is where both approaches to treatment can work to support each other and be truly "complementary".

In severe influenza, secondary infections can, in some situations, spread to other organs and lead to meningococcal infection (e.g. meningitis), or toxic shock syndrome (from a secondary staphylococcal infection).

Other, more rare complications can include kidney failure, muscle destruction (rhabdomyolysis), widespread and overwhelming clotting with subsequent haemorrhage (disseminated intravascular coagulation), paralysis (Guillain-Barré) and Reyes syndrome (a sudden, increased accumulation of fat in the liver, brain and other organs that mainly affects children who are recovering from a virus and this can be rapidly fatal).

In the influenza that we could consider "normal", these complications are very rare (<1%). However, they were prominent in the 1918 "Spanish Flu" pandemic.

CHAPTER 8

YOUR IMMUNE SYSTEM AND THE CYTOKINE STORM

WHY DO SOME PEOPLE DIE OF FLU?

Well, for a start, not everyone who gets flu dies from it. In most cases it is quite rare to die from flu, although some people do.

In order to understand why we can die of flu and particularly why the prospect of Swine Flu is so worrying, it will be useful to look, in more depth, at the pandemic of 1918.

We have good historical records of this illness – about the ways that the disease affected people, also from pathological reports from the time and also from recent histological reports from scientists who are using preserved tissues – recovered in recent years, from the permafrost of the frozen north, from people who died in 1918.

THERE WERE SEVERAL FACTORS THAT MADE THE 1918 PANDEMIC STAND OUT

The first of these was the incredibly high mortality rate of this influenza (20 times that of normal influenza). Although estimates vary, as we have seen, it is reckoned that around 50 to 100 million people died from it. But no one knows for certain just how many people actually died.

There was also an extraordinarily high level of infection. This was due to the high pathogenicity (disease causing) and virulence (powerfulness) of the H1N1 'Swine Flu' virus at the time. Instead of acting like a normal Influenza A, which usually just infects the respiratory tract, the H1N1 virus was, as discussed earlier, pantropic. This means it not only infected the mouth, throat and lungs of those who caught it – like normal influenza – it affected many other organs as well.

Unusual symptoms were reported that were very different to other influenzas seen by doctors at that time: there were phenomena such as heliotrope cyanosis – a deep lavender-blue discolouration of the skin and a blue-ish froth around the nose and the mouth. Ultimately, victims died due to overwhelming haemorrhaging into the lungs and the victims drowned as a result.

Those who did survive the initial assault of H1N1, were often killed by a rampant secondary infection from bacterial pneumonia.

As discussed briefly, another unusual characteristic of the 1918 pandemic was the age group that it attacked – most of the victims were aged between 20 to 50 years old. Normal Influenza A affects those who are more traditionally thought of as vulnerable – babies and young children and the elderly – i.e. those with immature (the young) or compromised (the elderly) immune systems.

Much is made of the fact that the people who were infected with and died from H1N1 were supposedly "healthy young people", but it should be noted, as above, that this age group was of military service age just as the First World War was coming to an end. Soldiers were grouped together in camps, barracks, transport ships and on the battlefield. Even if they didn't die at the front, or even serve in the forces, people were under enormous emotional strain.

Scientists also suspect that another of the reasons for the high mortality rates in the 1918 H1N1 influenza pandemic was due to the phenomenon known as a Cytokine Storm.

WHAT IS A CYTOKINE STORM?

The term "Cytokine Storm" is a somewhat graphic way of describing one of the ways the immune system reacts to a powerful attack from a threatening 'invader', like some forms of the influenza virus, for example. It is a metaphor that is able to evoke all sorts of frightening images and this is probably why the media have jumped upon this term – drama sells!

From a scientific point-of-view it is an odd term too, as no one really knows what is happening in this complex phenomenon. Even now, it is only just beginning to be partially understood. It is important to remember that an immune response is a process and not a single phenomenon and it is this series of processes, or 'cascade' of effects that causes extreme levels of damage to our internal organs – leading to multiple organ failure.

Essentially, a Cytokine Storm is an enormous over-reaction. These over-reactions are very rare events, which means that scientists don't know a great deal about them as they can rarely be studied. Furthermore, because of this lack of Conventional Medical knowledge, doctors do not know how to treat this problem successfully. What we do know is that this overwhelming immune response is very dangerous. Cytokine Storms can happen rapidly and patients who suffer them experience high mortality rates.

WHAT ARE CYTOKINES?

Cytokines are intra-cellular chemical messengers that are in fact soluble, hormone-like proteins. The hormones that we are perhaps more familiar with are the sex hormones such as testosterone and oestrogen that signal from organ to organ via the blood stream.

Many cytokines send signals over a very short distance, however others can travel to distant sites via the blood stream and act upon other organs. One example of this is the effect that cytokines have on the hypothalamus area of your brain. Among other things, your hypothalamus is responsible for "homeostasis" – maintenance of your body's status quo. This includes making sure that important things, like your blood pressure, body temperature, fluid balance etc. are kept between very fine tolerance points. In infection, cytokines can get the hypothalamus to "up-regulate" your body's temperature to cause a fever – which can help to create an inhospitable, hot environment for the virus.

Another action of cytokines on the hypothalamus is to cause you to feel overly tired and sleepy when you have an infection. This forces you to lie down and rest – thus providing your body with greater energy reserves to fight the invader. Cytokines also act on your liver, where they are instrumental in causing infection-fighting substances called 'complement' to be made.

Names of cytokines can be confusing and some even have many names as researchers in different labs didn't realise that they were working on the same cytokine – so made up a name for it – only to find that someone else had already named it differently. Even more confusingly – one particular type of cytokine may have different roles and will behave differently, according to the circumstances.

It is all very much based upon the context that the cytokine finds itself in. One particular context elicits one response and another elicits a totally different response – just as might happen if you had a conversation with a tennis player and a couple of newly-weds; you could legitimately talk about "love" to both, but due to the differences in their 'world understanding', the context and their 'emotional environment', their understanding of "love" has a totally different meaning.

Cytokines are important components of your body's immune system. Your immune system is enormously complex, so vastly complex in fact, that there is still much that is not yet understood. However, in the context of the latest outbreak of Swine Flu (H1N1) and in order to gain a better understanding of how you can prepare yourself to stand the best chance of combating this virus, we need to chunk down and consider the particular aspects of your immune system that are most relevant. This will help us to understand where cytokines sit in the greater scheme of things.

So, just taking a quick overview we know that your immune system protects you from infection (from viruses, bacteria, parasites, fungi). Your immune system can be described as being made up of two separate systems – your Natural or Non-Specific Immunity – sometimes called your Innate Immunity and your Specific Immunity, sometimes called your Adaptive Immunity or Acquired Immunity.

NATURAL OR NON-SPECIFIC IMMUNITY; YOUR INNATE IMMUNITY

You are born with your Innate Immunity already in place and functioning. It produces a non-specific reaction to attack 'invaders' like viruses, bacteria and other pathogens and is not directed against specific targets. Moreover, it is a 'fast-reaction' answer to an infection – and is a 'generalised' response i.e. "There's something wrong – let's go and attack it/sort it out!"

This protection system is activated immediately upon contact with a foreign object, which could be a bacteria, virus, or any foreign agent that your body recognises as not being part of you – or "non-self".

SO, YOUR FIRST LINE OF DEFENCE INCLUDES:

1. Your Skin – Your skin is your body's largest organ. Doctors consider this to be your first line of defence against any invader – it keeps the "bad guys" out.
2. Your Glands – the glands in your skin secrete substances that create an acidic environment that keeps bacteria under control. (These are different from the glands in your neck and groin for example, called lymph nodes which aren't really glands at all as they do not secrete anything – these are home to immune cells called lymphocytes – which also circulate in your blood.)
3. Mucous Membranes – These make up the lining of your nasal, oral and gastrointestinal tracts. Your Mucosal Membranes produce mucus that helps to trap any foreign invaders and also helps to expel them.
4. Cilia – Your respiratory tract is lined with these extremely tiny "hairs" which use a wave-like, sweeping motion to clear any debris away from the respiratory tract.
5. The Phagocyte System – The white blood cells; neutrophils, monocytes and macrophages (from Greek – macro = big, phage = eater) are all involved in killing invading foreign agents by phagocytosis – or "cell eating" target cells – that may contain a foreign body such as a virus. Phagocyte cells also produce free-radicals during oxidative bursts that occur as part of the cell eating process. The free-radicals that they produce kill the target cell.
6. The Reticulo-Endothelial System – This is made up of mononuclear (single nucleus) phagocyte cells in the lymph, spleen, bone marrow, lungs and liver. The reticulo-endothelial system acts a mechanical "filter" for catching invading micro-organisms in blood.
7. Natural Killer Cells – (NK Cells) are large granular lymphocytes – different from B and

T cells that can destroy a variety of target cells – without prior stimulation – they do this naturally and do not need to have "seen" a problem cell previously in order to target it. (More on this in the next section "Acquired" or "Adaptive" Immunity.) The cells that NK cells can kill will have undergone a cancerous transformation through a cytotoxic (toxic to cells) reaction. They also target and kill cells infected with viruses.

8. The Complement System – 20 proteins make up the Complement System. They are made in your liver and they are found in their greatest concentrations in your blood plasma. They are precursors to enzymes that are activated in order to destroy bacteria and tumour cells. They also play a role in inflammation as they increase the ability of phagocyte (cell eating) cells to surround and destroy infected cells or foreign objects.

9. Cytokines – As discussed, these are "chemical messengers" produced by the cells of the immune system and they affect the growth and activities of other cells. They have many functions and act as both messengers and regulators that affect various immune functions, without which the fight against foreign invaders would be very difficult. Cytokines have unusual names and abbreviations such as IL-beta, IL2 RANTES, IL-4, IL-10, TGF, TNFα and so on. One of the best known groups of cytokines are the Interferons. When these were first discovered and made into medicines it was thought that they would be a cure-all for cancers and other serious illnesses. While Interferons have proved useful in some diseases, they are not the magic potion that was hoped for. Interferon is just one small part of the immune system which, as we have seen, is enormously complex.

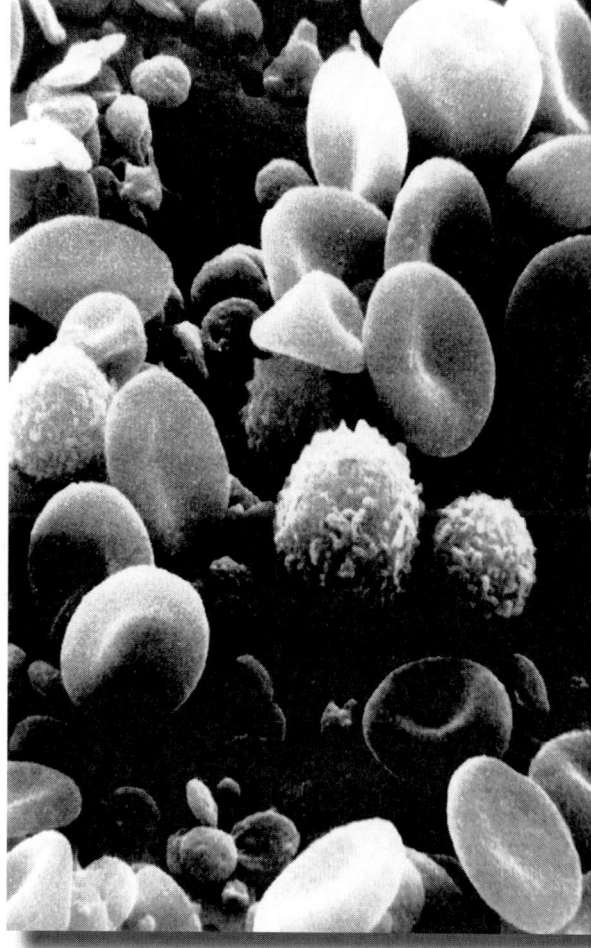

A scanning electron microscope image from normal circulating human blood showing red blood cells, several white blood cells including lymphocytes, a monocyte, a neutrophil, and many small disc-shaped platelets. Red cells are non-nucleated and contain haemoglobin, an important protein which contains iron and allows the cell to carry oxygen to other parts of the body. They also carry carbon dioxide away from peripheral tissue to the lungs where it can be exhaled. The infection-fighting white blood cells are classified in two main groups: granular and agranular. Granulocytes are formed in bone marrow; agranulocytes are produced by lymph nodes and spleen. There are two types of agranulocytes: lymphocytes, which fight disease by producing antibodies and thus destroying foreign material, and monocytes. Platelets are tiny cells formed in bone marrow and are necessary for blood clotting.
Source Image and description: National Cancer Institute; Author Bruce Wetzel (photographer). Harry Schaefer (photographer)

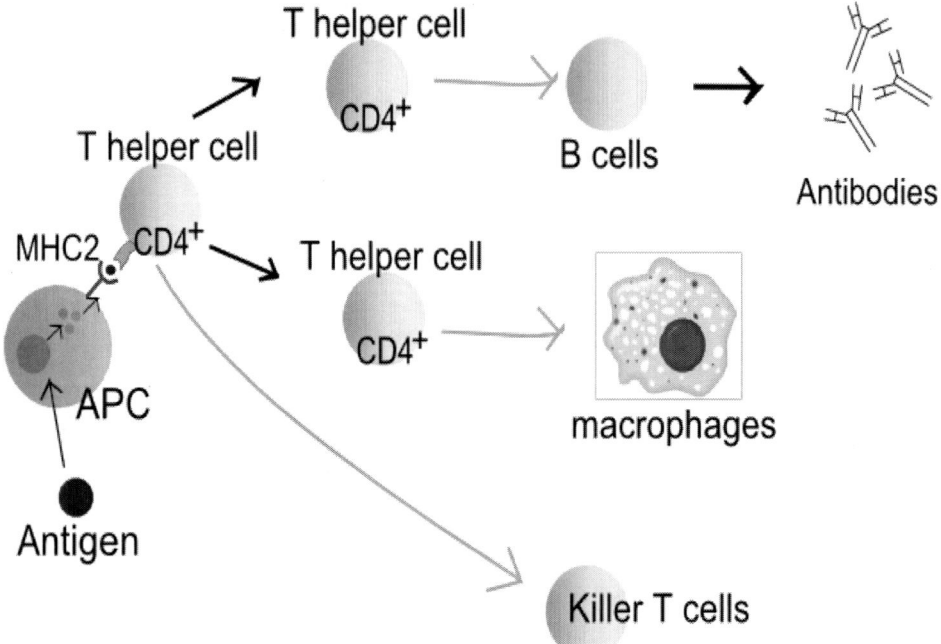

Function of T helper cells: Antigen presenting cells (APCs) present antigen on their Class II MHC molecules (MHC2). Helper T cells recognize these, with the help of their expression of CD4 co-receptor (CD4+). The activation of a resting helper T cell causes it to release cytokines and other stimulatory signals that stimulate the activity of macrophages, killer T cells and B cells, the latter producing antibodies. The stimulation of B cells and macrophages succeeds a proliferation of T helper cells. Diagram: Mikael Häggström

ACQUIRED OR ADAPTIVE IMMUNITY

Scientists believe that as we grow older (5 or so years and upwards), our Adaptive (or Acquired) Immune system develops and this is a "learned response".

What happens is that your immune system – through repeated exposure to them – learns to recognise particular pathogens (viruses, bacteria, fungi, parasites) and "remembers" them for the future, so it can respond to them far more quickly and effectively – with a specific response.

In contrast to Innate Immunity that responds immediately, Adaptive Immunity takes a while to develop – i.e. your immune system has to first of all recognise that there is a problem and then formulate a response to that particular problem and this can take days or weeks. (Adaptive Immunity is the mechanism by which vaccines work.)

YOUR ADAPTIVE IMMUNITY HAS TWO PARTS

The first part of this – your humoral immunity system acts against bacteria and viruses in your blood and other body liquids and develops through antibodies – also known as immunoglobulins. These are produced by B cells which originate in your bone marrow.

The second part of this system – your cell-mediated immunity is dependent upon cell-to-cell contact between a target cell (in Influenza A, your cells are infected by a virus and so become a "target") for one of a group of immune system cells called T-cells (which also originate from your bone marrow but which mature and reside in your thymus gland).

Overall, to be effective, your immune response is often violent and cells will kill each other and even "commit suicide" as long as this is for the greater good of the being (you). Thus in "cell-mediated immunity", a common strategy is to kill your infected cell to save the rest of the body, i.e. your other cells.

In humoral immunity, your antibodies will prepare an invader for destruction by "flagging" them, a bit like posting a sign on them that says "I'm an invader, kill me". After this has happened, special killing cells (cytotoxic) cells and other mechanisms can recognise and kill them. If left to their own devices, antibodies, cytotoxic cells and so on would run riot if not controlled – and this could cause terrible collateral damage – i.e. damage to your cells and organs. So, your body has a number of ways of turning down, or turning off (down-regulating) these aggressive mechanisms.

TO BETTER UNDERSTAND THE ACTIONS AND ENORMOUS COMPLEXITY OF YOUR IMMUNE SYSTEM, IT IS HELPFUL TO IMAGINE THE FOLLOWING SCENARIO:

> A person's house catches on fire. At first, they may not notice much but after a while, they will smell smoke. They'll investigate and realise that they have to summon the fire brigade. So, they make the 999 (911) call and tell the phone operator that there is an emergency and that they need the fire service. The fire-fighters are mobilised and jump into their fire engine and speed to the site of the fire. They then assess the situation and decide upon a plan of action. They need to put out the fire but must cause as little damage to your property as possible. Once they have managed to quench the fire, they then have to clean up, go back to the fire station and begin to file reports and so on. All of this has to happen in a particular order, if this response is to be useful – if things got out of order and the firemen filled in their reports before driving to the scene of the fire, then the whole situation would be in disarray. So it is with your immune system.

For your immune system to produce a meaningful and useful response – certain things have to happen in a particular order – rules are needed. Furthermore – there has to be communication throughout the system in order for things to work properly – just as with our fire-fighter analogy.

Cytokines are chemical messengers that your immune system cells use to talk to each other, in order to produce useful actions (i.e. "jump in the fire engine and drive to the fire") and also to 'down-regulate' activity (i.e. "stop spraying water") when the desired outcome is reached (i.e.

the fire is put out). They are a bit like commands given by the fire chief to the officers in order to co-ordinate their efforts. However, while fire-fighters do a great job, your immune system can sometimes get out of control.

WHAT ACTUALLY HAPPENS IN A CYTOKINE STORM?

As cellular messengers, one of the jobs of the cytokines is to summon your immune cells to the site of an attack. Once the immune cells arrive there, they may be encouraged by the first set of cytokines to produce more cytokines so that these can go off and summon yet more immune cells. This feedback loop could go on forever if it weren't dampened down by still other cytokines telling them to stop production.

Usually, in most viral illnesses this all works well and the viral invasion is halted and the cytokines slow down and stop what they are doing – however this can go wrong and it is thought that this is what happens in a Cytokine Storm.

The cytokine feedback loop is highly complex and as in all highly complex situations there are many factors that can go wrong. Sometimes it just takes one very small problem to wreck an entire system. Think about what happens if someone breaks down on the motorway.

The fact that one car has simply broken down – not crashed or anything dramatic, should not be a problem. However, human nature being what it is, dictates that other drivers will slow down to have a look. This has a knock-on effect that ultimately can cause major traffic jams and ten-mile tailbacks.

What does this have to do with the Cytokine Storm? Well, it is simply an illustration of the way that when a tiny thing goes only slightly wrong, it can have an overwhelming effect on the 'bigger picture'. Given that cytokines and their cascades are so incredibly complex, interrelated and interdependent it is not hard to appreciate that things can indeed go very wrong.

Apart from infections like Swine Flu, cytokine dysregulation plays a role in conditions including toxic shock syndrome and gram negative sepsis. In both of these, the problem is related to an activation of certain T-cells which fails to be down-regulated – so production accelerates. Scientists strongly suspect that the horrendous problems seen in the Spanish Flu outbreak are related to this over-activation of some of the key T-cells that get stuck in a loop of continuous production.

However, the strongest case for the role of an overwhelming cytokine response in influenza comes from research done with mice. In a recent experiment, they were infected with influenza virus that carries the 1918 genetic viral code – the same H1N1 variant as in Swine Flu - and this did produce a very strong cytokine response that actually stimulated immune cells to produce more than half a dozen different cytokines.

As most scientists tend to agree that the Cytokine Storm is to blame for the ravages of H5N1, this led medical practitioners to treat some of those infected with Bird Flu with steroids – because of their anti-inflammatory effects. However, there is no evidence that this helped any of the patients.

Interestingly though, cancer patients – who can produce a Cytokine Storm – are treated, often very successfully, with steroids. Of course, there is no infectious agent such as a virus at play here.

Complementary and integrated medical practitioners would not tend to advocate the use of steroids in the treatment of a Cytokine Storm, since the guiding principles underlying complementary medical approaches would suggest that steroids would down-regulate all aspects of the immune system (e.g. both the beneficial parts and the unhelpful parts) and this would allow the virus to run riot doing even more damage and potentially causing an even more overwhelming cytokine response. This would be a bit like using a steamroller to crack a nut.

THE APPROACH TO CONTROLLING A CYTOKINE STORM THAT WE RECOMMEND IS FIRSTLY PREVENTATIVE

Initially, we seek to dampen down the potential for a cytokine response by αgetting people to follow an anti-inflammatory lifestyle programme that includes an anti-inflammatory diet and supplementation. You can read more about this later in the book.

In the event that a person catches Swine Flu, history shows us that the most successful treatments were homeopathic medicines. Although homeopathic medicines must, by inference, have dampened down the cytokine response and led to a very high survival rate compared to people who were not treated – or were treated using the medicines of the day – we have no firm idea of how homeopathic medicines actually did this – we still lack a plausible mechanism of action.

In addition to homeopathy, nowadays, we also have large quantities of excellent, well-researched data about herbs and nutritional supplements that have antiviral, anti-inflammatory and anti-pyretic (fever-reducing) properties and may be of benefit to people with Swine Flu. However, it is important to appreciate that this hypothesis is only based upon scientific theory at the moment – albeit compelling, excellent research – as apart from the research evidence on the success of homeopathy in treating Spanish Flu, neither scientists nor complementary medical practitioners have used these herbal or nutritional supplementation approaches on anyone with serious H1N1 in controlled trials. Also, unlike the use of homeopathy in 1918 and other severe pandemics, there isn't much reliable historical data for the successful use of herbs to combat serious diseases like pandemic flu. However, going by the enormous amounts of research that supports the use of TNFα-a suppressing herbs like curcumin for example – these approaches show much promise.

THE CYTOKINE STORM AND SWINE FLU

TUMOUR NECROSIS FACTOR ALPHA

Recent research indicates that a particular cytokine called Tumour Necrosis Factor Alpha (TNFα for short or simply written as TNF), is particularly important in humans infected with viruses like Swine Flu, in particular. Tumour Necrosis Factor does what it name suggests – it is useful in fighting some cancers and is also secreted by your body to fight pathogens such as viruses, bacteria and fungi.

In Swine Flu (H1N1), the levels of most pro-inflammatory cytokines will be extremely elevated – TNFα especially so.

Research on Bird Flu has shown that TNFα is elevated in a particular way that is not a characteristic of other types of Influenza A. In all types of Influenza A, TNFα is elevated, but in H5N1 in particular, TNFα strongly stimulates the MAPK pathway (Mitogen Activated Protein Kinase), particularly MAPK p38, according to researchers at the University of Hong Kong and reported in the August 2005 copy of the Journal of Virology. The MAPK pathways represent key routes through which extracellular (outside cells) stimuli are transmitted into responses within cells – and these are translated into an inflammatory "vicious circle", which involves the up-regulation of the inflammation causing substance, NF-kappa B. (For more information about inflammation and NF-kappa B please see this book's sections on nutrition and herbal medicine.) MAPK p38 has been shown to be responsible for the Cytokine Storm seen in people who have contracted H5N1 Bird Flu. The good news is that there are a number of compounds which suppress the MAPK p38 pathway which in turn leads to a marked reduction in the amount of TNFα released in infected cells. H1N1 should, in theory, respond the same way.

There are a number of anti-TNFα drugs available however, these are expensive and would not be available in the quantities required if Swine Flu should spread virulently - also there has been no research on the use of anti-TNFα drugs on the current H1N1 virus. This is one of the reasons why we have researched alternatives in such great depth.

CHAPTER 9

THE CONVENTIONAL APPROACH TO THE TREATMENT OF SWINE FLU

"WHAT CONTROLS ARE IN PLACE TO PROTECT US?"

Countries affected by Swine Flu have all seen a regional prevalence of the virus, as is the case with seasonal flu outbreaks. In the US the key states affected in the initial phase were Wisconsin, followed by Texas and Illinois. In the UK, the West Midlands, London and Scotland accounted for the majority of the early cases.

In this phase, most countries did not attempt to isolate specific flu 'hotspots' and it is difficult to see how this would be effective.

Some countries who were not initially affected, did put in place checks on passangers entering their country who appear to have flu-like symptoms. Some still have these, and will place potential carriers into quarantine, or refuse them entry.

As we have seen Italy recommended travellers not to visit the UK, the most infected country in Europe, and travellers to China are being checked on entry, with anyone with Swine Flu being put straight into quarantine together with other members of their group. Some air passengers are being required to complete in-depth Health Questionnaires whilst in flight, which they then have to submit upon entry to a country. There are reports of some international airports – in France and Turkey using Infra-Red heat sensors to take temperatures of passengers at entry.

However, it does not appear that procedures are yet in place to quarantine any other passengers on the same flights who do not appear to have flu-like symptoms.

Some online commentators have pointed their fingers at airlines who continue to recirculate the air in cabins for economy reasons rather than filter it and/or bring in clean air. Almost all airlines have the ability to remove contaminants, such as bacteria and viruses, from the air, in flight. However, they continue to simply re-circulate air that is potentially infected, as this is a far cheaper option. Ironically, when they allowed smoking on flights, the airlines had to clean the air properly.

In most countries people appear to be relying on a general request that those who have flu-like symptoms should not go to work, or school. In the UK, the Government has issued all households with a pamphlet giving specific advice on what to do, and run TV campaigns on how to contain the spread of Swine Flu.[1] Various online website exist for advice from your particular Government on Swine Flu, e.g. this one from the US Government.[2]

"CAN WE TREAT SWINE FLU WITH CONVENTIONAL MEDICINE?"

At the outset of the pandemic in April, the US Government made 25% of its stockpile of flu drugs available to the most affected states at the time (California, Kansas, New York, Ohio and Texas).

Eighty percent of this US stockpile was made up of Tamiflu (Oseltamivir). The UK Government has stockpiled enough Tamiflu to treat about half of the UK's population.

As we have mentioned earlier, there are questions being asked about the resistance of H1N1 to Tamiflu.

Concerns over the reliance on stocks of Tamiflu (Oseltamivir):

Health authorities around the world followed each other in building up stocks of Tamiflu. However concerns are beginning to emerge that there is the start of a resistance to this drug, meaning that it may no longer work in controlling the H1N1 virus in people.

These reports are spasmodic at present, from countries like Denmark, Japan, Hong Kong and Norway (which reported 75% resistance: January 2008) and the WHO continues to insist that these are, as yet, rare cases.[3]

The WHO's own statistics, from earlier in 2009 appear to imply that this Tamiflu (Oseltamivir) resistance may be more prevalent than currently accepted. The WHO tested Tamiflu on strains of H1N1, from various countries from around the world, and reported that around 95% per cent of all H1N1 viruses tested worldwide, were resistant to Tamiflu.

In March 2009 (Dec – Jan 2009 data), the WHO issued another Official Report on Tamiflu resistance. It sampled H1N1 flu viruses from 30 countries – and found that there was almost

TOTAL resistance to Tamiflu (95% resistance) (98% UK: 98% US; 100% Canada; 100% France; etc with China at just 14%).

WHO REPORT: 18TH MARCH 2009:

...during this period, a total of 30 countries from all WHO regions reported oseltamivir resistance for 1291 of 1362 A(H1N1) viruses analysed.

During weeks 1-4 (28 December 08 – 24 January 09), the level of overall influenza activity in the world increased. In Europe, most countries reported regional or widespread activity with influenza A (H3) viruses predominating. Widespread influenza A activity (H1 and H3) was reported in Japan. In Canada, Hong Kong SAR and the United States, influenza activity increased but remained relatively low. Sporadic influenza activity was observed in Brazil (A), Croatia (H1,H3, B), Greece (H1, H3, B), Iran (H1, H3), Mongolia (A), Portugal (H1, H3, B), Serbia (H1, H3, B), Singapore (H1, H3, B), Slovakia (H3) and Turkey (H3, B).

During this period, a total of 30 countries from all WHO regions reported oseltamivir resistance for 1291 of 1362 A(H1N1) viruses analysed. [That's 94.787%: ed].

The prevalence of oseltamivir resistance was very high in the following countries/territory: Canada (52 of 52 tested), Hong Kong SAR (72 of 80), Japan (420 of 422), the Republic of Korea (268 of 269) and the United States of America (237 of 241). The resistance prevalence was relatively low in China (6 of 44 tested).

In Europe, H1N1 circulation was low during this period while the resistance prevalence was high: France (12 of 12 tested), Germany (66 of 67), Ireland (9 of 10), Italy (16 of 16), Sweden (11 of 12) and the United Kingdom (61 of 62).

http://www.who.int/csr/disease/influenza/H1N1webupdate20090318%20ed_ns.pdf

It would appear that the explanation for this, is that the strains of H1N1 tested were from 'seasonal flu', which is a different strain to the H1N1 strain in the current Swine Flu pandemic?

So, the WHO continue to stress that there has been little Tamiflu resistance found, in regard to Swine Flu, at present.

It would appear that only the Canadian Government, whilst not abandoning their stockpiles of Tamiflu, did, following the publication of these statistics, decide to "adjust" the mix of antiviral drugs in their emergency pandemic stockpile early in 2009.

SIDE EFFECTS OF TAMIFLU

On the Tamiflu website, the only side effects reported are "nausea and vomiting", however the USA's FDA website reports that "diarrhea, bronchitis, stomach pain, dizziness, asthma, sinusitis, aggravated asthma, insomnia and headache are a few of the side effects but this is not a complete list." There have been incidents of severe allergy to Tamiflu (anaphylaxis) and also Toxic Epidermal Necrolysis (TEN) which is a life-threatening skin disorder characterised by a blistering and peeling of the top layer of skin.

In November, 2006, the FDA ruled that the label had to be changed to show that possible side effects like delirium, hallucinations and other abnormal behaviour may occur after taking them.

Following reports that 15 people aged 10 – 19 had been injured, or jumped from buildings after taking Tamiflu, the Japanese authorities banned the prescribing of Tamiflu for teenagers (aged 10 – 19) in March, 2007, having already made the local manufacturers change the accompanying literature to explain the possible neurological and psychological side effects.[4,5]

A further investigation showed that 128 patients had reported 'abnormal behaviour' after taking Tamiflu since 2001.

A lengthy study of this problem was finished in April, 2009, in Japan. It found that children who took Tamiflu were 54 per cent more likely to exhibit abnormal behaviour than those who did not take the drug. When the team limited its analysis to children who had displayed serious abnormal behaviour that led to injury or death, it found those who had taken Tamiflu were 25 per cent more likely to behave unusually.

South Korea also issued safety warnings against prescribing Tamiflu to teenagers except in special cases in April, 2007. You can find out more about Tamiflu and its contraindications on the FDA's website.[6]

OTHER FLU-FIGHTING DRUGS: AMANTADINE AND RIMANTADINE

Amantadine is a drug that was developed to treat the symptoms of Parkinson's disease.

Its anti-flu properties were first discovered when elderly people taking it for Parkinson's disease did not get flu, although it was rampant in their nursing homes. It is known to have a number of 'problematic' side effects.

Rimantadine is a chemically-related compound that has fewer side effects than Amantadine and is also effective against normal Influenza A.

SIDE EFFECTS OF THESE FLU FIGHTING DRUGS

The known side effects of both Amantadine and Rimantadine include nervousness, anxiety, insomnia, difficulty concentrating, light headedness, nausea and anorexia.

Some of the more severe side effects include marked behavioural changes, delirium, hallucinations, agitation and seizures. Both of these drugs are considerably easier and cheaper to manufacture than the neuraminidase inhibitors.

The neuraminidase inhibitors are Oseltamivir (Tamiflu) which is a tablet, and Zanamivir (Relenza) which is an inhaler.

According to the USA's Center for Disease Control (CDC), Relenza (Zanamivir) side effects include, "diarrhea, nausea, sinusitis, nasal signs and symptoms, bronchitis, cough, headache, dizziness, and ear, nose, and throat infections".

Furthermore, the CDC states that Relenza should not be used by anyone who has "underlying airway disease (e.g., asthma or chronic obstructive pulmonary disease)"

Furthermore they state:

> "No definitive evidence is available regarding the safety, or efficacy, of zanamivir for persons with underlying respiratory or cardiac disease, or for persons with complications of acute influenza."

Unfortunately, the Bird Flu strains that have been affecting humans in Southeast Asia are resistant to both Amantidine and Rimantadine.[7] It is believed that this resistance developed because Chinese farmers feed sub-therapeutic doses of Amantidine to their chickens, against advice.

There is no evidence to date on whether Swine Flu will also prove resistant to these drugs.

"IS THERE A SWINE FLU VACCINE FOR PEOPLE YET?"

On 8th May the WHO reported that it was sending out 'wild-type' H1N1 viruses (H1N1 'California') to a number of potential vaccine manufacturers, on request, including Baxter, CSL, GlaxoSmithKline Biologicals, MedImmune, Microgen, Nobilon International, Novartis, Omninvest Vaccines, Pasteur, Solvay and Vivaldi.

From mid-year onwards, all of these companies began to develop a vaccine against H1N1.

The Conventional Medical Approach to Swine Flu

Baxter International, the only US-based manufacturer, who patented their vaccine in August, 2007, is one of these and has already (July) had to stop taking any further orders as it can't keep up with demand. Interestingly, Baxter has no orders from the US for its vaccine, as it has not received FDA approval, and it is only fulfilling orders to the UK, Ireland and, in theory, New Zealand. The safety of Baxter's vaccine has already been questioned in New Zealand and the Minister of Health has called for a full investigation into its potential use bacause of the legal proceedings instigated against it over the 'mishap' it had with the handling of the lethal H5N1 virus earlier in 2009. (Over the years, the company has been involved in several controversies. In 2001, malfunctioning dialysis machines resulted in several deaths; in 2008 the company supplied contaminated heparin; in 2009 the wrong strain of H5N1 avian flu virus was transported to laboratories across Europe: Supplies of Influenza A virus subtype H5N1 provided by Baxter were erroneously sent to a series of European laboratories. The deadly H5N1 strain was mixed with the less harmful H3N2 subtype of the seasonal flu virus, and was detected after it killed test animals more quickly than expected in a lab in the Czech Republic. Though there was a risk of serious consequences, Baxter strangely claimed the controls over the distribution of the virus were stringent and there was little chance of the virus harming humans.)

As with all major health scares like this, despite the fact that there is no evidence whatsoever behind the stories, the conspiracy theorists have already started to question the role that Baxter's award-winning, manufacturing plant in Cuernavaca, Mexico, outside of Mexico City might have, inadvertently, played in this outbreak. (Cuernavaca is just a few miles from the original H1N1 outbreak.)

Baxter estimates that it will start to send vaccines out in August, if not before.

Another drug company; CSL began testing on humans in July (22nd July), amongst 240 volunteers, in Australia.

Novartis expected to start trials of its vaccine in July, and Sanofi said that it expected to start tests in August - and to start delivering vaccines by November, or December.

As with all major outbreaks like this, as these vaccines are produced, we assume that "First Responders" will get the first vaccines – i.e. key personnel such as doctors, nurses, police and soldiers.

NO 'EFFECTIVE SWINE FLU VACCINE' "UNTIL SEPTEMBER, 2009, AT THE EARLIEST"

The WHO's official position throughout the early stages of this pandemic - and that of the US and UK Governments - has always been that a Swine Flu vaccine wouldn't be ready until September, 2009. And that this would provide a robust line of defence against the Swine Flu pandemic, should it worsen.

The WHO said it expects up to 4.9 billion doses to be produced over the next 12 months.

"ARE THERE ANY PROBLEMS WITH VACCINE ADDITIVES?"

Most new vaccines must go through an extensive testing period – to ensure that they work – **and that they do not have major side effects.** In this case, it appears that a number of new vaccines will be fast-tracked into use, with approval to use on humans.

One major concern with this reliance on vaccination to treat Swine Flu, especially given the 'fast-track' approach being taken towards testing, is that in order to make the vaccine 'go further', it is proposed that an adjuvant is added to it.

An adjuvant essentially prompts your immune system into being more reactive to the vaccine being injected.

The thinking behind adding an adjuvant to the vaccine is that you will also, theoretically, require a smaller dose of vaccine - thus making it go further - and making more doses available to more people.

This is especially useful, since scientists are reporting that the H1N1 that they are trying to grow in eggs is growing at a really slow rate - about 50% more slowly than they had anticipated. (At current rates of growth highly respected scientists, including Michael Osterholm, Director of the Center for Infectious Diseases Research and Policy at the University of Minnesota, estimate that we won't be vaccinating people in any reasonable quantities in September, 2009, as planned and they anticipate that it will be closer to December before required quantities of vaccines are generally available.)

There are a variety of chemicals used in vaccines as preservatives and as adjuvants. One of the more notorious of these was the Thimerosal (mercury) preservative used in the MMR vaccine.

This is not being proposed as the adjuvant in these Swine Flu vaccines - the adjuvants being proposed are aluminium and squalene.

ALUMINIUM AS A VACCINE ADDITIVE

Aluminium exposure in humans is thought by some researchers to be implicated in the development of Alzheimer's Disease and the British Medical Journal has also reported (17th March, 2009) that clinicians have noticed that injections which contain an aluminium adjuvant cause abcesses at the injection site.

SQUALENE AS A VACCINE ADDITIVE

It is well known that squalene causes auto-immune responses in rats injected with squalene experimentally.

A study conducted at Tulane Medical School and published in the February, 2000, issue of Experimental Molecular Pathology included the following statistics:

> " ... the substantial majority (95%) of overtly ill deployed Gulf War Syndrome (GWS) patients had antibodies to squalene. All (100%) GWS patients immunized for service in Desert Shield/Desert Storm who did not deploy, but had the same signs and symptoms as those who did deploy, had antibodies to squalene.
>
> In contrast, none (0%) of the deployed Persian Gulf veterans not showing signs and symptoms of GWS have antibodies to squalene. Neither patients with idiopathic autoimmune disease nor healthy controls had detectable serum antibodies to squalene. The majority of symptomatic GWS patients had serum antibodies to squalene."[8]

According to Dr. Viera Scheibner, Ph.D., a former principle research scientist for the Government of Australia:[9]

> "... this adjuvant [squalene] contributed to the cascade of reactions called **"Gulf War Syndrome,"** documented in the soldiers involved in the Gulf War.
>
> The symptoms they developed included arthritis, fibromyalgia, lymphadenopathy, rashes, photosensitive rashes, malar rashes, chronic fatigue, chronic headaches, abnormal body hair loss, non-healing skin lesions, aphthous ulcers, dizziness, weakness, memory loss, seizures, mood changes, neuropsychiatric problems, anti-thyroid effects, anaemia, elevated ESR (erythrocyte sedimentation rate), systemic lupus erythematosus, multiple sclerosis, ALS (amyotrophic lateral sclerosis), Raynaud's phenomenon, Sjorgren's syndrome, chronic diarrhoea, night sweats and low-grade fevers."

BUT SQUALENE OCCURS NATURALLY IN THE BODY:

Squalene is naturally found throughout your nervous system and also in your brain - and therefore your immune system recognises it as being 'safe'. Squalene is also found in a variety of food sources - including olive oil and it has enormous anti-oxidant properties. However, if you inject squalene into your body (as opposed to eating it) this is perceived by your immune system to be an attack. The problem then is that your body becomes primed to attack all squalene that it finds - including that found naturally in your immune system and brain.

"HAVE THERE BEEN PROBLEMS WITH MASS VACCINATION PROGRAMMES IN THE PAST?"

The Global Advisory Committee on Vaccine Safety met on July 7th, 2009, and concluded that the risks of causing Guillain-Barré Syndrome (GBS), or other serious health conditions by vaccinating populations with a new vaccine, were extremely low and that there were no significant safety concerns to the development of a vaccine against H1N1. [10]

During a threatened flu outbreak (H1N1; 'New Jersey' strain) in 1976, the US Government rushed a mass vaccination programme through, with President Gerald Ford being featured 'getting a shot' on TV, to encourage everyone to go and get vaccinated.

Commentators put this rush to get things done, down to the fact that Ford had been seen as an indecisive President, and it was a 'political' statement to show that he was capable of decisive action.

On 10th March, 1976, the Advisory Committee on Immunization Practices of the United States Public Health Service (ACIP) reviewed the evidence about the 'New Jersey flu (H1N1) and concluded that this new strain could be transmitted from person to person and that a pandemic was a possibility.

The ACIP recommended that an immunisation programme be launched to prevent the effects of a possible pandemic. One ACIP member summarised the consensus by stating:

> *"If we believe in prevention, we have no alternative but to offer, and urge the immunisation of the population."*

The US Government pushed the measures through and immunised 45 million people in just 10 weeks. During this time no evidence of H1N1 transmission was found and the programme stopped **as health concerns began to emerge.**

Over the next few years several hundred cases of Guillain-Barré Syndrome (GBS) were thought to have been caused by this vaccination programme. (Nationwide surveillance for GBS in 1976 covered a total of 1098 patients with onset of GBS from October 1, 1976, to January 31, 1977. A total of 532 patients had recently received an A/New Jersey influenza vaccination prior to their onset of GBS (vaccinated cases), and 15 patients received a vaccination after their onset of GBS. 543 patients had not been recently vaccinated with A/New Jersey influenza vaccine and the vaccination status for 8 was unknown. Epidemiologic evidence indicated that many cases of GBS were related to vaccination).

The Conventional Medical Approach to Swine Flu

"WILL MY ANNUAL FLU SHOT PROTECT ME AGAINST SWINE FLU?"

No. Current vaccines only protect you from viruses that are currently circulating so the usual annual flu vaccination will not provide any protection against this particular strain of Swine Flu yet.

There are conflicting reports that either there will be no seasonal flu vaccine produced for the 2009 flu season, or that a combined vaccine will be produced. Unfortunately, the capacity to produce enough of either, or both, vaccines, is limited by the production facilities available.

REFERENCES:
1. http://www.direct.gov.uk/en/Swineflu/DG_177884 SWINE FLU ADVICE LEAFLET
2. http://www.pandemicflu.gov/plan/index.html US Govt advice on Swine Flu
3. http://search.who.int/search?q=oseltamivir+resistance+2009&entqr=0&output=xml_no_dtd&sort=date%3AD%3AL%3Ad1&Search=Search&ie=utf8&client=WHO&sitesearch=&ud=1&site=default_collection&oe=UTF-8&proxystylesheet=WHO
4. http://en.wikipedia.org/wiki/Oseltamivir
5. http://www.timesonline.co.uk/tol/news/world/asia/article1549260.ece
6. http://www.fda.gov/Drugs/DrugSafety/PostmarketDrugSafetyInformationforPatientsandProviders/ucm107840.htm
7. Handbook for Zoonotic Diseases of Companion Animals By Glenda Dvorak, Anna Rovid Spickler, James A Roth
8. Adverse Effects of Adjuvants in Vaccines, by Viera Scheibner, Ph.D., 2000
9. http://docs.google.com/gview?a=v&q=cache:Kmjk2IdwmSEJ:www.who.int/immunization/sage/6.Midthun_H1N1_influenza_vaccine_safety_for_SAGE.pdf+H1N1+influenza+vaccine+safety+update+and+current+issues&hl=en&gl=uk
10. http://www.unis.unvienna.org/unis/en/news/2006/27April.html?print

CHAPTER 10

WHAT IS COMPLEMENTARY MEDICINE?

THE COMPLEMENTARY MEDICAL APPROACH TO THE PREVENTION AND TREATMENT OF SWINE FLU

In the UK, the term "Complementary Medicine" is used to describe any form of treatment that is not necessarily part of the Conventional Medical remit, but which uses an holistic approach in dealing with patients – taking all their symptoms into account – thus treating the "complement" of the person.

The term is also used in another, but highly relevant way, as these approaches can often be used to "complement" Conventional Medicine – ensuring that Complementary Medicine is used to support Conventional Medicine.

In the USA people use the terms "Alternative Medicine", or "Integrative Medicine", to describe much the same approach. In many cases the catch-all term "CAM" (Complementary and Alternative Medicine) is used.

Essentially, Complementary Medicine is "holistic", in so far as practitioners will take all of a patient's presenting symptoms into account when devising a treatment plan. This means that Complementary Medical practitioners view the mind, body and emotions as a whole and not as separate disconnected entities.

Conventional Medicine tends to metaphorically "chop people up" into discrete sections and believes that mind, body and emotions are not connected in any greatly meaningful way.

Thankfully, this approach is changing, due to the discoveries that are being made in the mind/

What is Complementary Medicine?

field of psycho-neuroimmunology and its sister disciplines of psycho-neurology (nervous system) and psycho-endocrinology (mind/hormonal system). (An excellent book on the subject is "Molecules of Emotion" by Candace Pert - the brilliant pioneer of mind-body medicine).

CAM disciplines include therapies that are not generally part of Conventional Medicine – with a very few exceptions. These exceptions tend to have been discovered in the Complementary Medical field and then adopted by Conventional Medicine. These include approaches, such as the use of Omega 3 essential fatty acids to combat high cholesterol levels and CoQ10 to extend and enhance the lives of those suffering from congestive heart failure.

More and more Complementary Medical approaches are being absorbed into Conventional Medicine and within a few years it is fairly certain that we will see both Complementary and Conventional Medical techniques being used together – thus creating an Integrated Medical approach.

WHAT ARE THE MAIN PRINCIPLES OF CAM?

- CAM practitioners base their prescriptions upon a "totality" of symptoms. Practitioners aim to understand what it is that makes the patient uniquely different from any other patient and it is this individualised approach that is unique to CAM and is not utilised in Conventional Medicine.

So, whether a practitioner is a massage therapist, acupuncturist, homeopath or nutritionist – the underlying common thread is that each practitioner is making their therapeutic recommendations for the patient, based on a complete analysis of that person's individual presentation.

- CAM practitioners aim to find out why the body produces certain symptoms, i.e. what the underlying cause of an illness is. Practitioners will then treat the underlying cause, thus enabling the person to return to a state of well-being. Conventional Medicine differs from CAM insofar as it generally treats patients by suppressing symptoms. For example, Conventional Medicine views symptoms as "undesirable things" that need to be eliminated and this often leads to a mere suppression of symptoms, and the underlying reasons for the appearance of symptoms in the first place are often not taken into consideration. For good examples of this approach, consider the conventional treatments for eczema, asthma, inflammatory diseases and so on. In Conventional Medicine, steroids will often be prescribed, even though conventional practitioners know that these are not curative and simply suppress symptoms.

- CAM practitioners see things differently and view symptoms as 'information' that can help to guide them to understanding more about what the underlying health problem is. Practitioners will often achieve complete cures for these problems by treating these underlying issues. In the case of asthma and eczema for example, these will often include allergies and sensitivities. Thus, CAM practitioners view symptoms as signs and signals given by the body/mind that there is something amiss.

• CAM approaches have been around for a very long time. Tibetan Bön (pronounced '*burn*') medicine has an 18,000 year history. Traditional Chinese Medicine (TCM) has been around for at least 4,000 years and it is thought by scholars that the Indian Vedas were written 6,000 years ago and most intriguingly, these reflect many current philosophies in the quantum science field. Much of the Conventional Medical pharmacopoeia used today is identical to that of an 18th century herbalist.

BUT IS CAM "SCIENTIFIC"?

• Complementary Medical disciplines, which are based on molecular science, are easily tested and proven. Nutrition and herbalism fall into this category and both perform outstandingly well in scientific trials, as it is easy to perform conventional Double-Blind trials using these approaches. In fact, Conventional Medicine is beginning to acknowledge that many nutritional and herbal medicines outperform their pharmaceutical counterparts (Omega 3's, gingko biloba, Vitamin E complex, St John's Wort, to name but a few).

• Manipulative techniques such as osteopathy and chiropractic can both be subjected to placebo trials and have been proven to work. The reason for this is that it is possible to perform 'sham' interventions to test osteopathy and chiropractic.

* However, it is not so easy to do 'sham' treatments with approaches like massage for example, as a person does know that they are, or are not, being massaged.

• Energy medicine – homeopathy, acupuncture/qi gong, Traditional Chinese Medicine (TCM), ayurveda, healing: These approaches truly treat the "totality" of symptoms. They are also the most difficult to test given the complex and individualised nature of prescribing. There is plenty of good research to support the effectiveness of ayurveda and TCM in their native countries and increasingly in the West. These approaches seem to have a commonality insofar as they aim to restore homeostasis (the body's natural balance) by manipulating the body's innate energetic systems known in various cultures as Vital Force/Qi/Chi/Prana etc. Homeopathy is tending to do well nowadays in trials, as scientists are finally beginning to understand that, in order to test an approach that is specifically designed to treat individuals, they need to design specific trials that take this into account. So, we are now beginning to see very well-conducted homeopathy trials which are reporting success rates of 78% and above. (For further evidence see "**Scientific Research in Homeopathy Conference**"; available as a DVD (2008): from The-CMA.Org. UK).

What is Complementary Medicine?

- **"Complementary and Alternative Medicine; the Scientific Verdict on What Really Works"**; is an encyclopaedia drawing on over 10,000 scientific research papers and covers all the scientific evidence – solely from Random-Controlled, Double-Blind, Placebo trials.: edited by Jayney Goddard (The-CMA.Org.UK),

And, surprisingly enough, for most people, it is now officially recognised that what we all take for granted as Conventional Medicine is nowhere near as 'scientific' as most people have thought:[1]

The British Medical Journal's website - ClinicalEvidence.BMJ.com - disclosed that **only 15% of medical tratments are known to be of any benefit.** The remaining 85% of them are of unknown efficacy (and thus safety - Ed.)

WHAT CAN CAM BE USED TO TREAT?

- Complementary Medicine is an ideal treatment and support option for "chronic", or long-term, conditions that do not spontaneously resolve themselves. This is especially useful in cases where there is very little to offer in conventional terms. Many doctors now recognise that Complementary Medicines are extremely valuable in treating chronic disease (long term illness) and nowadays, most are happy to refer their patients to qualified Complementary Medical practitioners, and many hospitals now have acupuncturists working in their pain clinics, for example.

- Acute illness – CAM approaches, such as homeopathy and herbalism, can be used to treat certain acute conditions such as cuts and bruises, toothaches, colds and "normal flu" and so on. Situations where CAM is not used include those where it is obvious that Conventional Medical techniques are necessary, e.g. trauma, severe injuries, broken bones etc. Of course, once the trauma, or injury, is resolved and bones set etc, then CAM techniques can enhance and speed up healing.

- CAM can act preventatively, remedially and even curatively.

WHAT TRAINING DO CAM PRACTITIONERS UNDERTAKE?

It depends upon the type of discipline: Massage will generally take about a year for both the anatomy and physiology and the massage training; osteopathy and medical herbalism are degree courses taking the usual 3 years; homeopathy is also a degree course, but can take up to 5 - 6 years, as many practitioners decide to go on to do post-graduate training.

HOW SAFE IS COMPLEMENTARY MEDICINE?

Very safe – to date there have been 5 recorded deaths across the entire CAM field in the UK since records began about around 40 years ago. Four of these were as a result of pneumothorax (air in the lung cavity), caused by wrongly placed needles in acupuncture. (These deaths were caused by conventional doctors who had taken it upon themselves to try to do acupuncture, based upon the idea that they thought that they had enough anatomical knowledge, due to their medical training).

The fifth death was a small child whose parents chose, on religious grounds, to give their child homeopathic treatment for an intestinal obstruction – against the advice of their homeopath. However, this tragic death is still attributed to homeopathy.

In Conventional Medicine, in the UK alone, there are, by comparison, over 40,000 deaths per annum as a direct result of completely avoidable 'medical blunders' and incorrect drug prescriptions which could have been totally avoided. This information comes directly from the British Medical Association.

In the US, the official annual figures for deaths due to 'medical blunders' are around 200,000.[2] It is well recognised and openly acknowledged by doctors that these figures are a gross under-representation of the true state of things - as many medical blunders are never reported.

The current fad of 'jumping on the Complementary Medical bandwagon' by some doctors – who will take a very brief training course in a particular Complementary Medical discipline – (some as short as a weekend or two), is of great concern to The Complementary Medical Association. It takes many years to train to become a practitioner of Complementary Medicine and just because a doctor has an excellent knowledge of anatomy and physiology, this doesn't mean that they are in any way capable of working within a specific area of Complementary Medicine, without years of extra training. Any form of medicine, Conventional or Complementary, requires that its practitioners be properly trained and this takes time and dedication.

There are some organisations that take this issue seriously, like the excellent British College of Integrated Medicine (BCIM), which trains doctors on how to integrate Complementary and Conventional approaches, over a 2 year course.

Naturally, if a substance or treatment has the power to heal then it makes complete sense that it may, possibly, have the power to do harm – although the vast majority of Complementary Medical approaches, when practiced by qualified practitioners, are safe. For example, there are certainly particular herbs that will interact with Conventional Medicines sometimes in a positive manner and sometimes in a negative one.

What is Complementary Medicine?

If you are concerned about this, The Complementary Medical Association has a full database of drug/vitamin/mineral/supplement interactions, both positive and negative. (The-CMA.Org.UK)

For the purposes of this book and in an attempt to devise beneficial prevention and treatment strategies for Swine Flu, the three Complementary Medical disciplines that we cover – in depth – are homeopathic medicine, herbal medicine and nutritional medicine. We also cover aromatherapy, as the essential oils (aromatic plant extracts) used in this discipline have been shown, in well conducted trials, to have anti-viral properties.

However, from the preventative medicine point of view, there are many Complementary Medical disciplines that have been scientifically proven in robust, well conducted trials, to contribute to your overall well-being. These include disciplines as diverse as massage, acupuncture and energy medicine techniques such as medical qi gong (chi kung), yoga and Bi-Aura therapy.

It is beyond the scope of this book to go into any of these to any great degree, but should you want to read more about these approaches - or if you wish to find a qualified practitioner - or even a training course - go to The Complementary Medical Association's website: The-CMA.Org.UK

COMPLEMENTARY MEDICINE AND SWINE FLU – WHAT WORKS?

It is entirely possible and indeed probable, that Complementary Medical approaches will be of great use in preventing and combating Swine Flu. This is based upon historical evidence gathered from the last two hundred years of pandemics and epidemics, and also upon the rigorous scientific research that supports the recommendations in this book.

We have spent the last 6 years researching a vast amount of data to see whether a viable Complementary Medical prevention and treatment option exists for potential pandemic-type flu outbreaks. We have discovered that it does indeed exist.

The preparation and prevention routines recommended in this book have not yet been clinically tested on anyone who has contracted serious Swine Flu, so we do not know for certain whether our prevention and treatment recommendations will work. However, based on our research, previous successful use of these approaches, and the excellent work being done in the field of immunology and microbiology by leaders in these fields whose discoveries support our approach, we feel confident in proposing these methods.

HOW THIS PARTICULAR COMPLEMENTARY MEDICAL APPROACH CAN WORK FOR YOU

As we have seen, the very essence of Complementary Medicine incorporates individualised forms of treatment, that's why we believe it is absolutely vital that you see your qualified practitioner at this time, in order to address any individual underlying health issues that you may have. You can discuss the recommendations in this book with them and they should be able to support you in implementing the recommended changes.

THE CORRECT APPROACH TO NUTRITION, SUPPLEMENTATION AND THE USE OF HERBAL MEDICINE

One of the problems faced by most people who will read this book, is that they are highly likely to be following a "Western Diet" that provides us with too much sugar, the wrong kinds of fats and a lack of fruit and vegetables. Scientific research has shown this Western Diet to be extremely deleterious to health and devastating to the immune system.

Because of the way that Swine Flu attacks our bodies, you are at even greater risk of contracting the H1N1 virus if you stick to the Western Diet and if you do contract Swine Flu, the effects of the virus could be even more dangerous for you. Given that most people reading this book may well be eating this Western Diet, we have had to develop a preventative medical approach, based on nutrition, herbal medicine and supplementation, to help as many people as possible.

Although this generic, preventative approach is not adhering strictly to the central principle of Complementary Medicine, that of individualisation, we have felt it necessary to devise this regime to provide people with a set of recommendations that will be applicable to virtually everyone.

These recommendations which centre around a healthy diet, a specific nutritional approach and the use of certain herbal supplements, have all been scientifically proven to be beneficial, and, in most cases, even necessary, for your health – regardless of any underlying health issues you may have. You could think of this as a basic health insurance policy. We believe – and scientific evidence confirms – that our preventative approach, which supports the immune system, will help the vast majority of people. The suggestions in this book are sensible, practical steps that we can all take – easily.

This particular approach to supporting the immune system is recommended by a number of eminent medical experts, including Professor Luc Montagnier, winner of the 2008 Nobel Prize in Physiology or Medicine for co-discovereing HIV:

> *"We have learned a lesson from AIDS, that a good immune system is important to fight the virus and also to prevent infection. So if we have a good system, in terms of immunity, both antibody immunity and cellular immunity, we can eliminate or eradicate many beginnings of infections like the Avian Flu for instance."*

What is Complementary Medicine?

GENUS EPIDEMICUS

Aside from our recommendations for a generalised preventative Complementary Medical approach, tailored to suit the vast majority of people, it has also been possible to formulate a generalised recommendation for the homeopathic treatment of Swine Flu symptoms.

This is, of course, an unusual approach to take since, as mentioned above, the essence of Complementary Medicine is "individualised" treatment. However, history shows that in previous pandemics, homeopaths have found that very often, one particular remedy is vastly more effective than all the others.

In the case of the 1918 Spanish Flu pandemic, the remedy was Gelsemium. The reason that a single remedy can be used to treat enormous numbers of people is because the disease is so virulent, and the symptoms of the disease are so powerful, that each person is affected in the same way and produce virtually identical symptoms. When a single remedy is found to suit the majority of people it is called a "Genus Epidemicus".

We have carefully looked at the symptoms shown by people in the current H1N1 outbreak – where the data exists – in order to ascertain exactly what the common symptoms actually are, and we have been able to use this information to create a Genus Epidemicus for Swine Flu.

This has not been tested on anyone with serious Swine Flu in this current outbreak, although many homeopaths have very successfully treated mild cases and have noticed that the duration of the illness is much shorter than in untreated people. Historical evidence of the success of this approach robustly supports our recommendations.

Furthermore, should this pandemic become more serious, we do not believe that anyone – Complementary Medical practitioner or Conventional Medical doctor – will have the luxury of being able to prescribe medicines on an individual basis. It would be time-consuming and impractical and this would be of no use whatsoever to the vast majority of people.

As we have seen in July in the UK, the health authorities are already directing people away from seeing their GP and towards various online, or telephone Hotlines (manned by people as young as 16 and without any medical qualifications).

Whether you follow the approach outlined in this book, or not, it will at least provide you with the information you need to make an 'informed' opinion on how you want to protect yourself – and what you can do if you do catch Swine Flu.

"WHAT IF SWINE FLU DOESN'T AFFECT ME?"

If you follow our recommended plan of action – to improve your health and Swine Flu doesn't affect you directly, you will be far healthier than you were when you started. You will be less susceptible to chronic degenerative diseases associated with long-term inflammation, such as cancer, heart disease, diabetes, arthritis and neurological problems such as Alzheimer's disease.

In addition, you'll look better and feel better because the suggestions in this book – coincidentally – have been proven to have a positive impact on the ageing process too.

AS THE WHO SAYS; FURTHER INTERNATIONAL SPREAD OF SWINE FLU IS UNSTOPPABLE

So whether Swine Flu is a flash in the pan and does not prove to be as deadly as it might have been, there are plenty of other viruses around that do have the potential to become highly virulent.

The WHO has been warning us for years, against "Bird Flu Fatigue", where we just get fed up with the warnings and give up the fight to protect ourselves. What Keiji Fukuda, former (2006 - 2008) Director of WHO's Global Influenza Programme and currently Assistant Director-General - Health Security and Environment, has said about Bird Flu, is just as applicable to a number of other diseases like Swine Flu:

> *"The world must prepare for a long-term fight against Bird Flu and not give in to fatigue that seems to have set in . . . it is the H5N1 virus's tenacity rather than geographical spread that has raised the risk it could evolve into a form that moves more easily among humans."* (Apr 27th 2006)

SO, WHAT DO YOU HAVE TO LOSE?

GET HEALTHY AND WELL AND PROTECT YOURSELF AGAINST SWINE FLU THE NATURAL WAY!

REFERENCES

1. http://www.telegraph.co.uk/health/3536981/40000-die-every-year-after-hospital-blunders-MPs-are-told.html
2. http://www.medicalnewstoday.com/articles/11856.php ; 2006

PREPAREDNESS

The following sections contain information based upon tried and tested SAS survival techniques and also from lessons learned from the Hurricane Katrina disaster.

No one actually knows just what will happen should Swine Flu adapt into a more lethal strain, so we have no idea just how long any disruption to essential supplies could last. However, in order to write this section of the book, we have looked carefully at the advice given by Governments and other official bodies and also researched what happened to societies, cities, towns and even countries during the 1918 Spanish Flu outbreak.

However, now that you know the scope and magnitude of the potential threat to society and the potential disruption and civil unrest that may occur in the event of a more serious flu pandemic, it is vital to make certain preparations.

It is a well-established fact that in emergency situations people who are well prepared, have put a lot of thought into their survival strategies and actually know how to implement them smoothly and effectively have a much greater chance of survival.

One simple example of this is the data that airlines produce regarding the types of people who do well in emergency situations – they are the kind of people who do pay attention to the emergency procedures, do understand how to evacuate and also know exactly where their nearest exit is.

Similarly – hotels back this up by stating that people who know where the fire exit is stand a much better chance in the event of an emergency.

You can prepare for a more serious influenza pandemic right now. This will lessen its impact on you and your family. The following information will help you gather the information and resources you may need should Swine Flu – or indeed Bird Flu - actually cause economic chaos or civil unrest and a temporary breakdown of normal life.

CHAPTER 11

PREPAREDNESS

WHAT TO DO IF THIS PHASE 6 PANDEMIC BECOMES MORE SERIOUS: SURVIVING A PANDEMIC

1. YOUR SURVIVAL UNIT

YOUR "SURVIVAL UNIT"

In true emergency situations, as in Hurricane Katrina in New Orleans (and should this phase 6 pandemic become more serious), peoples' behaviour changes and it is likely to turn into a 'survival of the fittest' scenario – with the fittest inevitably doing best. However, in today's environment, 'fittest' doesn't necessarily mean 'physically strongest'.

In fact, the term 'fittest' actually means those who are best prepared. Also, the 'fittest' are those who are the most adaptable and those who can flexibly adjust to the demands of their situation. This is where some really hard decisions have to be made.

In extreme situations like this you do need to think about how you should form what is known as a 'Survival Unit'.

WHAT IS A SURVIVAL UNIT?

Your Survival Unit is a group of people who will join together to help ensure your group's best chance of survival. Who would be in your Survival Unit? Who are you able to care for? Children, elderly people, the sick? What happens if you get ill? Can someone else in your

Preparedness: Your Survival Unit

Survival Unit look after you?

FIND A "FLU FRIEND" SAYS UK GOVERNMENT

The UK Government recommends you find a 'Flu Friend', someone, or a group of people who you can work with to help each other. They say you need a Flu Friend – and need to be other peoples' Flu Friend, so that you can pick up prescriptions for each other, go shopping for each other and generally look out for each other.[1]

CARING FOR OTHERS CAN BE DEEPLY STRESSFUL:

Researchers at Ohio State University found that people who were caring for loved ones with Alzheimer's disease got twice as many colds as people who are not caregivers. This led researchers to conclude that the enormous amount of emotional stress in dealing with a loved one with a disease as devastating as Alzheimer's can lead to people becoming immuno-compromised.

If this pandemic becomes far more serious in nature, we believe that you are far more likely to survive it best by forming a Survival Unit, rather than just having a few Flu Friends to support you.

ETHICAL ISSUES TO CONSIDER

Terrible ethical issues raise their ugly heads here. If you have managed to prepare your stockpiles and have an efficient and adaptable Survival Unit, will you be willing to let others in?

Consider the following scenario – your teenage daughter has been going out with a boy for a month. They are "serious" and totally "in love". So, can you tell your daughter that her boyfriend can't come and share your stockpiles, etc? What about his brothers and sisters, parents, grandparents?

If they are all starving on your doorstep and you are inside your well-protected and well-provisioned home, what do you do?

This group of people may not be content with just sitting on your doorstep – they may also be trying to break in to steal your stocks with a greater or lesser degree of violence.

This is why it is absolutely essential to decide in advance who is in your Survival Unit.

It is also essential to keep your preparedness plans top secret. Do not flaunt your supplies; do not boast about your preparations. Make sure that everything is well hidden.

Don't invite problems by making a delicious, aromatic roast dinner – just because you can, when everyone else is starving. It is the quickest way of getting yourself into very serious trouble indeed.

Consider ways in which you can successfully protect yourself and your Survival Unit and your supplies. In addition, consider how you are going to store your food and water. These are bulky items and must be kept cool and away from sunlight.

REFERENCES

1. http://www.independent.co.uk/life-style/health-and-families/health-news/network-of-flu-friends-could-help-says-health-ministry-1679713.html

CHAPTER 12

PREPAREDNESS

WHAT TO DO IF THIS PHASE 6 PANDEMIC BECOMES MORE SERIOUS:
SURVIVING A PANDEMIC

2. THE PSYCHOLOGY OF SURVIVAL

We hear a lot about the benefits of a "Positive Mental Attitude" and this is never more important than in a situation where your very survival is at stake. Survival is so much more than just applying the knowledge that you may learn from books and websites, it is so much more than being able to find food and water, build shelter, make fires and so on. It takes a huge amount of bravery, determination and a positive mental framework to confront and overcome the types of issues that you may be faced with in a serious pandemic situation.

If the H1N1 virus does mutate to become more lethal, there will be overwhelming stressors for you to come to terms with – illness, death of loved ones, fear of disease, the breakdown of society, self protection etc.

It's well known that some people with little or no survival training have managed to survive life-threatening circumstances. However, others with advanced survival training have not used their skills and died. The key issue that differentiates these two groups is the mental attitude of the individual(s) involved. Of course, having survival skills is vitally important and preparation for survival in the face of an impending disaster is essential. However, having the will to survive is also essential. Without a desire to survive, any skills and knowledge that you do manage to acquire will be wasted.

There is a "psychology" to survival. Anyone in an extreme survival environment such as might arise when faced with a serious flu pandemic, faces many stresses that ultimately impact on the mind and body. These stresses can produce thoughts, emotions and feelings that, if poorly understood, can transform a confident, well-prepared individual into an indecisive, ineffective individual which will severely compromise his or her ability to survive. Thus, it is essential to learn about and to recognise the stresses commonly associated with survival situations.

It is also vital to recognise the types of reactions that one might produce in a highly stressful situation. By recognising sources of stress and your reactions to them and arming yourself with coping strategies, you manifestly increase your chances of survival and that of your loved ones.

STRESS

It is helpful to learn a little bit about stress and our reactions to various stressors that one might encounter in a severe pandemic crisis survival situation. This will help us to understand the types of stress responses that we might experience and help us to develop coping strategies that will give us a better chance of survival. Stress is not a disease that you cure and eliminate. Instead, it is a condition we all experience. Stress can be succinctly described as our reaction to "pressure".

We experience the sensations and physical reactions associated with "stress" when the demands upon our various resources, be they mental, physical, spiritual or emotional, outstrip our innate resilience and coping abilities. More commonly, "stress" is the name given to the experience we have as we physically, mentally, emotionally, and spiritually respond to life's tensions – if they are beyond our "comfort zones" in each area.

THE NEED FOR STRESS

Stress is in fact paradoxical as we need stressors (things that challenge our coping abilities – mental, physical, emotional, spiritual etc.) because they have many positive benefits. Positive forms of stress – sometimes known as "eustress" actually provide us with challenges that we respond to in a positive way. These events will often give us the chance to learn about our values, strengths and abilities.

Certain types of stress can show our ability to handle pressure without collapsing; it tests our adaptability and flexibility. Furthermore, certain stressors can stimulate us to do our best.

Stress also provides us with a gauge that helps highlight what is important to us. An example of eustress, for instance, could be the enormous excitement that some people derive from doing well at an extreme sport, cheering their favourite sports team to victory or watching their child win in the nail-biting finalé of the egg and spoon race. All these examples are undoubtedly positive, albeit, tense, experiences for those undergoing them. Eustress, is then, a matter of perspective. (e.g. the supporters of the losing team will be suffering from "distress").

We need to have some stress in our lives, but too much of anything can be bad. The goal is to have stress, but not an excess of it. Too much stress – known as distress, exacts a high price from people and organisations. Distress causes an uncomfortable tension and the natural tendency is to try to avoid it in the first place and if it does occur, to escape from it. The following list is a group of symptoms that may become apparent if you, or your Survival Unit are faced with stress:

- Depleted energy levels
- Constant worrying/anxiety
- Difficulty in making decisions or making poor decisions
- Angry outbursts
- Forgetfulness
- Mistakes
- Thoughts about death or suicide
- Social problems/can't get along with others
- Withdrawal from social groups
- Abstaining from responsibilities
- Inattention
- Carelessness
- Compromised health

"Perspective" is key when it comes to reacting to stressors. Those who do survive in extreme situations are able to take control of their reactions to stressors. Those who perceive stressors as eustress – i.e. a situation that is a positive challenge that can and will be overcome, will inevitably do better than those who perceive stressors as predominantly overwhelming and destructive.

One of the most important tools to cultivate in an extreme survival situation is a positive attitude, this incorporates goal-setting and acknowledgement of achievements, no matter how small. Any soldier will tell you that good morale is vital to the success of any campaign.

SURVIVAL STRESSORS

In a serious pandemic situation, there may be many stressors – some enormous and some small. Sometimes, the tiny little stressors can be the straw that breaks the camel's back in a survival situation, as they are insidious and they mount up almost imperceptibly. However, the one guarantee in any survival situations is that stressors are not courteous – they do not turn up in an orderly fashion and present themselves to you one by one. On the contrary – by their very nature – stressors are disorganised and come at you left, right and centre – this is what makes them stressful events – if we could plan for them we would not perceive them as stress-inducing.

Once your body recognises the presence of a stressor, a series of reactions, or "cascades" are thrown into motion. This is the way that your body acts to protect itself. Generally, in response to a stressor, your body prepares itself for what is loosely termed "fight or flight." (This is of course a simple and brief overview of the stress response, which is, in reality, an incredibly complex set of mind/body actions and reactions which are way beyond the size and scope of this current book.) The preparations involved in "fight or flight" responses include hormonal "SOS" messages being sent through your body, in order to prepare it to deal with a stressor.

A few of the many reactions that take place include the release of stored fuels (sugars and fats) to provide quick energy; muscle tension increases to prepare for action; your breathing rate increases so that blood is more oxygenated; blood clotting chemicals are released to reduce bleeding from cuts. Furthermore, your senses become heightened (your hearing becomes more sensitive, your pupils widen and your sense of smell becomes more acute) so that you are more aware of your surroundings. In addition, your heart rate and blood pressure both rise in order to provide more highly oxygenated blood to your muscles.

All of these amazing preparations are extremely "costly" in energetic terms and they are impossible to maintain for any length of time. The stress response is intended to get you out of an emergency and is not "designed" to cope with ongoing, relentless situations such as you might find in a pandemic emergency.

So, the cumulative effect of many stressors, both large and small can lead to enormous and overwhelming problems for your body/mind and because these all require such enormous energy reserves to service these responses, a state of exhaustion can quickly set in. At this stage you lose the ability to cope with stressors (or the ability to turn them to your advantage) and at this point signs of distress appear.

However, it has been shown time and again that preparation for, and anticipation of, potential stressors greatly reduces the deleterious effects of stressors and thus reduces the exhaustion levels that you might otherwise experience. It is therefore essential that anyone in an extreme survival setting should be aware of the types of stressors that they may encounter.

ILLNESS OR DEATH

Illness, either your own illness, or those of your loved ones – even culminating in death – are real possibilities when faced with a serious phase 6 pandemic. As we know, Bird Flu has a lethality of around 60% amongst the people who have contracted it and we have yet to discover the true lethality of Swine Flu. Even if it has a low lethality, if it is as virulent as it was when it started (and comes in waves, like most flu outbreaks) the sheer number of people infected – and the numbers of fatalities could be large enough to cause stress on a vast scale.

Perhaps nothing is more stressful than being subjected to large numbers of deaths, perhaps of your loved ones and of course having to live with the notion that you are virtually powerless to do anything about this. In addition, there is the constant fear that you too might become ill.

It is only by controlling the stress related to the vulnerability to illness and death that one can have the courage to take the risks associated with survival tasks. Maintenance of this courage will have an enormous impact upon your ability to make good decisions about survival issues for you and all those around you. Taking time now to think about coping strategies that you would use when faced with illness and death that you fear, will enable you to plan for these eventualities and this very planning activity will assist in reducing the impact of these stressors. This will in turn help to maximise your chances of survival and that of your loved ones.

UNCERTAINLY AND LACK OF CONTROL

Many people have trouble coping in situations where everything is not clear-cut. In an extreme survival situation such as one that might occur should a severe flu pandemic ensue, the only guarantee is that there will be enormous upheaval and that, for a short time at least, society and our environment will be very different. Given the economic changes we have been through in recent times an upheaval like this added to it would certainly be likely to be traumatic for most people. One would need to operate on limited information and knowledge about many matters that we normally take for granted. In addition, the sense of lack of control of your situation, environment and outcomes are all stressors.

ENVIRONMENT

Your environment may present you with stressors – electricity and water may not function, normal communications such as telephones and radios may not work. You may be faced with discomforts arising from being too cold, too hot, outside your usual environment (should you be forced to leave your home for any reason) and so on. Again, thinking this all through and preparing for these possibilities reduces the burden of potential stressors.

HUNGER AND THIRST

Hunger and thirst are both stressors. Without food and water a person will weaken and become susceptible to illness and of course may eventually die. Therefore, ensuring that you have adequate supplies of food and water is essential – both from the physical perspective, in so far as these items are essential to survival, but also from the point of view that you are reducing your potential burden of stressors – and there is an enormous psychological booster-effect in simply knowing that at the very least, you are equipped to look after yourself and your loved ones on the purely physical level.

FATIGUE

Overwhelming tiredness is a problematic factor in survival. It occurs for many reasons, including sheer physical tiredness that may come about from exertion. There is the stress-induced exhaustion to contend with but also it is important to understand that overpowering stressors will cause us to produce a sensation of overwhelming tiredness as one tries to psychologically "escape" from the dire situation one is in. Trying to stay awake is in itself a stressor – physically and mentally and it is important to realise that you may need to stay awake in order to nurse a loved one. Don't forget that should a small child or particularly vulnerable adult fall ill, you will need to be vigilant 24 hours a day to ensure that you are keeping them properly hydrated.

ISOLATION

If you have a Survival Unit you may do better – humans are social animals and are very often reliant upon others for support – be it mental, emotional or physical. Of course, having others around that you can trust also helps should you fall ill. Just knowing that someone will be there for you is a great help – even better if you have taught them what to do to care for a person with Swine Flu.

Loneliness is a significant stressor in its own right and one that can usually be addressed. In addition, it is helpful for a Survival Unit to work together to ensure the survival of the group. The stressors mentioned above may all sound very negative and frightening. This is not the intention. It is vital that you be as prepared, physically, mentally and emotionally as it is possible to be.

Preparation is key to reducing the number and severity of potential stressors. The fewer and less significant the stressors you encounter, the better your chances of surviving. Remember – the object of this is to change the things that you can control and to cope with the things that you can't control, or do anything about.

The more knowledge that you have and the more anticipatory preparation you invest in doing this – right now – will increase your chances of survival. Obviously, we can't cover every potential stressor that one may encounter in a survival situation but it would be wise to spend some time thinking about the issues that may crop up and what you would do to cope with them. A mental exercise such as this pre-primes your emotional responses so that you can react to such stressors as and when they do occur in a calmer fashion, making good, appropriate, life-saving decisions.

As with the principles of Complementary Medicine – it is important to remember that we are all individuals and situations that are stressful to one person may not be stressful to another. Your experiences, morale, personal view of life, your emotional, mental and physical fitness and your self-confidence all contribute to what you will find stressful in a pandemic emergency. You won't be able to avoid all stressors certainly, however the key to survival is managing those stressors and making them work in your favour as an impetus to your survival.

You now have a general knowledge of stress and the stressors common to survival; the next step is to examine your reactions to the stressors you may face.

PREPARING YOURSELF

Your number one priority is to stay alive. Your next priority is to keep your loved ones alive. In an extreme survival situation you will experience an extreme range of emotions and thoughts. Your choice is to decide whether you are going to let these work for you – or against you. Your morale is of the utmost importance and it is vital to keep a positive attitude. Granted – it may not be possible not to be sad, angry, upset, guilty, fearful, lonely, depressed and so on, at times – these are normal human emotions and you must expect to experience these. In fact, if something very sad happened to you and you did not experience appropriate sadness there would be a very good chance that you are suffering from a psychological disorder.

As emotions of various forms occur, feel them, acknowledge them and then decide whether they are going to work for you or against you. Even the most devastating sadness can be used to spur one on to survive and even achieve great things. Soldiers – who have been trained to cope with extreme survival situations – report that the knowledge that they will, in the course of their work, experience the whole gamut of the so called "negative" emotions, actually prompts them to prepare themselves more diligently when training. These emotions also push them to fight back against odds more aggressively and to take brave actions to ensure their survival and the survival of their unit.

If our responses to negative or debilitating emotions cannot be controlled, they can be absolutely paralysing. You lose the ability to summon up your internal resources and instead begin to listen to the negative mind-chatter that will debilitate and dramatically reduce your chances of survival.

It is a well known military tactic to defeat an enemy psychologically – by using mentally and emotionally weakening mind games such as propaganda and other misinformation to depress, frighten and diminish the opposition's morale. A mentally defeated soldier is a beaten soldier. It is exactly the same in a survival situation that might arise as a result of a more severe flu pandemic.

Remember, survival is your natural response to the most challenging situations. The circumstances that would arise from the chaos of a serious flu outbreak will not be normal, or natural in any way, and you will have reactions that may be overwhelming – the key is to prepare physically, mentally and emotionally to rule over these situations so that they serve you and spur you on towards achieving your goal – your survival and that of your loved ones.

Preparedness: The Psychology of Survival

PSYCHOLOGICAL PREPARATION TIPS

Research and history show that people can and do survive extreme situations and that there are certain traits that they have in common. The first of these is an unswerving belief that they will survive. This comes about because these people have deeply integrated the following into their minds and emotions:

- Know Yourself – Take the time to discover who you are on the inside. Friends and family who have your best interests at heart can probably help you with this.
- Get Strong – Strengthen your positive strong qualities and identify any areas that are less well-developed and work on these to improve them.
- Anticipate Fears – Everyone has fears – everyone! Identify and analyse those issues that would frighten you the most if faced with a highly lethal pandemic. Learn as much you can about the types of things you might be faced with and plan your response to them. You cannot eliminate fears but you can increase your ability to function in spite of your fears. Bear in mind that one of the most fear-provoking things is fear of the unknown. By doing research and thinking about possibilities deeply, you familiarise yourself with them and fears are lessened. By focussing on fears in a detached manner, you are effectively "shining a psychological flashlight" on them and this helps you to "see" the issues at hand more clearly – this makes them less frightening.
- Be Rational But Adopt A Positive Attitude – A clear-headed appraisal of situations will work in your favour. It is essential to see circumstances as they are and not endow them with things that you would prefer to see. Staying positively realistic is difficult but possible. This entails taking stock of the circumstances and realistically appraising them while simultaneously remembering that you have to make the situation work to your advantage. If you find yourself in a survival setting with unrealistic expectations, you may be laying the groundwork for bitter disappointment – which is a stressor as it is demoralising.
- Stay Rationally Positive – Positivity is about training yourself to see the highest good or potential in everything – people, situations, etc. It boosts your morale and that of others in your Survival Unit and it is also a highly creative and imaginative mind game which is a psychologically healthy and energy-giving pastime.
- Never Give Up – this is also known as "the will to survive". Plan, prepare and plan again so that you are at your peak of mental, physical and emotional endurance should a pandemic hit. These skills are never wasted and are always positive attributes in any given situation. Furthermore the strengths and skills outlined above will benefit every person who learns them in every area of their lives.
- Remember the 6 "P"s – a saying oft quoted in the Army and now adopted by the corporate world, also applies to survival:

PRIOR PREPARATION PREVENTS P*** POOR PERFORMANCE!

CHAPTER 13

PREPAREDNESS

WHAT TO DO IF THIS PHASE 6 PANDEMIC BECOMES MORE SERIOUS: SURVIVING A PANDEMIC

3. SHELTER

Most Governments and official bodies estimate that if a more virulent strain of Swine Flu emerges we will all need to make sure that we can survive for around three months as this is the length of time that they think essential supply chains could be disrupted. So, it is important to plan ahead so that you know what you will need to do to ensure that you have a safe shelter.

Something to bear in mind is that, as far as preparedness plans are concerned, back in 1918 people were in a better position to weather the pandemic storm than we are in modern society. This was because back in 1918, societies did not rely as heavily as we do today on imported supplies. Countries as a whole were far more self-sufficient and generally grew their own foods and thus had more supplies available to people.

Of course, there are many factors at play here and the vastly bigger population numbers of today do mean that supplies such as food and fuel must be imported - or certainly transported vast distances. This is not a great help when faced with a possible pandemic, especially as the things that we take for-granted in our homes, such as light, heating, cooling and water are so reliant upon electricity and gas to function.

Generally speaking, in the case of a serious phase 6 pandemic, finding a remote country retreat would be the best option. In the Great Plague of 1665 the people who did best were the wealthy who could retreat to the country and the people who lived in the countryside. However, this is unlikely to be practical or possible for most people. So, the next best option is to stay put at home – where you can ensure that your survival supplies are protected and easily available to you.

Preparedness: Shelter

One of the first things to consider regarding shelter is whether you need to stay indoors all the time – in order to avoid infection. Will you have to go out? Will you want or need to see friends and family?

LET'S TRY TO ANSWER EACH OF THESE IMPORTANT POINTS

It is probably best to stay inside as much as you possibly can – it is also sensible to try to avoid other people as much as possible. This will help to limit your exposure to the virus. Certainly, in 1918 the Spanish Flu virus was transmitted by breathing in air that contained viruses that people had sneezed or coughed out.

When you consider that a sneeze travels at around 100 mph and a cough can travel at up to MACH 1 (the speed of sound), you will realise that it is possible that air that you breathe, may well be contaminated with viruses, if you go outside and mix with others. So, it is probably best to stay in as much as possible and certainly to avoid others.

On another note, it is entirely possible that people may be infectious before they start to show symptoms – this is common in other diseases. So, even if a person looks perfectly well, they may in fact be sickening for the flu. It is currently estimated that a person can harbour the Swine Flu virus for around 1 to 12 days before they actually show symptoms. (Scientists really don't know the exact incubation periods yet.) In addition, it would be easy to mistake early Swine Flu symptoms for a "normal" tummy bug or a simple cold as opposed to a manifestation of H1N1.

YOUR ENVIRONMENT

It is essential to make sure that you know how to heat and cool your environment, should a major disruption to normal services such as electricity and gas supplies occur. Investigate whether it will be practical to have a fireplace. If so, you will need fuel for this. Also, if you need heat, consider purchasing a propane heater and perhaps a Calor gas stove for cooking. (Hot food is a great morale booster). Generators too, are a great idea in principle; however they are heavy and noisy and may attract unwanted attention. Also, they emit toxic exhaust fumes which could be lethal in an enclosed space. You would also have to consider how and where you would store the necessary petrol or diesel.

Should you need to, you can heat water. Although very makeshift, water can be heated in dark containers in the sun (not ideal for anyone in the Northern Hemisphere, but even on a cold, but reasonably sunny, day, this will still work fairly well).

Dark colours retain heat, so a dark bucket will retain heat, thus warming the contents, in this case, water. The kinds of containers to use could be a large black, or other very dark colour, plastic bucket. A large dark-coloured water butt could work well for example. Remember – the darker the colour – the more efficient the heating ability. If you are considering drinking this water then it is absolutely essential to make certain that the container has not been used to store any toxic material whatsoever.

Cooling your environment is best achieved by creating through-breezes. Experiment by opening different combinations of windows and doors. Security is of course of paramount importance, so do make sure that it is safe to do this. Also, if there is any likelihood that airborne viruses could get into your home, e.g. if you live very near to others who are coughing and sneezing, then you have to consider that viruses could enter through open windows, so caution is advised.

While heating and cooling of your environment may seem trivial at first glance, certainly when compared to all the other very serious things that could be going on should Swine Flu spread more virulently, it is important to realise that temperatures and other environmental circumstances that are uncomfortable to us are sources of stress. As we have seen, stress compromises and badly affects your immune function, and can make you more susceptible to disease – thus more vulnerable to Swine Flu.

To maintain morale and optimum well-being in a difficult environment, it is essential to make your surroundings as comfortable as they can possibly be. To see how important this really is, take a look at the psychologist Maslow's "Hierarchy of Needs" (below). Shelter is the one of the most important basic, underlying "Human Need".

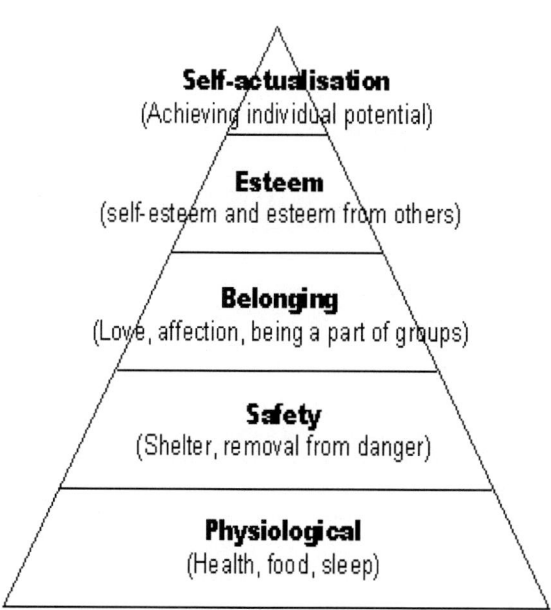

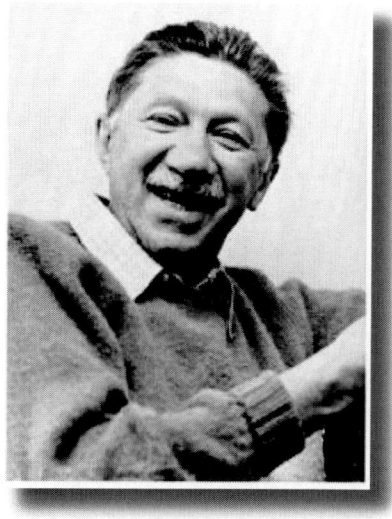

Abraham Maslow
http://z.hubpages.com/u/298635_f260.jpg

Preparedness: Shelter

NURSING PEOPLE AT HOME

If Swine Flu does become a far more serious problem, it is highly likely that you will need to nurse members of your 'Survival Unit'. The best way to do this is to set up one room that is an isolation room and to make sure that only one designated member of the unit is allowed to go in and out at a time, and to ensure that they observe strict hygiene rules – such as correct hand-washing techniques (see chapter Cleanliness and Sanitation) and the ill person stays in the isolation room, away from the other members of the Survival Unit, so as not to infect them.

Much has been written about using flu masks, but there is no real hard evidence that these will prevent you from contracting the disease. However they may be of some value in helping to prevent the spread of the disease if worn by an infected person. They could possibly reduce the amount of virus that the infected person could sneeze or cough into the air and onto others.

An isolation area will require various supplies. Use this checklist:

- Bed or blow up mattress e.g. a lilo if no bed is available in the designated isolation room
- Sheets
- Large black bags (for rubbish and also to use if plastic bed covering is required)
- Towels
- Toilet facilities (see how to make a field toilet in our "Sanitation" section)
- Water (drinking and washing)
- Clothing
- Thermometer
- Toothbrush and toothpaste
- Medicines
- Masks
- Torches
- Batteries
- Candles
- Matches
- Entertainment; books, radio, cards etc.
- Potential 'Complementary', and/ or Conventional treatments/ medicines
- Vitamins, herbs and other supplements

CHAPTER 14

PREPAREDNESS

WHAT TO DO IF THIS PHASE 6 PANDEMIC BECOMES MORE SERIOUS: SURVIVING A PANDEMIC

4. WATER SUPPLIES

One of the most important survival considerations is access to drinking water. It is bulky to store but an absolute necessity. People can survive for weeks without food, but only a number of days without water. Furthermore, dehydration severely weakens people and also compromises thinking ability – so, if severely dehydrated, you may make serious survival errors. So, if your supplies run low – never ever ration water – drink the water you have available and search for more tomorrow. For more information about the dangers of dehydration and ways to treat it see the next Chapter on Hydration.

HOW MUCH WATER WILL I NEED TO STORE?

The average adult will require 4 to 6 pints of drinking water each day – more if the weather is hot or they are exerting themselves. Women who are breastfeeding and people who are ill will require more than this. Children's requirements are generally fairly high and are similar to adult requirements. Because you also need water for food preparation and hygiene, it is recommended that you store a total of one gallon (4 litres) of water per person, per day.

AS AN ABSOLUTE <u>MINIMUM</u> YOU REALLY NEED TO STORE TWO WEEKS SUPPLY OF WATER FOR EACH MEMBER OF YOUR FAMILY I.E. 14 GALLONS PER PERSON (63.5 LITRES).

Most Governments and official bodies tell us that they expect society to be severely disrupted

Preparedness: Water Supplies

and supply chains compromised for a period of three months, if a truly severe pandemic sets in, so store three months supply of water if you possibly can.

It is vital to try to do this as soon as possible, over a period of days or weeks, as it is heavy to carry and difficult to store such large amounts of water – so work out where you will keep it. Ninety gallons per person (410 litres) – three months supply – takes up a lot of space. A gallon is eight pints and a large bottle of water usually contains about two to three pints (1.5 litres) so, 90 gallons is around 270 bottles per person!

HOW TO STORE WATER

If you are taking your water from your tap, a well, or a stream you need to ensure it is OK to drink and you need to store it in thoroughly washed plastic (but please read notes at the end of this Chapter), glass, fibreglass or enamel-lined metal containers. It goes without saying that you should never use a container that has held toxic substances – if in doubt don't use the container.

Remember too, that any water that you stockpile must be kept dry and cool – ideally in the dark. When considering your storage location, make sure that your supplies are not near any toxic substances as these can "leach" through plastic and have contaminated drinking water in the past – with serious consequences.

Make sure that you date your water stores – and start to use them straight away – replacing the amount of water used with new purchases/refills on a regular basis – just like you normally do. Store newer supplies at the back of your storage area and move older supplies to the front to be drunk, thus ensuring that you are constantly rotating your stock. If you keep bottled water for a long period and don't use it, you will need to replace it after 6 months. It doesn't 'keep' forever. So don't just lock it away and store it – remember to use it as your normal supply every day and replace stocks as you go.

If you deplete all your water supplies then you will need to find other sources and will also need to make sure that these can be purified.

OUTDOOR WATER SOURCES INCLUDE THE FOLLOWING:

- Rainwater
- Streams, rivers and other moving bodies of water – check to ensure that this is not potentially infectious – i.e. are there no dead bodies – human or animal – floating in it.
- Ponds and lakes

- Natural springs
- Wells

If water has an odour, has anything floating in it that is not immediately identifiable as safe or is dark do not drink it. (One exception to this is if you live in an area where rivers are very "clay-ey". This water can be absolutely safe, but will need to be filtered. You can use sea-water only if you distill it first, but this can be difficult in emergency conditions. Never drink floodwater.

FOUR WAYS TO PURIFY WATER

Contaminated water can contain micro-organisms that cause diseases such as dysentery, typhoid and hepatitis and it is possible that influenza viruses could be present in it too. In addition, it can taste awful. If in any doubt about the purity of water that you wish to drink, you should always err on the side of caution and purify it – just in case. Remember – it is also necessary to purify water that you intend to use for food preparation and hygiene i.e. tooth brushing, bathing, hair washing and so on.

There is no "failsafe" way of making sure that your purification process is perfect so it is often a good idea to take a "belt and braces" approach, i.e. to use two or more forms of purification. The second and third methods of water purification outlined below will kill microbes but none of the following methods will remove other potentially dangerous contaminants such as chemicals and heavy metals.

1. STRAINING

First strain the water you wish to use through clean cloth. If the particles in the water are very tiny you may need to double the cloth over to make a finer sieve. At a pinch, a paper towel will be reasonably useful but will tend to disintegrate and also paper towels may have been treated with chemicals that you might not want to ingest.

2. BOILING

Boiling water is one of the best methods of purifying water – allow the water to boil rapidly for one minute and remember to cover the top of the utensil that you are using to boil the water in, or your precious water supplies will evaporate. Naturally, water must be allowed to cool before drinking.

One excellent tip from survival experts is that boiled water will taste better if you put oxygen back into it. This can be achieved by pouring the water back and forth between two clean containers, or putting it into a clean bottle and shaking it. This is also a good tip for improving the taste of stored water – but if shaking water in a bottle, you need to make sure that it is not full to the brim otherwise there is not enough air available to properly oxygenate the water.

Preparedness: Water Supplies

3. BLEACH

Household bleach will kill micro-organisms. It is safe to use if the following points are strictly observed: Use only ordinary household liquid bleach that contains 5.25 % sodium hypochlorite.

Do not use any other "water purifiers" such as the types that you may find in camping shops, unless they contain the minumum of 5.25 % sodium hypochlorite.

Do remember that most bleaches contain numerous other ingredients to "improve" the bleach i.e. scents, colours and thickeners. You need to buy the very cheapest bleach that you can as this is often the plain variety. Make a point of checking the label.

The correct purification dosage is 16 drops of bleach per gallon (8 pints; 4 litres: 4 quarts) of water. Remember to proportionally reduce the dosage of bleach for smaller amounts. Use a dropper for accuracy. Stir this and let stand for 30 minutes. If the water does not have a slight bleachy smell, repeat the dosage and let stand another 15 minutes. Use caution and measure your doses very carefully. You are aiming for only a very slight smell of bleach.

4. DISTILLATION

A more complex but also ultimately more effective purification process is distillation which will kill microbes and also remove toxins such as heavy metals, chemicals and salts. The process of distillation condenses steam from boiling water and feeds this purified water into another receptacle for use.

A GOOD HOMEMADE STILL CAN BE RIGGED UP AS FOLLOWS:

Fill a saucepan halfway with water. Tie a cup to the knob or handle on the top of the saucepan lid, so that the cup will hang right-side-up when the lid is upside-down. Make sure the cup is not dangling into the water in the saucepan and it may be useful to have a cup that has two handles for stability – like a child's beaker. Put the upside-down saucepan lid with the cup hanging underneath onto the saucepan and boil the water for 20 minutes. As the steam rises, it collects on the upside-down saucepan lid and drips down to the handle. Next it will drip down into the cup. The water that drips from the lid into the cup is distilled.

It is worth having a practice run at rigging this up correctly before you need to use this technique in an emergency. Of course, this technique is only going to work if you have a way of boiling water – so think about getting a gas stove or other cooking equipment of the type used for camping.

The Survivor's Guide to Swine Flu

UTILISING THE UNSEEN WATER SUPPLIES IN YOUR HOME:

In an emergency, there are a number of hidden water stores in most houses. For example:

- There is water in your hot water tank.
- Most houses also have a cold water reservoir too.
- You may have ice cubes in your freezer.
- There is also a store of water in your toilet cistern – not the bowl!

Make sure you know the location of your incoming water supply "shut off" tap or stop-cock. You will need to shut this off if you hear that contaminated water or sewage is coming into homes. If you live in a house with more than one storey you may be able to drain your pipes and use the water in them. Turn on a tap at the highest point in the house. A small amount of water will trickle out – save it. Then turn on a tap at the lowest point of your house and gravity will do the rest for you.

If your house has a hot water tank, you may be able to drain this too but remember that you must not turn on any electricity or gas supply to it if it has been drained.

URINE

One last but vital point to note is that in an absolute emergency, it is possible to drink your own urine. This is a horrible thought for most people but well worth knowing. Although probably a last resort for many people, in true survival situations, urine has kept people alive for what could be a couple of extra vital days. Contrary to popular belief, urine is not a dirty and toxic substance rejected by the body. In fact, urine is a by-product of blood filtration, not waste filtration. Medically it is referred to as "plasma ultrafiltrate".

Therefore, it becomes apparent that urine is a purified derivative of the blood itself, made by the kidneys, whose principal function is not excretion but regulation of all the elements and their concentrations in the blood. While there is much controversy over whether a branch of alternative health practice called urotherapy (drinking your own urine for its possible health

BEWARE OF USING 'PLASTIC' PRODUCTS CONTAINING BISPHENOL A (BPA)

Background: Bisphenol A, commonly abbreviated as BPA, is an organic compound with two phenol functional groups. It is a difunctional building block of several important plastics and plastic additives. With an annual production of 2–3 million metric tonnes, it is an important monomer in the production of polycarbonate.

Suspected of being hazardous to humans since the 1930s, concerns about the use of bisphenol A in consumer products were regularly reported in the news media in 2008 after several governments issued reports questioning its safety, and some retailers removed products made from it off their shelves.

In the last 30 years well over 100 studies have linked bisphenol-A to breast cancer, obesity, heart disease, diabetes, liver abnormalities and implicated it in problems of brain function and mood disorders in monkeys and to behavioural changes in children and to developmental defects, including abnormalities of the brain and prostate glands in developing fetuses and infants.

Where would we be without plastic containers and bottles? Most people use them all the time – and without even thinking about it. Ongoing controversies over the inclusion of bisphenol-A (BPA) – have centred on getting this ingredient removed from baby's bottles.

However the contamination from bisphenol-A is so great in the Western world that it can even be measured by taking samples from rivers and estuaries.[1]

The CDC in the US estimates that 93% of all Americans have detectable levels of BPA in their urine.

It is all around us – used not just in baby's feeding bottles – but in 'plastic bottles', ones we use for water and soft drinks, as well as in food storage containers, PVC water pipes and as a lining inside metal cans. It's used in films, sheets, and laminations; in enamels and varnishes; adhesives; artificial teeth; nail polish; compact discs; and a whole lot more products. It's all around your home, it's in your car, it's in your workplace. It's everywhere.[2]

Although scientists have known about its dangers since the 1930's, Government bodies like the US FDA, have accepted the reassurances made by scientists that the harmful effects of bisphenol -A – were minimal, as it passes through your body "so quickly".[3]

But a study published in January, 2009, in the journal - Enviromental Health Perspectives (Jan 28th, 2009), undertaken at the Rochester Medical Center in New York state, challenges this assumption and says that it takes AT LEAST 8 times longer for bisphenol-A to pass through your body than previously thought.[4]

Dr Richard Stahlhut, the lead researcher said:

"In our data, BPA levels appear to drop about eight times more slowly than expected – so slowly, in fact, that race and sex together have as big an influence on BPA levels as fasting time."

In addition, he theorised that BPA may seep into fat tissues, where it would be released more slowly.

benefits) actually works, it is certain that urine is a potentially valuable source of fluid that may make the difference between death and survival.

REFERENCES

1. http://www.ourstolenfuture.org/NewScience/oncompounds/bisphenola/bpauses.htm
2. Takahashi and Oishi 2000
3. The journal Environmental Health Perspectives published the research online January 28, 2009.
4. http://www.urmc.rochester.edu/pr/news/story.cfm?id=2361ls,

CHAPTER 15

PREPAREDNESS

WHAT TO DO IF THIS PHASE 6 PANDEMIC BECOMES MORE SERIOUS: SURVIVING A PANDEMIC

5. HYDRATION: AND THE DANGERS OF DEHYDRATION

Dehydration is one of the biggest dangers in any emergency situation. It can be defined as "the excessive loss of water from the body".

Dehydration can be caused in a number of ways; diarrhoea, excessive sweating and vomiting can all cause problems. In babies, dehydration caused by an otherwise mild disease can actually lead to enormous and potentially life-threatening problems. It's a straightforward equation – if we take in less fluid than we use this equals "dehydration".

There are general guidelines about the treatment of dehydration that you should be aware of, but each person is an individual, and therefore their own particular needs should be taken into account. Normally, if a person was suffering from severe dehydration, they would generally be admitted into hospital and put onto a rehydration drip, however, in a severe pandemic situation it may be unlikely that this necessity, that we normally take for granted, would be available.

CAUSES OF DEHYDRATION

Bacterial, or viral, infection can lead to the intestines becoming inflamed and this can cause the lining of the intestines to produce more water than can be absorbed. This liquid is then expelled from the body as diarrhoea.

Other causes of dehydration include a decrease in oral liquid intake, due to feeling sick (nausea), or loss of appetite. This loss of water may be exacerbated by an inability to keep things down (vomiting). Certain medications such as diuretics can also cause increased fluid loss. People who have had a bowel resection (ileostomy) are more susceptible to dehydration.

SIGNS AND SYMPTOMS OF DEHYDRATION

Some obvious signs of dehydration include; a dry mouth, lack of saliva, no tears, sunken eyes, a reduction in urination, and skin that stays compressed when pinched. Increasing thirst, dry mouth, weakness or light-headedness (particularly if worsening on standing). Darkening of the urine, or a decrease in urination are also potential pointers to dehydration. In babies, the fontanelle (soft spot on the top of the baby's head) may be sunken.

Another reliable clue is a rapid drop in weight. A reduction of 10% of body weight is considered a sign of severe dehydration. This loss may equal several pounds in a few days (or at times hours). Top athletes experience this often and are well aware of how to hydrate properly to compensate for this, however, in illness, it is absolutely essential to understand how to recognise the signs of dehydration and to act very quickly to address the issue.

One of the problems faced by those looking after sick people is that the symptoms of dehydration may be difficult to distinguish from those of the original illness.

TREATMENT PROTOCOLS

First of all – don't let dehydration happen. Prevention is always better than cure.

Certain foods and drinks promote dehydration and these include any food or drink that contains caffeine, such as coffee, tea, chocolate, cola etc. Also, salt and salty foods dehydrate people. Another serious dehydration culprit is alcohol and this needs to be completely avoided as aside from dehydration it also impairs immune function dramatically, making you more susceptible to catching flu. Anti-histamines and decongestant medication can also cause dehydration as can diuretics.

WHEN DEALING WITH A PATIENT, YOU NEED TO MAKE SURE THAT YOU OBSERVE THE PERSON CAREFULLY AND IMPLEMENT THE FOLLOWING STRATEGIES AS SOON AS POSSIBLE IF DEHYDRATION IS SUSPECTED:

In order to rehydrate people in a situation where H1N1 has caused a pandemic so severe that your access to normal help mechanisms is not possible (where you may not have access to hospitals and intravenous drips), it is possible to rehydrate people by mouth (orally), by getting them to drink, or helping them to drink, a rehydration solution. The following rehydration solution was developed by the WHO in the 1960's, and its use has saved countless lives since.

HOW TO PREPARE AND ADMINISTER YOUR OWN ORAL REHYDRATION SOLUTION (ORS)

Mix together the following:

> 1. Sea Salt – 3/4 teaspoon (table salt can be used in an absolute emergency but it usually contains other chemicals which can be harmful and may contribute to further dehydration. Never use salt substitutes - these won't work).
> 2. Baking Powder – 1 teaspoon.
> 3. Sugar – 4 tablespoons.
> 4. Orange Juice – 1 cup (for palatability and improved electrolyte balance – long life juice is fine and feel free to substitute other juices. Note that beverages sold as Fruit "DRINK" are often dilute juices, and are full of sugar, and are not to be used as an ORS).
> 5. Water – 1 quart/litre/2 pints.

(NB Throughout this book we advise against the use of refined sugar. ORS is the one exception to this rule. The sugar in the solution actually assists and improves the absorption of the salt and water.)

This ORS drink can be taken in small, frequent sips, and is often well tolerated in the face of nausea and vomiting. There are several excellent rehydration solutions available commercially but they achieve basically the same effect. This solution outlined above is certainly much less expensive.

Try to get an adult or larger child to drink 2 pints (one litre) of this solution per hour until the frequency of urination begins to increase and the urine colour turns light or clear.

A smaller child or infant should be given 1.5 fluid ounces (44 millilitres) of the ORS above, per pound (.45 kilograms) of body weight over the first four hours, then 1 fluid ounce (30 millilitres) of ORS per pound of body weight per eight-hour period, until it is apparent that the dehydration has improved and the symptoms of dehydration they were showing have resolved.

If the patient is unable to drink this solution by themselves then you, or someone else, will need to administer it by dripping it into their mouths. If they are not swallowing, you need to massage their throats gently to get them to swallow. Make certain that the patient is in a reasonably upright position to avoid the danger of them aspirating the fluid – i.e. it "going down the wrong hole" and into the lungs.

You will need to monitor the patient carefully and make changes in the amount of fluid replacement that may be needed as symptoms improve.

Most health practitioners advise that food intake should be continued if at all possible, except for high fibre fruits and vegetables which may irritate the intestines. Milk ought to be avoided as the lactose that it contains may also cause problems, which can exacerbate diarrhoea.

COMPLEMENTARY MEDICAL ADVICE ABOUT DIET DURING AN ATTACK OF DIARRHOEA

During an attack of diarrhoea you need to maintain your hydration levels and it is important to try to stop the diarrhoea as soon as possible, as it can lead to very rapid dehydration.

- Eat and drink plenty of fluids, especially fruit juices and carrot juice if possible, along with lots of water. Drinks high in protein are good for treating diarrhoea so consume drinks made with Whey protein supplement.

- Boil half a cup of brown rice in 750 ml of water for 45 minutes, eat the rice and drink the water. Brown rice helps to form stools and also supplies essential B vitamins.

- It is also good to eat oat bran (if you are not intolerant to this), raw foods, and yogurt (with live bacteria).

AVOID THE FOLLOWING

The enzyme needed to digest lactose – a sugar in milk – is lost for a while during an attack of diarrhoea, so avoid dairy products for a few days, even if you are not lactose intolerant. It is fine to eat low-fat soured products though like yogurt with live bacteria for example.

Reduce your intake of foods containing gluten as this can exacerbate diarrhoea. Gluten is found in wheat, rye, oats, barley, spelt.

SUPPLEMENTS TO TAKE THAT WILL HELP WITH TREATING DIARRHOEA

ACIDOPHILUS
Replaces 'good' bacteria that may be lost due to diarrhoea. It is especially good to take after a bout of diarrhoea because 'good' bacteria get flushed out of the digestive tract, leaving it vulnerable

to new infections. Take 1 teaspoon in distilled water twice daily on an empty stomach. Note: some probiotic bacteria preparations need to be kept cold, which may not be possible during a serious pandemic situation, so look for products that still maintain their potency without the need for refrigeration.

SB (SACCHAROMYCES BOURLARDII)

Another form of pro-biotic has been proven in trials to prevent diarrhoea. It should be taken particularly if the diarrhoea is a result of taking antibiotics. It has also been used in studies on other forms of infectious diarrhoea. Travellers' diarrhoea treated with "Sb" showed positive results.

MULTI-VITAMINS

Should be taken as directed on the label. The body finds it hard to absorb vitamins and minerals when you have diarrhoea, so it is good to supplement with multi-vitamins as an extra precaution. 'Food-state' vitamins are best – these are vitamin supplements that closely match vitamins which occur naturally in food.

It is not wise to take the cheapest multi-vitamins that you can find as these often are either a waste of time as many of these are synthetic and therefore are not recognised by the body and can pass straight through you or can even be harmful. Take a look at the Nutrition section in this book for more information.

CHARCOAL TABLETS

These absorb toxins in the bloodstream and colon. Take 4 tablets every hour until diarrhoea subsides. These are available from chemists. Do not take at the same time as other supplements as charcoal can inhibit the absorption of beneficial vitamins and other supplements.

GARLIC

Capsules kill bacteria and other pathogens and also enhance immunity. Ideally take the equivalent of a clove of raw crushed garlic two to three times each day.

KELP:

Helps to replace minerals lost in loose bowel movements. Good mineral balance is essential to health.

POTASSIUM

Potassium is lost in a diarrhoea attack and needs to be replaced.

ESSENTIAL FATTY ACIDS: (OMEGAS 3 & 6)

Take as directed on label as Essential Fatty Acids help form stools. Please see the Nutrition section in this book for much more in-depth information about the Omega family of Essential

Fatty Acids.

HERBS THAT WILL HELP TO CONTROL DIARRHOEA

PSYLLIUM HUSKS OR SEEDS
Take 4 capsules or 9–30 grams of the seeds daily at bedtime with at least one large glass of water as they expand in the intestines. Psyllium Husks help make the stools more solid and in cases of non-infectious diarrhoea, have been proven to alleviate symptoms. (Interestingly, aside from treating diarrhoea, Psyllium Husks are also an excellent way to treat constipation.) Psyllium Husks are best avoided by those with IBS since they may aggravate this problem in some people. Start with a low dose and work up as your body learns to tolerate the Psyllium Husks.

CAROB
Carob is usually bought as a brown powder and is derived from carob seeds. It is very often used as a chocolate substitute. It can be used quite successfully for treating diarrhoea in children and can also be used for adults. Although not ideal, given its high sugar content and the impact that sugar has on the immune system, the usual way of taking Carob is as follows: Mix 15 grams of Carob with jam (for taste) and take daily. (Be aware that the sugar in jam may act as a laxative and that Sorbitol – sometimes used in low-sugar jams and other confectionary is known to produce loose stools).

CHAMOMILE
Steep 2–3 grams of dried Chamomile flowers in boiling water for 10 minutes or use a Chamomile tea bag. You can buy loose Chamomile flowers from health-food stores and also on the internet but there is not much difference between using the flowers or teabags from a therapeutic point of view.

This tea reduces intestinal cramping and eases irritation and inflammation. (Do not take Chamomile on an ongoing basis, and do not take if you are allergic to Ragweed).

OTHER HERBS THAT CAN BE DRUNK AS TEAS AND ARE USED TRADITIONALLY FOR DIARRHOEA INCLUDE

Blackberry Root Bark, Pau d'Arco and Raspberry Leaf.

Traditionally, Barberry herb has been used in the successful treatment of diarrhoea although there haven't been many scientific studies supporting its effects, either positive or negative. It can be bought from health-food stores or from reputable herb suppliers.

The traditional dosage is; tincture of 2–3 ml 3 times daily, 15–20 minutes before a meal. Because of the lack of research on Barberry we would advise that it should not be taken by pregnant or nursing women until more information is available.

HOMEOPATHIC REMEDIES THAT CAN HELP TREAT DIARRHOEA

When making any herbal tea, remember to cover the container with a saucer to stop the therapeutic essential oils from evaporating while brewing and drink the tea 3 or more times a day.

The following remedies are very often prescribed by homeopaths for diarrhoea and you can read more about homeopathic medicine in the Homeopathy section of this book – including how to actually take the remedies. It is important to make sure that you do this correctly as they are easily anti-doted. Generally, the dosage for people with diarrhoea is one "30c" tablet each hour until symptoms subside.

ARSENICUM

This is the remedy of choice in treating most forms of diarrhoea – especially if caused by food poisoning. One of the main guiding symptoms for Arsenicum is that the person will be thirsty but will only be able to take small sips of water. They are restless, anxious and have a cold sweat. Usually, treatment with Arsenicum is extremely rapidly successful and often symptoms will subside within the half hour after taking the remedy.

CROTON TIG

The patient's stools are copious and watery, they gush out of the body and they look yellowish and may look like yellow water. There is lots of gurgling and urging to "go" before the actual diarrhoea attack. Croton diarrhoea can be painful and this pain can be in the umbilical (tummy button) region. The person feels worse and symptoms are also worse if they take any food or drink. Moving around also exacerbates symptoms. The person feels better if they can sleep.

GRATIOLA

Gratiola is indicated if stools just gush out of the body and are green and frothy but painless and after evacuation and there may be a burning sensation around the anus. Eating, drinking and motion all make the patient feel worse and fresh air makes them feel better.

COLOCYNTHIS

One of the guiding symptoms of a Colocynthis diarrhoea is that the patient will be in a lot of pain and will need to bend double to relieve it. They may rub their abdomen and might rock back and forth in an attempt to relieve the pain. All of the pains come in waves over the person. Stools are frothy, watery, yellowish and the person may be very flatulent. The person is very thirsty and they feel worse if they eat any food.

Preparedness: Hydration

CHINA

The symptoms that China treats very well are those associated with Giardia – an amoebic parasite that is often picked up by people travelling in developing countries. However, regardless of whether you are treating Giardia or diarrhoea with similar symptoms the guiding symptoms remain the same:

The stools are frothy and watery and may contain undigested food. The main characteristics of the conditions that this remedy is used for are: a great deal of wind associated with passing the diarrhoea and lots of spluttering and foul smelling stools. The person becomes weakened and dehydrated and they cannot stand being touched and they are adverse to noise. If they bend double, they will feel better and they are also comforted by warmth. The remedy 'China', has a marked periodicity so that symptoms get better and worse again on alternate days.

DEHYDRATION IN CHILDREN

Oral fluid replacement may be needed, depending on severity of fluid loss:

- For diarrhoea with no dehydration, feed the child normally and give the Oral Rehydration Solution (ORS) as directed above.
- If a dehydrated child is breast-fed, keep nursing (offer the breast more often). If the child is fed on baby formula, stick with this and then change to a soy-based formula, or the ORS, if the diarrhoea persists. It is essential to make sure that the mother is also properly hydrated if she is breastfeeding more frequently.
- If dehydration is severe, this can be life-threatening and the child may need intravenous hydration in a hospital or medical centre. This may be difficult to get in a pandemic situation so ORS should be continued on an ongoing basis. You may even need to use a dropper to drip feed the child constantly. (This is extremely debilitating for the carer and the carer needs to make sure that his or her energy levels are kept up.)

HYDRATION IN NON-EMERGENCY SITUATIONS

Correct hydration is vitally important for all people as a means of staying healthy and enabling your body to be optimally resistant to illness, including viruses. As outlined above, you need to make sure that you are drinking adequate amounts of water.

There is also evidence that demonstrates that taking a small amount of Sea or Rock Salt with your water improves its absorption into your body.

Some practitioners recommend that you drink 1/2 your body's weight in ounces of water, per day, adding 1/4 teaspoon of Sea or Rock Salt to your diet for each quart (2 pints/litre) of water consumed. Another useful tip that many practitioners recommend is to put a little Rock or Sea Salt on your tongue after drinking a glass, or two, of water.

However, you may want to check with your health professional before adding salt to your diet, as there are a few conditions which will not benefit from salt consumption. Do not use common table salt for this procedure as this contains various chemicals that do not benefit the body and may possibly be quite toxic.

The theory behind the Rock Salt regime, specifically, is that Rock Salt is composed of many minerals other than sodium chloride (plain table salt) and it is this mineral complex that is beneficial to optimum absorption.

Although we have not been able to find any scientific studies that come up to the standards required by The Complementary Medical Association (The CMA), we have looked into this regime in detail. Our findings are that in practice, people do report that they are certainly better hydrated and that they feel much better too. A number of US based doctors who use advanced body composition measuring equipment have reported that this regime measurably improves hydration. We realise that this is anecdotal evidence but we are sufficiently convinced of the benefits of this regime to include it in this book.

CHAPTER 16

PREPAREDNESS

WHAT TO DO IF THIS PHASE 6 PANDEMIC BECOMES MORE SERIOUS:

SURVIVING A PANDEMIC

6. CLEANLINESS AND SANITATION

In a serious pandemic situation, it is entirely likely that severe disruption will occur and things that you take for granted, like your water supply and sewerage, will be affected to a greater or lesser extent. If the worst should happen it is vital to consider how you and your family will cope with things like keeping clean and using the toilet etc.

CLEANLINESS

Cleanliness is an absolute necessity for many reasons. First of all, you need to make sure that you are clean so that you reduce the chances of the flu virus spreading on your clothing, or on your unclean body. Cracks and crevices which are all but invisible to the naked eye, such as the tiny ridges of our finger prints, are enormous mountains and valleys, when compared to the size of a virus. So these mountains and valleys can easily hide viruses, bacteria and other infectious matter.

Do follow the hand washing procedures outlined below. Get a hand sanitiser gel (preferably a low or non–alcoholic one) and use it.

The reason that we recommend low, or ideally non-alcoholic, hand sanitisers is because the alcohol contained in the most commonly available products is very high and this is absorbed through the skin. There have been reports of surgeons being found to be 'over the limit' - not due to alcohol consumption but due to their constant use of alcohol based hand sanitisers.

Preparedness: Cleanliness & Sanitation

Attend, immediately, to cuts and scrapes as these can become infected easily. You must clean any wound thoroughly and then apply antibiotic ointment, or homeopathic Hyper-cal (a mixture of Hypericum and Calendula) – known for its disinfectant and wound healing properties.

HAND-WASHING – PROPERLY

One of the first things you need to consider when it comes to Swine Flu, is how to avoid contracting it in the first place. Various official bodies give mixed and sometimes confusing advice, e.g. don't go out at all, don't mix with people and so on.

While suggestions like these are eminently sensible, it is highly likely that if a more serious pandemic situation does occur, you will have already been mixing with people who are infectious, but who are not yet displaying symptoms. However you may need to go out, to work, deal with people, look after sick loved ones, travel etc. So, the best way of protecting yourself is by taking preventative action.

One of the biggest medical breakthroughs of all time is simple and straight-forward and has saved countless lives – hand-washing!

Even in a non-pandemic situation it's very sensible to get into proper hand-washing habits.

Even if you are out and about and can't avoid people, you absolutely must wash your hands before eating, touching your mouth, nose or eyes, before preparing food, after using the bathroom, tending to sick people. Well, the list is endless!

HAND-WASHING; A BRIEF HISTORY

The importance of hand-washing really came to light in 1847, thanks to the discovery made by Hungarian doctor, Ignaz Semmelweis.

At that time, vast numbers of women (30%) who had just given birth died from "childbed fever", or "puerperal fever". These were the names given to the condition that doctors, at that time, believed caused these deaths.

As there were so many dead bodies available in the various "lying-in", or maternity hospitals, they were also great centres of learning for doctors, who used to dissect cadavers to discover more about anatomy and illness.

Semmelweis observed that after a dissection, a doctor would go to deliver a baby – without washing his hands - and that many of these women would die. All other doctors at the time attributed the high death rate to "miasmas", something unfavourable in the atmosphere.

Semmelweis thought differently and got his colleagues to start washing their hands. The death rate dropped rapidly to 1% of patients.

Shortly after this, Semmelweis' friend cut his finger while doing an autopsy and also died. For Semmelweis, this was overwhelming evidence that "something" was being "transferred" from cadaver to patient. In spite of his brilliant discovery and the countless lives he saved as a result, Semmelweis was totally rejected by society and died a horrible death in an asylum for the insane.

So, one important question is – why do we still have problems in hospitals today with infection being caused by some members of staff not washing their hands? Well, possibly one reason was that Semmelweis was a really poor politician and attacked influential colleagues aggressively – calling them "murderers" and "fiends" in response to their non-adoption of his suggestions – that they turned against him and actually ordered their staff not to observe Semmelweis' cleanliness procedures.

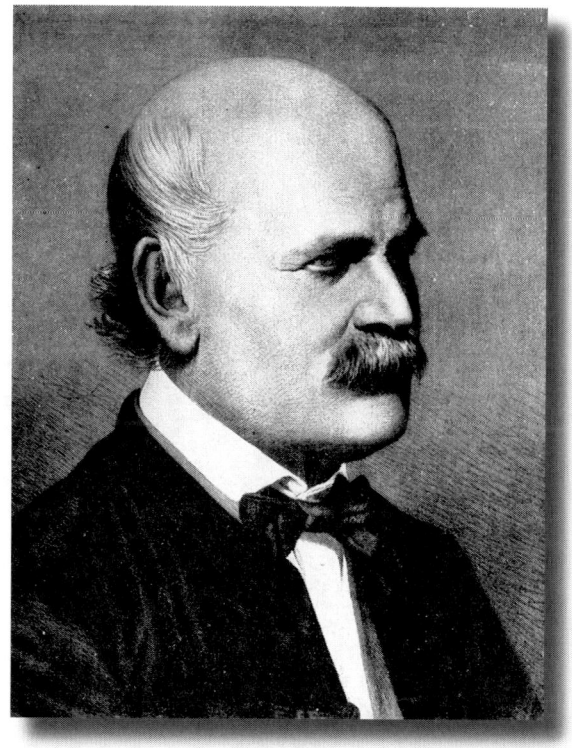

Ignaz Semmelweis 1860
(Copper plate engraving by Jenő Doby)

Upon researching historical data on this odd series of events, it becomes apparent that it is entirely possible that the great aggression towards Semmelweis and the rejection of his procedures may be contributing to the lack of hand-washing that we still see today. (In the UK the authorities have admitted to over 8,000 deaths caused by MRSA and C-diff infections – mainly caught in hospitals (2006)[1]. All of these are completely avoidable deaths.)

A term that describes the dismissal or rejection, out of hand, of any information, as an automatic knee-jerk reaction, without taking time to think about it, look deeper or experiment is called "The Semmelweis Reflex". The phrase elegantly describes many people's personal experiences with the phenomena and it illustrates the reactions of anyone who engages in such behaviour. There are hundreds of examples of this behaviour throughout history and poor Semmelweis was not alone in not being believed, or being rejected for his beliefs.

Preparedness: Cleanliness & Sanitation

HERE'S HOW TO WASH YOUR HANDS PROPERLY

It is absolutely vital that you remember that the sink, tap, soap dispenser and any areas that others might touch are contaminated by potential pathogens such as viruses, bacteria and fungi.

Try to avoid touching them.

• Turn on the taps – if your supply is still on – using a paper towel and then wet your hands – right up to the wrists and higher if your arms have been in contact with potentially contaminated surfaces, e.g. have you been leaning on your desk, for example? (Tip – take a note of the type of paper towel dispenser that you are using – are you going to need to dispense more paper towels for later on? See below.)

• Use soap (anti-bacterial soap is ideal) and work it into a rich lather.

• Now – here's the bit that most people get wrong – vigorously rub together all the surfaces of your soapy hands for 20 seconds each. (A good tip is to sing "Happy Birthday" all the way through, more or less quietly depending on your circumstances – it's about 20 seconds long.)

The rubbing action will help to remove dirt and micro-organisms such as viruses and bacteria.

Don't forget that your cuticles, nails and rings may well harbour pathogens so pay special attention to these. Also, don't forget to scrub away between your fingers.

• Rinse your hands under running water – if you have it – and make sure that you are rinsing everything off "downwards" so that contaminated water doesn't run up your arms towards your elbows.

• Use the paper towel to turn off the tap.

• Use a fresh paper towel to dry your hands. (Here's the tricky bit – if your paper towel dispenser is one of the types where you have to push a lever down to get a bit of paper out you will need to push this lever down with a paper towel – one that you dispensed earlier while getting your paper towel for the taps!)

• Dry your hands completely.

• You might need paper towels to open the door of the bathroom area – especially if you are in a public location. Remember that other people may not have washed their hands properly – so the exit door may be contaminated.

- Dispose of the towels in the nearest bin.

This is all pretty time consuming but well worth the effort. However it is reasonably complex – especially if you are in a location where correct hand-washing is difficult because of a lack of paper towels for example. One option is to carry with you an anti-viral/anti-bacterial hand sanitiser and use this as needed. Remember to wash your hands properly as outlined above as soon as you possibly can.

It is important not to become paranoid about pathogens but at the same time, sensible cleanliness precautions are useful and have been proven to reduce illnesses caused by the transfer of pathogens via hands.

(In advice given to businesses who are attempting to plan for how they might cope with a severe flu pandemic, many advisors are telling them to ensure that their staff get used to NOT shaking each other's – or client's – hands when they meet).

The UK Government undertook a telephone research survey in May 2009 to check whether people were taking any notice of the messages they were putting in their advertising and advice pamphlets about changing their behaviour because of the Swine Flu outbreak.

They found that 38% of people surveyed said that they had, in fact, changed their behaviour at some time in the previous 4 days because of Swine Flu (increased their hand washing, cleaned their work and home surfaces more thoroughly, etc).[2]

CLEANLINESS WITH COMPLEMENTARY MEDICAL ANTI-FUNGALS

It is also important to clean your body thoroughly - in order to avoid fungal infections. If these fungal infections occur, one of the best Complementary Medical anti-fungals to use to get rid of them is Tea-tree essential oil. This is one of the few essential oils that you can apply directly to your skin.

Tea-tree also has anti-viral and anti-bacterial properties and the good news is that bacteria are not resistant to Tea-tree oil in the way that some bacteria such as MRSA and clostridium are resistant to antibiotic drugs. Increasingly, viruses too are mutating in ways that render them immune to anti-viral medication and again, Tea-tree does not seem to have this problem.

Make sure your body is clean. In the absence of a water supply you will need to use the kind of wipes sold to campers – and baby wipes work well too. Make it a rule never to go to sleep dirty. Sticking to rules like this are, as we have seen, important morale boosters – they make you feel more "in control" of the situation.

It is possible to rig up a "field shower" if you have the facilities. Fill a strong, heavy-duty, 3-6 gallon black bag with water and hang it in the sun for a few hours. It will heat up well and should provide water for two to three people to shower under. (In the "Shelter" section we have described how to heat water in a dark container such as a large black bucket.) The reason that a black bag is recommended is that the black colour will absorb the sun's rays better than any other colour and will therefore heat up the water inside it.

Tooth-brushing is also an absolute necessity for cleanliness and to avoid tooth problems while disruption caused by a pandemic situation exists. It is also a major morale booster – again it is about feeling that you are in control and making "good" and "self-supportive" decisions to care for yourself.

Shaving is also very important – not just to look nice, but more importantly, to feel good. In the absence of large supplies of water, shaving oils work really well and are very good for your skin.

One absolutely vital but often overlooked aspect of cleanliness is the morale-boosting effect of simple tasks, such as tooth brushing, shaving, washing etc. In fact, one of the common themes in all the reports from people faced with on-going, enormously stressful situations (i.e. holocaust, kidnapping, etc.), is that a high level of morale is essential for survival. According to American journalist, Steve Lipman, who researched the use of humour during the Holocaust;

> *"Wit produced on the precipice of hell was not frivolity but psychological necessity. Humor is one of the greatest gifts God gave mankind to pull itself out of despair."*

MORE ABOUT THE PSYCHOLOGICAL BENEFITS OF CLEANLINESS

The elite military force – the British SAS, are taught that tooth-brushing is an essential survival aid. One feels so much better with a clean mouth, coupled with the fact that you are actively making a decision to "look after yourself". As discussed, this decision making process, however small, puts you "back in control" of your situation.

One of the biggest sources of fear in any situation is that of the "unknown". By feeling "in control" and going through particular decision-making processes, people are less prone to fear and can make much better decisions – you can read more about this in the "Psychology of Survival" section of this book.

The best of all the morale boosting, cleanliness options is, of course, a hot bath but this would probably be virtually impossible to achieve in a serious pandemic situation, if society is severely disrupted. Nevertheless, as we've said, it is essential to keep clean – as much as possible – for both health and morale boosting purposes.

And never underestimate the power of luxuries such as cosmetics, perfumes and the like.

There were many reports from the Balkan War about how the various contents of the Red Cross packages were received. Obviously, people were grateful for much needed necessities such as food, blankets and so on – all the essentials. However, one of the items that made the biggest impact was lipstick. The women were happy to have this non-essential, luxury item – perhaps a symbol of a return to normality – and as a result general morale in society was increased exponentially.

OTHER GREAT HABITS TO GET INTO – NOSE BLOWING
As well as taking hand-washing and overall cleanliness more seriously, there are a number of other good habits you need to get into, to help you stay healthy. One of these is - nose blowing.

Instead of sniffing, it is essential to blow your nose.

Sniffing forcibly drives pathogens up high into your nasal passages and bypasses many of your nose's natural defence mechanisms. Instead, blow your nose and use an anti-viral tissue.

Paper products' manufacturers have really come up trumps in this area and have already produced some excellent anti-viral products. As sniffing is an ingrained tendency for most people, the sooner you start to break this habit and start blowing your nose – the better.

Remember to dispose of your tissue immediately and safely – it's contaminated with millions of potential pathogens. It's not good practice to leave used tissues in your rubbish bin at work, or in other public locations. Put used tissues into a plastic bag – a re-sealable sandwich bag will do, you can dispose of this carefully when convenient and you know that you are not going to expose others to your viruses or bacteria.

Don't use a handkerchief as this can harbour billions of bacteria/viruses and other pathogens. Remember – to avoid spreading disease, coughs and sneezes must be covered by an anti-viral tissue. If you do not have a tissue available, sneezing and coughing into your hands is a good way of preventing the spread of viruses but this is only useful if you can clean your hands properly – immediately. Always carry an anti-viral hand sanitizer with you and wash your hands properly at the earliest opportunity.

DO NOT STIFLE SNEEZES – SOME PEOPLE DO THIS AS THEY CONSIDER IT "POLITE".

Sneezing is your body's way of getting pathogens out of your body. By stifling a sneeze you are not allowing your body to do what it needs to do to protect you. But do sneeze into a paper towel/ tissue and dispose of it properly straight away.

Preparedness: Cleanliness & Sanitation

SEWAGE

In extreme emergencies, sewage systems may not be functioning. During these times it may be necessary to create a temporary, emergency toilet for safely collecting and handling human waste until normal sewage systems can be restored.

How to make a temporary toilet:

1. Line the inside of a toilet bowl, 5 gallon bucket, or another appropriately sized waste container with two heavy-duty plastic rubbish bags.

2. Place cat litter, fireplace ashes, or sawdust into the bottom of the bags.

3. At the end of each day, the bagged waste should be securely tied and removed to a protected location such as a garage, basement, outbuilding, and so on, until a safe disposal option is available.

4. You may be able to dispose of the waste in a properly functioning public sewer, or septic system, or you could bury the waste on your own property. Human and animal waste matter is a potential source of disease – take great care to observe the following:

• Locate the toilet away from food preparation or eating areas.

• Locate latrines and portable toilets at least 100 feet away from surface water bodies such as lakes, rivers, streams, and at least 100 feet downhill or away from any drinking water source (well or spring), home, or campsite in case of leaks which could contaminate water supplies.

• Ideally, provide a place next to the emergency toilet to wash hands that offers soap, running water, and paper towels. In the absence of this it is essential to provide effective hand sanitisers. Always clean your hands after using the toilet.

• Keep doors and covers closed (if you have them) when the toilet is not in use to keep out insects and animals, to prevent injury.

• Always supervise small children when they are using the emergency toilet.

REFERENCES

1. http://www.healthdirect.co.uk/2008/06/superbugs-mrsa-and-clostridium.html
2. Public perceptions, anxiety, and behaviour change in relation to the swine flu outbreak: cross sectional telephone survey: BMJ. 2009;339:b2651: Authors: Rubin GJ, Amlôt R, Page L, Wessely S: PMID: 19574308

CHAPTER 17

PREPAREDNESS

WHAT TO DO IF THIS PHASE 6 PANDEMIC BECOMES MORE SERIOUS: SURVIVING A PANDEMIC

7. FOOD STORAGE AND STOCKPILING

Just in case food and other essentials should be in short supply during a severe pandemic outbreak it will be essential for you to have a good store of essential items. You can always use these supplies for other types of emergency too – apart from a potential pandemic, so they are a good investment and a sensible safety precaution.

SUGGESTIONS FOR ITEMS TO STOCKPILE

Ready-to-eat foods are excellent as there may not be power available for cooking. These include: canned meats, canned fish, canned fruits, canned vegetables, and canned soups. Note that canned vegetables and fruits are also a valuable source of fluids.

It is also essential to make sure that any canned foods you use are low in salt, or salt free This will help you avoid getting dehydrated from the high level of salts that these items usually contain. Canned fruits should be in water, or natural juice, as high levels of sugar impair immune response and make people more susceptible to illness - for more on this see our section on Nutrition and Supplements. Canned foods can be heated up over a gas camping stove if you have one and it is impossible to overestimate the morale-boosting effects of hot food.

YOUR STOCKPILE LIST

• Protein and fruit bars – compact and easy to store, these are highly recommended.

• Dry cereal or muesli/granola – a good source of much needed fibre.

• Peanut butter or nuts – make sure that these are kept cool and don't buy large packages, unless you can use them quickly, to avoid spoiling.

• Dried fruit.

• Canned Fruit

• Canned Vegetables

• Canned Soup

• Canned Meat

• Canned Fish

• Crackers/biscuits/cookies – view these as "occasional treats" as they are often high in sugar content and as mentioned previously, this can impair your immune response.

• Canned/ Boxed Long Life juices – the lower the sugar content the better.

• Bottled water – (see chapter on Water for how to store water safely).

• Canned or jarred baby food and formula, should this be necessary.

• Seeds for fast growing herbs, cress and other seeds, such as beans and peas that can be "sprouted". These are a rich source of vitamins and protein. You may also wish to buy a "Sprouter" from your local health-food store. This will help you to grow a variety of sprouts easily. Sprouters are cheap and are properly "set up" so that the water that you need to use to grow the sprouts drains correctly and minimises the risk of your sprouts going mouldy.

• Pet food – if planning to use dried food, ensure that you have enough clean water for your pet as too much dried food, without water to accompany it, will quickly dehydrate your pet and this could lead to serious problems.

• Prescribed medical supplies such as glucose and blood-pressure monitoring equipment, insulin, etc. Plan in advance how you will keep insulin cool.

• Soap and low-or non-alcohol-based hand sanitiser.

• Water-free body wipes as sold for campers, or baby wipes.

• Toothbrush and toothpaste.

• Luxury items such as lipstick and other cosmetics, razor blades etc. Great as barter items but essential for morale. Shaving oil – good for skin and useful if low on water supplies.

• Fuel: wood for fires, or other combustible material; Calor gas (with a stove); Propane heaters etc.

• Lighters, fuel, matches, candles.

• Complementary and Conventional Medical treatment/medicines.

• Anti-diarrhoeal remedies. (See our chapter on Hydration for Complementary Medical advice on treating diarrhoea).

- Thermometer
- Oral Rehydration Solution ingredients as outlined in our section on Hydration (Seas Salt, baking powder, sugar and orange juice if you can store it – or buy long life juice). These are also known as Electrolyte Preparations. (See chapter on Hydration).
- Vitamins/supplements. (See chapter on Nutrition).
- Household cleaners & cloths/wipes etc.
- Bleach – cheapest household bleach that you can get without any additives. Can be used to clean and also for water purification.
- Radio/Torch/Flashlight – consider buying a wind-up torch. There are also wind-up torch radios available which are inexpensive and they are energy efficient too, with about 90 turns (approx 1.5 minutes) of the crank equalling about 20 minutes of airplay. It is also possible to get hold of solar-powered/wind-up radios, again these are very reasonably priced. These are an essential morale booster and vital to keep abreast of pandemic developments. (A wind-up i-Pod is now available).
- Batteries – check which sizes you need for all important battery powered objects. Having access to music, radio, games and so on is vital for morale and as you know, good morale boosts your chances of survival.
- 2x manual can openers.
- Super strong black rubbish bags – invaluable items. There are so many uses for these.
- Tissues, toilet paper, disposable nappies/diapers, feminine hygiene products.
- Entertainment items such as books, jigsaws, games, packs of cards, sewing/knitting equipment (of practical value too!). Entertainment and practical project items are great morale boosters.
- Kids toys that do not run on batteries, books, dolls, teddys, etc.
- Spectacles – distance and near vision, as required.
- Antibiotic ointment – essential for cuts and grazes.
- A homeopathic remedy called "Hypercal" – it is extremely useful for cuts and grazes.
- Plasters/Band-Aids/bandages/slings.
- Safety pins of various sizes, needles, thread, pins.
- Scissors.
- Paper, pens, paperclips, staples, pencils.
- Sharp knives.
- Contraceptives (condoms etc. If on the pill, make sure you have enough supplies to last at least three months.)
- Consider your need to travel. If this will be essential for you then get a bicycle that is in good working order. Make sure that you also have a bicycle repair kit too. If you use your bicycle for fetching and carrying objects make sure that you have panniers on the bike that are up to the task. A bicycle would be a valuable item in a serious pandemic crisis and could render you vulnerable to attack, so use your bike as inconspicuously as possible – possibly at night, unless

curfews have been imposed. If no street lights are working you need to make sure that you can cycle safely – falling off your bike and injuring yourself would cause much more of a problem in a serious pandemic than at other times as you would not be able to just go to the hospital and get stitches for a cut for example. You'll also need a locking device to chain it up.

• Barter items – if the disruptions caused by a pandemic last for a while you may need to trade with other people. Remember though that you must be very careful about whom you trade with and also not let anyone outside your Survival Unit know about your stockpiles, as this could compromise your safety and survival chances.

• Protection Items – a hard decision for anyone. In the UK it is illegal for anyone to own a gun unless specifically licensed to do so following various police checks etc. In the USA, gun laws are much more relaxed. Given that a great deal of civil unrest is predicted by our Governments, if the situation worsens, it makes sense to protect yourself, your family and your supplies. How you go about this is a very personal decision and there is plenty of excellent information about this available on the internet and it is beyond the scope of this book to go into this issue in any detail.

One point that we found during our extensive research though, is that one of the best forms of defence is to not get into trouble in the first place and this means that you need to lie low and be as inconspicuous as possible. Don't invite trouble and work out how you and your Survival Unit will move around outside the home and not attract attention, if you do have to go out.

Many of the stockpiling lists found on the internet and in well-meaning books advise people to stock up on baking goods such as flour, cake mixes and so on. This seems to us to be somewhat superfluous, as, in a serious pandemic, it is likely that there will be interruptions to power sources, and this would make baking impossible. Also, we are concerned that bulky items like flour will take up valuable storage space, which would be better utilised for other, easier to prepare, items.

FOOD FOR FREE

Nothing can beat fresh food and it is highly likely that supply chains to grocery stores will be severely compromised, or may not exist at all for a while, should a severe pandemic hit. As well as tasting great, fresh food contains many nutrients that are essential to health. Take time now to do some research as to the types of foods that are available to you in your immediate surroundings. Be aware of what is available season by season, for example, it is no good hoping to forage apples and blackberries in Spring.

Finding food for free is somewhat more difficult for city dwellers, but edible stuff does exist virtually everywhere. (Sometimes though, you may have to broaden your gastronomic horizons somewhat.) Consider buying seeds for cress and fast growing herbs. These will fulfil your desire for something fresh and also are an extremely valuable source of vitamins, anti-oxidants and bioflavaniods.

A full breakdown of freely available food from nature is beyond the scope of this book as we would have to itemise what is available region by region and country by country. (That is a whole book by itself!)

Do take the time now to look at some of the excellent wilderness survival websites available. Consider buying the fabulous books by Ray Mears, the Extreme Survival expert. Another great book for all survival matters is the SAS Survival Manual. You'll be amazed at some of the things that we normally wouldn't consider eating, that are actually delicious, highly nutritious and possibly life-saving.

WHAT TO AVOID

Generally, even survival experts advise against eating wild mushrooms unless you really know what you are doing and even "mushroom experts" have been caught out in the past. Also, avoid anything that animals won't eat. This is not a definitive guide though, as there are certain things that animals can eat that humans can't. For example, cows can eat grass but humans lack the ability to digest it and it would make us very ill. (For example, cats eat grass too, but it's in an effort to make themselves vomit – it's a form of self medication and useful for self-treatment of fur-balls).

The general rule when attempting to eat any unfamiliar plant is DON'T!

In a survival situation it is just too risky and there is plenty of scope for finding things that you know to be safe.

Also, another consideration is the type of wood you should use for cooking upon. For example, although not a potential issue in the upper Northern Hemisphere, the wood from the beautiful, fragrant, oleander bush is highly toxic and will render any food cooked on it poisonous, due to the toxic smoke it emits. (Similarly, it would be a great mistake to use this wood for a fire to keep warm, as breathing the smoke could kill you). Of course it is not just oleander that causes problems and it is wise to learn as much as possible about trees and plants in your general vicinity if you plan to use these in any way.

CHAPTER 18

PREPAREDNESS

WHAT TO DO IF THIS PHASE 6 PANDEMIC BECOMES MORE SERIOUS: SURVIVING A PANDEMIC

8. EXERCISE AND YOUR IMMUNE SYSTEM – LESS IS MORE?

Exercise stresses your body. Moderate exercise provides you with physical challenges that help your body to become fitter and this has an overall benefit upon your immune system. However, over-exercise produces too much stress and this can adversely affect your immune system.

In fact stress – in any form – as we have seen, can do all sorts of deleterious things to your immune system and will render you much more susceptible to colds and flu. Aside from too much exercise, overstretching ourselves, mentally or emotionally too, can cause the release of the stress hormones cortisol and adrenaline and these impair your immunity.

MODERATION IS THE KEY

For anyone in a stressful situation ranging from caregivers to top athletes, moderation in stress levels is the key to good immune health. For people in any stressful situation – and let's face it, in today's world that accounts for most of us – there is clearly a physical benefit to moderate, regular exercise.

Moderate exercisers' immune systems get a temporary boost in the production of macrophages

– the cells that attack and eat up bacteria, viruses and other foreign bodies. Research has found that regular, consistent moderate exercise can lead to substantial benefits in immune system health over the long-term. This means fewer colds, flu and other illnesses that scientists believe are connected to poor immune health, like some cancers, heart disease and diabetes.

During intense physical exertion, your body increases production of cortisol and adrenaline and these both temporarily lower immunity. As well as suppressing your immune system, these stress hormones raise your blood pressure and cholesterol levels and this effect has been linked to increased susceptibility to infection.

This susceptibility is particularly marked in people such as endurance athletes, in whom stress hormone levels are particularly high after extreme exercise such as marathon running or triathlon training. Their immune systems are suppressed as a result and this is why we often hear that endurance athletes so often get colds, flu and other viral infections.

WHAT AMOUNT OF EXERCISE IS BEST?

Current Government guidelines suggest that a healthy level of exercise for most people is about three times a week – on non-consecutive days – in order to give yourself time to recover. These exercise periods should last for about half an hour and you should be able to get yourself "moderately out of breath". This will have the effect of increasing your resistance to illness. However, if you are an endurance athlete and are training for ultra-endurance events, an important element of your training should be including enough rest and recovery days to allow your immunity to recover.

If you are feeling run-down or have other symptoms of over-training syndrome, you should consider toning down your training. Over-training symptoms include:
• Increased resting heart rate
• Slower recovery heart rate
• Irritability
• General heaviness and fatigue

LESS REALLY IS MORE

But, if you are ill, you should be careful about exercising too intensely. Your immune system is already taxed by fighting your infection and additional stress could undermine your recovery. Constantly over-stressing the immune system is extremely unhealthy and has been linked to long-term diseases like Chronic Fatigue Syndrome. The only time that exercise may be of benefit in aiding recovery from a viral illness is if you have a light cold – and that you are certain of this! If you have only very mild symptoms and absolutely no fever, then gentle – not intense – exercise may help to boost your macrophage production, which can speed up your recovery. Intense exercise is generally guaranteed to make you feel worse and could extend the period of time that you are ill for.

WITH SPECIFIC REFERENCE TO SWINE FLU AND BIRD FLU

The suppression of your immune system that excessive exercise can cause may render you vastly more susceptible to viral infection and this is a real cause for concern – should a very serious flu pandemic occur.

WHAT SHOULD YOUR TARGET HEART RATE BE AFTER EXERCISE?

THE AMERICAN HEART ASSOCIATION RECOMMENDS YOU TARGET THE FOLLOWING HEART RATES – DEPENDING UPON YOUR AGE – DURING EXERCISE:

Age	Target Heart Rate Zone 50–85 % Average	Maximum Heart Rate 100 %
20 years	100–170 beats per minute	200 beats per minute
25 years	98–166 beats per minute	195 beats per minute
30 years	95–162 beats per minute	190 beats per minute
35 years	93–157 beats per minute	185 beats per minute
40 years	90–153 beats per minute	180 beats per minute
45 years	88–149 beats per minute	175 beats per minute
50 years	85–145 beats per minute	170 beats per minute
55 years	83–140 beats per minute	165 beats per minute
60 years	80–136 beats per minute	160 beats per minute
65 years	78–132 beats per minute	155 beats per minute
70 years	75–128 beats per minute	150 beats per minute

Your maximum heart rate is about 220 minus your age. The figures above are averages, so use them as general guidelines.

http://www.americanheart.org/presenter.jhtml?identifier=4736

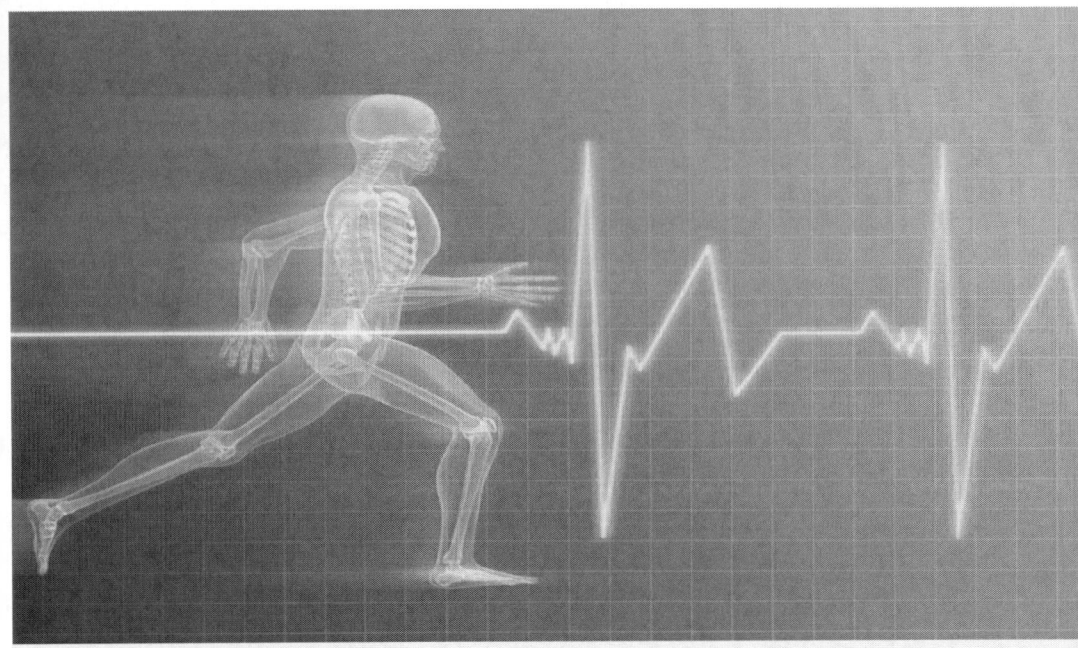

NEW BRITISH RESEARCH SHEDS LIGHT ON THE BENEFITS OF BRIEF INTENSIVE EXERCISE: WHAT HAPPENS IF YOU DON'T HAVE TIME TO DO THE RECOMMENDED 30 MINUTES THREE TIMES EACH WEEK?

New research suggests there may be an option: The health benefits of short, intense physical activity for reducing the risks of diabetes in later life have been studied at Heriot-Watt University. James Timmons, professor of exercise biology has studied the effects of quick exercise. In his study, published in the journal BMC Endocrine Disorders 16 men were put through a short, intense period of exercise three times a week for two weeks. All they did was a 30 second 'flat-out' sprint four times at each exercise period – with a few minutes rest in between.

At the end of the two week period he found a 23% improvement in insulin function. His study looks at the way our bodies break down the glycogen that it stores. Glycogen is stored in muscles - which is where it should be - but when it gets free into our blood system it can cause damage.

Timmons said that we should think about diabetes as being "glucose circulating in the blood rather than stored in the muscles where it should be".

Normal exercise allows our bodies to oxidise glycogen, but it doesn't deplete the stores of glycogen in our muscles. When we deplete these stores our muscles have to take the glycogen they need from our blood.

"The only way to get to this glycogen is through very intense contractions of the muscles. If we can get people in their 20s, 30s and 40s doing these exercises twice a week then it could have a very dramatic effect on the future prevalence of [type 2 - Ed.] diabetes."

So it is possible to gain significant health benefits without having to do the 30 minutes a day that is currently recommended.

"Only 7.5 minutes of exercise each week -- if that is all that you find the time to do," is all you need, says. Timmons.

SOURCES AND FURTHER READING:

http://news.bbc.co.uk/1/hi/scotland/edinburgh_and_east/7852987.stm

http://www.biomedcentral.com/1472-6823/9/3/abstract

COMPLEMENTARY MEDICAL APPROACHES TO PREVENTING AND TREATING SWINE FLU

CHAPTER 19

USING ESSENTIAL OILS TO MAKE YOUR ENVIRONMENT AS "VIRUS PROOF" AS POSSIBLE

As you know the Swine Flu virus, like all flu viruses, will be spread in many ways and, as it is often airborne, can infect people simply by being breathed in. It also lurks on surfaces that may be touched and then transferred to the eyes, nose or mouth (and even to ears, as proposed by some scientists), where it may gain entry to the body. With this in mind it is helpful to sanitise your direct environment in order to render it as virally "unfriendly" as possible. In the field of Complementary Medicine there are some amazingly powerful essential oils that are anti-bacterial, anti-viral and anti-fungal.

WHAT IS AN ESSENTIAL OIL?

An essential oil is a concentrated, hydrophobic (water-repelling) liquid, containing volatile aromatic compounds which are extracted from a wide variety of plants.

In fact, essential oils are not really oils at all but are highly concentrated, "essences" of plants. This aromatic essence can be produced by distillation, expression, or solvent extraction. Essential oils are used in perfumery, aromatherapy, cosmetics, incense, medicine, household cleaning products and for flavouring food and drink. Useful anti-viral and anti-bacterial

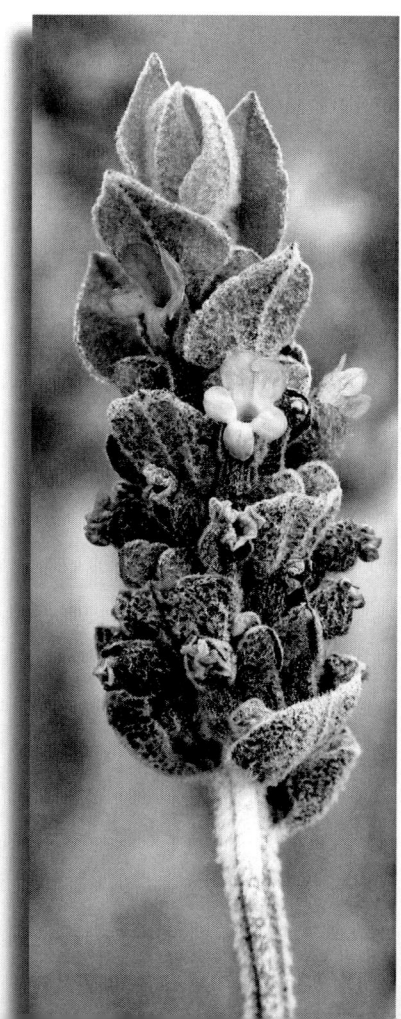

essential oils are commonly available and include oils such as Cloves, Tea-tree and Lavender etc.

HISTORICAL USE OF ESSENTIAL OILS

As discussed in an eariler Chapter, The Bubonic Plague (caused by the Yersinia pestis bacillus) decimated the European population in the Middle Ages and it is estimated to have killed over 30% of the population (see History of Pandemics). However, in the affected areas, it was noted that the people who worked in Lavender distilleries, and in jobs that incorporated the use of Lavender, rarely became ill.

As a consequence, recipes for preventing plague by using various essential oils became popular during this time. People carried bundles of dried herbs that were suffused with essential oils to ward off the plague.

There has been a steady accumulation of evidence – both anecdotal and research based – in recent years that supports the positive benefits of essential oils. Many oils are now accepted to have anti-viral and anti-bacterial properties.

France has long been a world leader in the practice of, and research into, essential oils in general, and the anti-infectious use of essential oils in particular. In studies of essential oils, specific components have been isolated and found to have anti-viral properties. These include anethole, carvone, beta-caryophyllene, citral, eugenol, limonene, linalool, and linalyl acetate.

"HOW CAN ESSENTIAL OILS HELP 'VIRUS-PROOF' MY ENVIRONMENT?"

Because of the increasing amount of research into essentials oils, scientists have discovered that different plant families and the essential oils extracted from them, exhibit varying degrees of anti-viral effectiveness [1,2,3,4,5,6,7,8,9,10,11,12,13,14], depending on the virus strain. This seems to be primarily due to the particular molecular structures found in each type of oil.

Researchers think that the different types of oils penetrate different viruses in different ways and to varying degrees. So, the effect on each virus strain depends also on the virus structure (enveloped, non-enveloped, molecular symmetry, etc.) Scientists propose that, one of the reasons for essential oils' anti-viral effectiveness, is their lipophyllic character (they are "attracted" to oils and fats).

Essential oils are easily absorbed into your body's tissues, where they can produce excellent results. Interestingly, when studying the anti-viral effects of essential oils, scientists have found that normal cells seemed to acquire a special resistance to viral penetration when treated with anti-viral essential oils, although the exact reason for this effect is not yet known.

"HOW DO ESSENTIAL OILS PROTECT US FROM VIRUSES?"

There are several reasons why essentials oils have a marked anti-viral effect. Scientists have proposed that some essential oils obstruct surface glycoproteins in the viral envelope, thus preventing attachment of the virus to host cells. Other essential oils seem to assail viruses in the host cells, possibly at the level of the cell membrane [15].

Some essential oils are also known for their ability to modify your immune response and may offer some indirect protection against viral infection in this way.

At the time of writing this book, there are no studies which have examined the effectiveness of essential oils against the Swine Flu virus, specifically. However, since essential oils have been shown to have effects against a very wide range of other similar viruses, the use of some of these oils is strongly recommended.

HOW TO USE ESSENTIAL OILS TO COMBAT ENVIRONMENTAL VIRAL HAZARDS

Essential oils can be dispersed with an atomizer (one to five drops essential oil for every 3 tablespoons of distilled water). For a very basic anti-microbial spray, mix a few drops of the essential oils of Lavender and Tea-tree with distilled water in a plant sprayer and spray liberally around your rooms.

Spritz the air regularly. Do feel free to add other oils as desired, as various oils do have differing anti-microbial effects – so there is a good rationale for using a mixture of any of the following essential oils: Clove [16,17,18,19,20,21,22], Cinnamon [23,24,25,26,27,28,29,30,31], Thyme [32,33,34,35,36,37,16,38], Oregano [39,40,41,42,43,44,45], Lavender [46,47,48,49,50,51], Sweet Marjoram [52,53,54,55,56], Peppermint [57,58,59,60,61,62,63,64,65,66], Tea-tree [67,68,69,70,71,72,73,74,75,76,77,78,79,80].

Of particular relevance to Swine Flu is one research study that has found that the essential oils mentioned above have specific properties which protect our respiratory tract from pathogens.

You can also evaporate essential oils into your environment using an "Oil Burner". This does not in fact, actually burn the oil. Rather, a candle is placed under a small water-filled reservoir to which the essential oils have been added. As the flame heats up the water, the oils evaporate into the atmosphere.

Viral spread in the work place is a real concern – so it is essential to make sure that surfaces such as desks, keyboards and door handles are wiped over regularly with a Lavender-Tea-tree solution and it is vital to remember to disinfect telephone handsets and mouthpieces.
Make your own essential oil inhaler by dropping your favoured anti-microbial essential oils onto cotton wool and enclosing these in a plastic bag – so as to slow down the evaporation of

Essential Oils

the oils. Sniff this as desired.

Note that for regular inhalation, Lavender and Tea-tree are both safe. Some essential oils must be used with caution and it is wise to check on The Complementary Medical Association's website The-CMA.Org.UK if you need more information about a particular essential oil.

REFERENCES

1 Reichling J, Koch C, Stahl-Biskup E, Sojka C, Schnitzler P. Virucidal activity of a beta-triketone-rich essential oil of Leptospermum scoparium (manuka oil) against HSV-1 and HSV-2 in cell culture. Planta Med. 2005 Dec;71(12):1123-7.
2 Duschatzky CB, Possetto ML, Talarico LB, Garcia CC, Michis F, Almeida NV, de Lampasona MP, Schuff C, Damonte EB. Evaluation of chemical and anti-viral properties of essential oils from South American plants. Antivir Chem Chemother. 2005;16(4):247-51.
3 Allahverdiyev A, Duran N, Ozguven M, Koltas S. Antiviral activity of the volatile oils of Melissa officinalis L. against Herpes simplex virus type-2. Phytomedicine. 2004 Nov;11(7-8):657-61.
4 Sinico C, De Logu A, Lai F, Valenti D, Manconi M, Loy G, Bonsignore L, Fadda AM. Liposomal incorporation of Artemisia arborescens L. essential oil and in vitro antiviral activity. Eur J Pharm Biopharm. 2005 Jan;59(1):161-8.
5 Vijayan P, Raghu C, Ashok G, Dhanaraj SA, Suresh B. Antiviral activity of medicinal plants of Nilgiris. Indian J Med Res. 2004 Jul;120(1):24-9.
6 Sokmen M, Serkedjieva J, Daferera D, Gulluce M, Polissiou M, Tepe B, Akpulat HA, Sahin F, Sokmen A. In vitro antioxidant, antimicrobial, and antiviral activities of the essential oil and various extracts from herbal parts and callus cultures of Origanum acutidens. J Agric Food Chem. 2004 Jun 2;52(11):3309-12.
7 Garcia CC, Talarico L, Almeida N, Colombres S, Duschatzky C, Damonte EB. Virucidal activity of essential oils from aromatic plants of San Luis, Argentina. Phytother Res. 2003 Nov;17(9):1073-5.
8 Minami M, Kita M, Nakaya T, Yamamoto T, Kuriyama H, Imanishi J. The inhibitory effect of essential oils on herpes simplex virus type-1 replication in vitro. Microbiol Immunol. 2003;47(9):681-4.
9 Schuhmacher A, Reichling J, Schnitzler P. Virucidal effect of peppermint oil on the enveloped viruses herpes simplex virus type 1 and type 2 in vitro. Phytomedicine. 2003;10(6-7):504-10.
10 Zhang B, Chen J, Li H, Xu X. [Study on the Rheum palmatum volatile oil against HBV in cell culture in vitro] Zhong Yao Cai. 1998 Oct;21(10):524-6. Chinese.
11 Primo V, Rovera M, Zanon S, Oliva M, Demo M, Daghero J, Sabini L. [Determination of the antibacterial and antiviral activity of the essential oil from Minthostachys verticillata (Griseb.) Epling] Rev Argent Microbiol. 2001 Apr-Jun;33(2):113-7. Spanish.
12 Schnitzler P, Schon K, Reichling J. Antiviral activity of Australian tea tree oil and eucalyptus oil against herpes simplex virus in cell culture. Pharmazie. 2001 Apr;56(4):343-7.
13 De Logu A, Loy G, Pellerano ML, Bonsignore L, Schivo ML. Inactivation of HSV-1 and HSV-2 and prevention of cell-to-cell virus spread by Santolina insularis essential oil. Antiviral Res. 2000 Dec;48(3):177-85.
14 Benencia F, Courreges MC. Antiviral activity of sandalwood oil against herpes simplex viruses-1 and -2. Phytomedicine. 1999 May;6(2):119-23.
15 J Appl Microbiol. 2000 Jan;88(1):170-5. The mode of antimicrobial action of the essential oil of Melaleuca alternifolia (tea tree oil). Cox SD, Mann CM, Markham JL, Bell HC, Gustafson JE, Warmington JR, Wyllie SG. Centre for Biostructural and Biomolecular Research, University of Western Sydney, Hawkesbury, New South Wales, Western Australia. s.cox@uws.edu.au
16 Phytother Res. 2000 Nov;14(7):510-6. Inhibitory effects of sudanese medicinal plant extracts on hepatitis C virus (HCV) protease.Hussein G, Miyashiro H, Nakamura N, Hattori M, Kakiuchi N, Shimotohno K. Institute of Natural Medicine, Toyama Medical and Pharmaceutical University, 2630 Sugitani, Toyama 930-0194, Japan.
17 J Appl Microbiol. 2000 Feb;88(2):308-16. Antimicrobial agents from plants: antibacterial activity of plant volatile oils. Dorman HJ, Deans SG. Aromatic and Medicinal Plant Group, Scottish Agricultural College, Auchincruive, South Ayrshire, UK.
18 Kurokawa M, Hozumi T, Basnet P, Nakano M, Kadota S, Namba T, Kawana T, Shiraki K. Purification and characterization of eugeniin as an anti-herpesvirus compound from Geum japonicum and Syzygium aromaticum. J Pharmacol Exp Ther. 1998 Feb;284(2):728-35.
19 Shiraki K, Yukawa T, Kurokawa M, Kageyama S. [Cytomegalovirus infection and its possible treatment with herbal medicines] Nippon Rinsho. 1998 Jan;56(1):156-60. Review. Japanese.
20 Cai L, Wu CD. Compounds from Syzygium aromaticum possessing growth inhibitory activity against oral pathogens. J Nat Prod. 1996 Oct;59(10):987-90.
21 Yukawa TA, Kurokawa M, Sato H, Yoshida Y, Kageyama S, Hasegawa T, Namba T, Imakita M, Hozumi T, Shiraki K. Prophylactic treatment of cytomegalovirus infection with traditional herbs. Antiviral Res. 1996 Oct;32(2):63-70.
22 Kurokawa M, Nagasaka K, Hirabayashi T, Uyama S, Sato H, Kageyama T, Kadota S, Ohyama H, Hozumi T, Namba T, et al. Efficacy of traditional herbal medicines in combination with acyclovir against herpes simplex virus type 1 infection in vitro and in vivo. Antiviral Res. 1995 May;27(1-2):19-37.
23 O'Mahony R, Al-Khteeri H, Weerasekera D, Fernando N, Vaira D, Holton J, Basset C. Bactericidal and anti-adhesive properties of culinary and medicinal plants against Helicobacter pylori. World J Gastroenterol. 2005 Dec 21;11(47):7499-507.
24 Matan N, Rimkeeree H, Mawson AJ, Chompreeda P, Haruthaithanasan V, Parker M. Antimicrobial activity of cinnamon and clove oils under modified atmosphere conditions. Int J Food Microbiol. 2006 Mar 15;107(2):180-5. Epub 2005 Nov 2.
25 Yang YC, Lee HS, Lee SH, Clark JM, Ahn YJ. Ovicidal and adulticidal activities of Cinnamomum zeylanicum bark essential oil compounds and related compounds against Pediculus humanus capitis (Anoplura: Pediculicidae). Int J Parasitol. 2005 Dec;35(14):1595-600. Epub 2005 Sep 15.
26 Cheng SS, Liu JY, Hsui YR, Chang ST. Chemical polymorphism and antifungal activity of essential oils from leaves of different provenances of indigenous cinnamon (Cinnamomum osmophloeum). Bioresour Technol. 2006 Jan;97(2):306-12. Epub 2005 Apr 13.
27 Lopez P, Sanchez C, Batlle R, Nerin C. Solid- and vapor-phase antimicrobial activities of six essential oils: susceptibility of selected

foodborne bacterial and fungal strains. J Agric Food Chem. 2005 Aug 24;53(17):6939-46.
28 Friedman M, Henika PR, Levin CE, Mandrell RE. Antibacterial activities of plant essential oils and their components against Escherichia coli O157:H7 and Salmonella enterica in apple juice. J Agric Food Chem. 2004 Sep 22;52(19):6042-8.
29 Friedman M, Buick R, Elliott CT. Antibacterial activities of naturally occurring compounds against antibiotic-resistant Bacillus cereus vegetative cells and spores, Escherichia coli, and Staphylococcus aureus. J Food Prot. 2004 Aug;67(8):1774-8.
30 Kalemba D, Kunicka A. Antibacterial and antifungal properties of essential oils. Curr Med Chem. 2003 May;10(10):813-29. Review.
31 Fabio A, Corona A, Forte E, Quaglio P. Inhibitory activity of spices and essential oils on psychrotrophic bacteria. New Microbiol. 2003 Jan;26(1):115-20.
32 Rasooli I, Rezaei MB, Allameh A. Ultrastructural studies on antimicrobial efficacy of thyme essential oils on Listeria monocytogenes. Int J Infect Dis. 2006 May;10(3):236-41. Epub 2006 Jan 10.
33 Lai PK, Roy J. Antimicrobial and chemopreventive properties of herbs and spices. Curr Med Chem. 2004 Jun;11(11):1451-60. Review.
34 Bagamboula CF, Uyttendaele M, Debevere J. Antimicrobial effect of spices and herbs on Shigella sonnei and Shigella flexneri. J Food Prot. 2003 Apr;66(4):668-73.
35 Kalemba D, Kunicka A. Antibacterial and antifungal properties of essential oils. Curr Med Chem. 2003 May;10(10):813-29. Review.
36 Dorman HJ, Deans SG. Antimicrobial agents from plants: antibacterial activity of plant volatile oils. J Appl Microbiol. 2000 Feb;88(2):308-16.
37 Cosentino S, Tuberoso CI, Pisano B, Satta M, Mascia V, Arzedi E, Palmas F. In-vitro antimicrobial activity and chemical composition of Sardinian Thymus essential oils. Lett Appl Microbiol. 1999 Aug;29(2):130-5.
38 Smith-Palmer A, Stewart J, Fyfe L. Antimicrobial properties of plant essential oils and essences against five important food-borne pathogens. Lett Appl Microbiol. 1998 Feb;26(2):118-22.
39 J Agric Food Chem. 2004 Jun 2;52(11):3309-12. In vitro antioxidant, antimicrobial, and antiviral activities of the essential oil and various extracts from herbal parts and callus cultures of Origanum acutidens. Sokmen M, Serkedjieva J, Daferera D, Gulluce M, Polissiou M, Tepe B, Akpulat HA, Sahin F, Sokmen A.
40 Mol Cell Biochem. 2005 Apr;272(1-2):29-34. Minimum inhibitory concentrations of herbal essential oils and monolaurin for gram-positive and gram-negative bacteria. Preuss HG, Echard B, Enig M, Brook I, Elliott TB. Department of Physiology and Biophysics, Georgetown University Medical Center, Washington, DC 20057, USA. preusshg@georgetown.edu
41 Bozin B, Mimica-Dukic N, Simin N, Anackov G. Characterization of the volatile composition of essential oils of some lamiaceae spices and the antimicrobial and antioxidant activities of the entire oils. J Agric Food Chem. 2006 Mar 8;54(5):1822-8.
42 Chami F, Chami N, Bennis S, Bouchikhi T, Remmal A. Oregano and clove essential oils induce surface alteration of Saccharomyces cerevisiae. Phytother Res. 2005 May;19(5):405-8.
43 Arcila-Lozano CC, Loarca-Pina G, Lecona-Uribe S, Gonzalez de Mejia E. [Oregano: properties, composition and biological activity] Arch Latinoam Nutr. 2004 Mar;54(1):100-11. Review. Spanish.
44 Sokmen M, Serkedjieva J, Daferera D, Gulluce M, Polissiou M, Tepe B, Akpulat HA, Sahin F, Sokmen A. In vitro antioxidant, antimicrobial, and antiviral activities of the essential oil and various extracts from herbal parts and callus cultures of Origanum acutidens. J Agric Food Chem. 2004 Jun 2;52(11):3309-12.
45 Elgayyar M, Draughon FA, Golden DA, Mount JR. Antimicrobial activity of essential oils from plants against selected pathogenic and saprophytic microorganisms. J Food Prot. 2001 Jul;64(7):1019-24.
46 Hammer KA, Carson CF, Riley TV. Antimicrobial activity of essential oils and other plant extracts. J Appl Microbiol. 1999 Jun;86(6):985-90.
47 Forbes MA, Schmid MM. Use of OTC essential oils to clear plantar warts. Nurse Pract. 2006 Mar;31(3):53-5, 57.
48 D'Auria FD, Tecca M, Strippoli V, Salvatore G, Battinelli L, Mazzanti G. Antifungal activity of Lavandula angustifolia essential oil against Candida albicans yeast and mycelial form. Med Mycol. 2005 Aug;43(5):391-6.
49 Edwards-Jones V, Buck R, Shawcross SG, Dawson MM, Dunn K. The effect of essential oils on methicillin-resistant Staphylococcus aureus using a dressing model. Burns. 2004 Dec;30(8):772-7.
50 Cavanagh HM, Wilkinson JM. Biological activities of lavender essential oil. Phytother Res. 2002 Jun;16(4):301-8. Review.
51 Inouye S, Watanabe M, Nishiyama Y, Takeo K, Akao M, Yamaguchi H. Antisporulating and respiration-inhibitory effects of essential oils on filamentous fungi. Mycoses. 1998 Nov;41(9-10):403-10.
52 Lopez P, Sanchez C, Batlle R, Nerin C. Solid- and vapor-phase antimicrobial activities of six essential oils: susceptibility of selected foodborne bacterial and fungal strains. J Agric Food Chem. 2005 Aug 24;53(17):6939-46.
53 Friedman M, Buick R, Elliott CT. Antibacterial activities of naturally occurring compounds against antibiotic-resistant Bacillus cereus vegetative cells and spores, Escherichia coli, and Staphylococcus aureus. J Food Prot. 2004 Aug;67(8):1774-8.
54 Lai PK, Roy J. Antimicrobial and chemopreventive properties of herbs and spices. Curr Med Chem. 2004 Jun;11(11):1451-60. Review.
55 Kalemba D, Kunicka A. Antibacterial and antifungal properties of essential oils. Curr Med Chem. 2003 May;10(10):813-29. Review.
56 Fabio A, Corona A, Forte E, Quaglio P. Inhibitory activity of spices and essential oils on psychrotrophic bacteria. New Microbiol. 2003 Jan;26(1):115-20. PMID: 12578319
57 Schuhmacher A, Reichling J, Schnitzler P. Virucidal effect of peppermint oil on the enveloped viruses herpes simplex virus type 1 and type 2 in vitro. Phytomedicine. 2003;10(6-7):504-10.
58 Logan AC, Beaulne TM. The treatment of small intestinal bacterial overgrowth with enteric-coated peppermint oil: a case report. Altern Med Rev. 2002 Oct;7(5):410-7.
59 Iscan G, Kirimer N, Kurkcuoglu M, Baser KH, Demirci F. Antimicrobial screening of Mentha piperita essential oils. J Agric Food Chem. 2002 Jul 3;50(14):3943-6. PMID: 12083863
60 Shapiro S, Meier A, Guggenheim B. The antimicrobial activity of essential oils and essential oil components towards oral bacteria. Oral Microbiol Immunol. 1994 Aug;9(4):202-8.
61 Edris AE, Farrag ES. Antifungal activity of peppermint and sweet basil essential oils and their major aroma constituents on some plant pathogenic fungi from the vapor phase. Nahrung. 2003 Apr;47(2):117-21. PMID: 12744290
62 Shkurupii VA, Kazarinova NV, Ogirenko AP, Nikonov SD, Tkachev AV, Tkachenko KG. [Efficiency of the use of peppermint (Mentha piperita L) essential oil inhalations in the combined multi-drug therapy for pulmonary tuberculosis] Probl Tuberk. 2002;(4):36-9. Russian.
63 Imai H, Osawa K, Yasuda H, Hamashima H, Arai T, Sasatsu M. Inhibition by the essential oils of peppermint and spearmint of the growth of pathogenic bacteria. Microbios. 2001;106 Suppl 1:31-9.
64 Pattnaik S, Subramanyam VR, Kole C. Antibacterial and antifungal activity of ten essential oils in vitro. Microbios. 1996;86(349):237-46.
65 Tassou CC, Drosinos EH, Nychas GJ. Effects of essential oil from mint (Mentha piperita) on Salmonella enteritidis and Listeria monocytogenes in model food systems at 4 degrees and 10 degrees C. J Appl Bacteriol. 1995 Jun;78(6):593-600.

Essential Oils

66 Pattnaik S, Subramanyam VR, Rath CC. Effect of essential oils on the viability and morphology of Escherichia coli (SP-11). Microbios. 1995;84(340):195-9.

67 Bagg J, Jackson MS, Petrina Sweeney M, Ramage G, Davies AN. Susceptibility to Melaleuca alternifolia (tea tree) oil of yeasts isolated from the mouths of patients with advanced cancer. Oral Oncol. 2006 May;42(5):487-92. Epub 2006 Feb 20.

68 Carson CF, Hammer KA, Riley TV. Melaleuca alternifolia (Tea Tree) oil: a review of antimicrobial and other medicinal properties. Clin Microbiol Rev. 2006 Jan;19(1):50-62. Review.

69 Wilkinson JM, Cavanagh HM. Antibacterial activity of essential oils from Australian native plants. Phytother Res. 2005 Jul;19(7):643-6.

70 Al-Shuneigat J, Cox SD, Markham JL. Effects of a topical essential oil-containing formulation on biofilm-forming coagulase-negative staphylococci. Lett Appl Microbiol. 2005;41(1):52-5.

71 Halcon L, Milkus K. Staphylococcus aureus and wounds: a review of tea tree oil as a promising antimicrobial. Am J Infect Control. 2004 Nov;32(7):402-8. Review.

72 Carson CF, Mee BJ, Riley TV. Mechanism of action of Melaleuca alternifolia (tea tree) oil on Staphylococcus aureus determined by time-kill, lysis, leakage, and salt tolerance assays and electron microscopy. Antimicrob Agents Chemother. 2002 Jun;46(6):1914-20.

73 Kulik E, Lenkeit K, Meyer J. [Antimicrobial effects of tea tree oil (Melaleuca alternifolia) on oral microorganisms] Schweiz Monatsschr Zahnmed. 2000;110(11):125-30. German.

74 Sherry E, Boeck H, Warnke PH. Percutaneous treatment of chronic MRSA osteomyelitis with a novel plant-derived antiseptic. BMC Surg. 2001;1:1. Epub 2001 May 16.

75 Gustafson JE, Cox SD, Liew YC, Wyllie SG, Warmington JR. The bacterial multiple antibiotic resistant (Mar) phenotype leads to increased tolerance to tea tree oil. Pathology. 2001 May;33(2):211-5.

76 May J, Chan CH, King A, Williams L, French GL. Time-kill studies of tea tree oils on clinical isolates. J Antimicrob Chemother. 2000 May;45(5):639-43.

77 Cox SD, Mann CM, Markham JL, Bell HC, Gustafson JE, Warmington JR, Wyllie SG. The mode of antimicrobial action of the essential oil of Melaleuca alternifolia (tea tree). J Appl Microbiol. 2000 Jan;88(1):170-5.

78 Harkenthal M, Reichling J, Geiss HK, Saller R. Comparative study on the in vitro antibacterial activity of Australian tea tree oil, cajuput oil, niaouli oil, manuka oil, kanuka oil, and eucalyptus oil. Pharmazie. 1999 Jun;54(6):460-3.

79 Carson CF, Riley TV. Antimicrobial activity of the major components of the essential oil of Melaleuca alternifolia. J Appl Bacteriol. 1995 Mar;78(3):264-9. PMID: 7730203

80 Inouye S, Yamaguchi H, Takizawa T. Screening of the antibacterial effects of a variety of essential oils on respiratory tract pathogens, using a modified dilution assay method. J Infect Chemother. 2001 Dec;7(4):251-4. PMID: 11810593

CHAPTER 20

WHICH HERBS SHOULD I TAKE?

Herbal medicine is enjoying more popularity than ever in Britain now, thanks mainly to the excellent BBC series "Grow Your Own Drugs", featuring ethnobotanist James Wong.

WHAT IS HERBAL MEDICINE?

Herbal medicine, also known as phytotherapy or herbalism, is the use of plants for medicinal purposes. Herbal medicine is said to be as old as mankind itself. Food and medicine have always been linked and Hippocrates, the "Father of Medicine", is often quoted as saying:

> "Let food be your medicine and medicine be your food."

Many plants make aromatic substances, most of which are phenols, or their oxygen-substituted derivatives such as tannins. The majority of these are actually known as "secondary metabolites".

These are substances that whilst not critical to the particular plant's growth, flowering ability, or reproductive capacity, are nevertheless important for things like rendering the plant unattractive to insects, animals and micro-organisms such as bacteria and fungi.

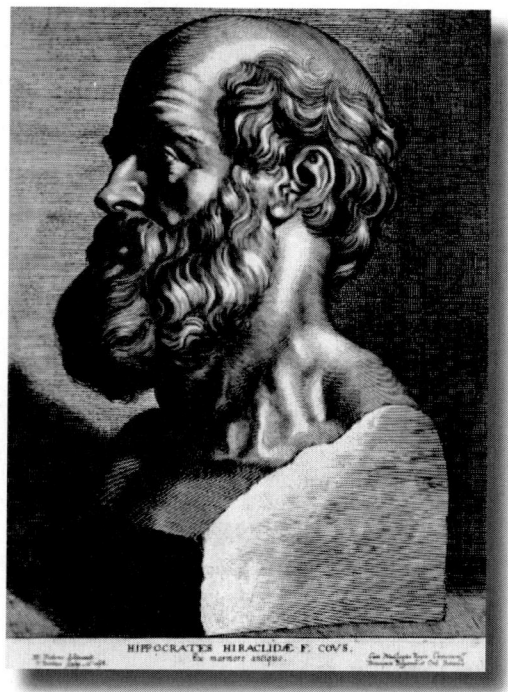

Hippocrates - Engraving by Reubens 1683
Courtesy: National Library of Medicine

Which Herbs Should I Take?

It is estimated that so far around 12,000 of these aromatic substances have been isolated but this is just the tip of the iceberg as it is thought that there are probably still another 120,000 or so, left to find.

Many of the pharmaceutical drugs currently available to Western physicians have a long history of use as herbal remedies, including opium, aspirin, digitalis, and quinine. So, the race is on to find more medicinal plants that may hold the key to the treatment of various diseases.

THERE ARE THREE MAIN "SCHOOLS" OF HERBAL MEDICINE:

- The Western School, based on Greek and Roman sources
- The Ayurvedic School, from India
- Traditional Chinese Herbal Medicine

THE HISTORY OF HERBAL MEDICINE

Our knowledge and medicinal use of herbs can be traced back to Egyptian texts dating from 1500 B.C.E. However, there is evidence that the Neanderthals living in the region that we now call Iraq used herbs as long ago as 60,000 B.C.E.

In ancient Egypt, slave workers were given a daily ration of garlic to ward off infection and fevers that were common at the time and one of the most ancient known uses of herbal medicine dates back to 16,000 B.C.E. in the Tibetan Bön (pronounced '*burn*') Tradition.

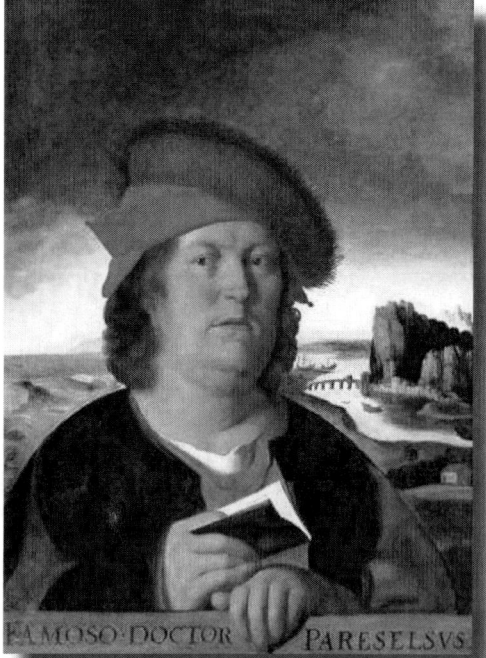
Paracelcus by Quentin Massys

The history of herbal medicine progressed through Hippocrates to the Greek physician Galen and through to the 16th century genius of Paracelsus.

Paracelsus (1493 - 1541), born Theophrastus Philippus Aureolus Bombastus von Hohenheim, was a famous physician who, like most other physicians of the day, was also an astrologer, alchemist and general occultist.

He had a rather high opinion of himself, probably well deserved, but he managed to rub people up the wrong way – especially when later in his life he took the name

"Paracelsus", to indicate that he was superior to the great Roman physician Celsus. We get the word "bombastic" from the "Bombastus" part of Paracelsus' name.

In spite of the fact that he was not well liked, Paracelsus was undoubtedly a brilliant doctor and he is often considered to be the "Father of Toxicology" (the study of toxins). He travelled the world, seeking out eminent doctors to study with and transformed our understanding of herbal medicine.

True to form, Paracelsus flew against the prevailing wisdom of the day and formulated some quite outrageous ideas for the time – one of his great breakthroughs was in the treatment of wounds. Paracelsus believed that wounds were capable of healing themselves – if kept clean and allowed to drain. This was a totally revolutionary concept for the time as the treatment of the day involved cauterising wounds with boiling oil or allowing them to turn gangrenous and then amputating the limb.

Paracelsus' was instrumental in influencing modern day toxicology and his work was also, no doubt, familiar to Samuel Hahnemann – the inventor of homeopathy. There are striking similarities in the following Paracelsian quote that has direct relevance for both modern day toxicology and homeopathy:

In the original German:

"Alle Ding' sind Gift und nichts ohn' Gift; allein die Dosis macht, das ein Ding kein Gift ist."

This translates as:

"All things are poison and nothing (is) without poison; only the dose makes a thing a poison."

In other words, the amount of a substance – or "dose" of a substance – a person is exposed to is as important as the nature of the substance. For example, small doses of digitalis (a drug derived from the common foxglove) can be beneficial to a person with heart disease but at higher doses, this medicine is poisonous.

In the 17th century the Englishman, Nicholas Culpeper, (1616 – 1654) was a botanist, physician and astrologer. He studied in Cambridge, and afterwards became apprenticed to an apothecary. He later ran a pharmacy in the Halfway House in Spitalfields, London. He was a radical republican and opposed to the "closed shop" of medicine. Culpeper believed that the use of Latin by doctors, lawyers and priests was a plot to keep power and freedom away from the "common people".

In order to bring knowledge to the public, Culpeper made an unauthorised translation of the

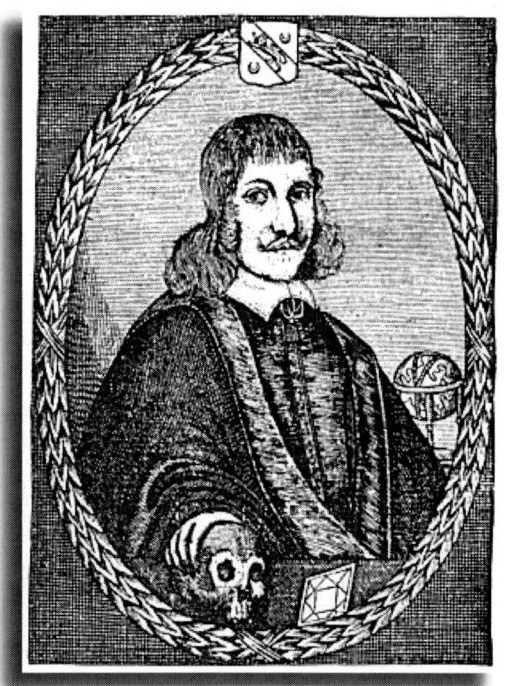
Nicholas Culpeper

'Pharmacopoeia' (the book of medicines used by doctors), which was, at that time, written in Latin. Another of Culpeper's major contributions to modern medicine was his "Herbal" which is still in print today.

HERBAL MEDICINE – THE UNDERLYING PRINCIPLES

The emphasis in Herbal Medicine is on the maintenance of good health and the prevention of disease. Partly because of this and the growing mistrust of pharmaceutical drugs, more and more people today are turning to herbal medicine. Globally, Herbal Medicine is three to four times more commonly practiced than Conventional Medicine.

HOW TO PREPARE MEDICINAL HERBS

Herbs can be prepared for use in several different ways. Certain herbs are only suitable to be taken in particular forms.

CAPSULES
These are often gelatine-coated and are swallowed whole with a little water, or chewed, according to directions. Vegetarian capsules are available. Only take capsules that have been recommended by a fully qualified herbal practitioner.

COMPRESS
This form of preparation is commonly made from a decoction, or an herbal infusion, by soaking a linen or muslin cloth in the mixture. Compresses are either hot or cold and the method involves placing the cloth over the affected area. They are especially useful where the herbs are too strong for internal use.

DECOCTION
This is an extraction produced by boiling the herbs in a measured amount of water for a determined length of time. These are especially useful where specific herbs are not soluble in water and for subsequent use with a compress. After this process the extract will contain the

essential minerals and alkaloids of the herb, which are the herb's active components.

EXTRACTS

Extracts are herb concentrates, which vary in strength and are made of a mixture of an appropriate herb and suitable dissolving agent, this usually being water or alcohol, or a mixture of the two. If left for a few days the mixture can become very potent and useful for the topical treatment of a number of conditions.

INFUSION

By pouring hot liquid onto the herbs and allowing the mixture to steep for a determined length of time, say about 20 minutes, you make an infusion. The infusion is an extract containing the herb's active constituents. Herb teas can be considered "infusions".

TINCTURE

These are herbal concentrates made using alcohol in the place of water, thereby extending their shelf life. They are suitable for application to the skin and the use of alcohol provides a cooling sensation on the skin as the liquid evaporates. Tinctures can also be taken by mouth and they would usually be diluted in water.

Of the modern medications currently used in Western Allopathic (Conventional) Medicine, 85% were originally derived from the natural herbs used since ancient times in traditional medicine, then later synthesised into various chemical analogues. So, it is fair to call herbal medicine "experience based medicine", given its successful use over the millennia. It is also important to acknowledge the immense body of scientific evidence that now supports the efficacy of Herbal Medicine.

A herbalist will use the principles of "holism" to make a prescription for a patient – by taking all the patient's symptoms into account. A careful analysis of these symptoms will help the herbalist to select the correct herb – or sometimes group of herbs that will cure the patient.

HOW LONG DOES HERBAL TREATMENT TAKE TO WORK?

This will vary according to the condition and the individual. Herbal medicines are very effective if taken with care and in the correct doses. Their effects can be immediate, or they may take several days or weeks to become noticeable.

CONTRA-INDICATIONS OR SIDE EFFECTS

A contra-indication is a situation in which a substance should not be taken. So, for example, if you look at a Conventional Medicine package, it will have a list of indications i.e. the conditions that the medicine is supposed to treat and also a list of contra-indications – those conditions in which it might be unhelpful or even dangerous to take the medicine. So it is with herbs. Many herbs have no contra-indications. However, as with all substances, it is never advisable to exceed the recommended dosage in any case. Always consult a fully qualified practitioner of herbal medicine before taking herbal treatments if you are pregnant, likely to become pregnant, or breast-feeding.

Also, if you are already taking Conventional medication, check The Complementary Medical Association website: The-CMA.Org.UK for a database of drug/herb/supplement interactions. Sometimes herbs can interact with drugs in various ways, some helpful, others unhelpful.

Occasionally, these interactions can enhance the ability of a drug to do its work. A good example of this would be gingko biloba, an extremely safe and effective herb that has many effects, one of which is enhancing circulation. This may however, increase the likelihood of haemorrhage when taken with blood thinning medication such as Heparin or Warfarin, although scientists disagree whether this is so[1].

CAN I TAKE HERBAL MEDICINES AT THE SAME TIME AS TAMIFLU OR OTHER ANTI-VIRAL DRUGS?

All that we can say with any certainty is that the herbs that we recommend you take, in the following section, are not known to interact with Tamiflu, either to boost its effectiveness or to lessen it. Tamiflu and its ilk are neuraminidase inhibitors and while some of the herbs that we recommend are also neuraminidase inhibitors, they have not been shown to interact with Tamiflu in either a positive or negative way.

HERBAL MEDICINE AND SWINE FLU

Herbal medicine works – beyond a shadow of a doubt – for many illnesses, when herbs are correctly prescribed. This has been proven in many excellent scientific trials the world over. China, in particular, with her rich history of Traditional Chinese Herbal Medicine provides much scientific evidence for the undoubted efficacy of herbs. However, herbal medicines are strong and effective and must therefore be judiciously used. One of the trends that The Complementary Medical Association finds very alarming is that many, ill-advised, experts with no real understanding of how the immune system actually works – especially if one is infected with Swine Flu – are suggesting that we all go and "boost" our immune systems.

Immune 'boosting' can be easily achieved with herbs such as Echinacea [2], Black Elderberry [3] extract etc. This is in fact the last thing one should do, as this is likely to increase the lethality of the disease for anyone who does take these herbs after they have been exposed to Swine Flu or Bird Flu.

Immune boosting herbs, such as Echinacea and Black Elderberry, actually increase the production of stem cells that then "differentiate" into immune cells that are implicated in the phenomenon known as the "Cytokine Storm".

There is some evidence to suggest that Black Elderberry, in particular, does have some anti-viral properties and that it up-regulates the production of various cytokines including IL-10, which helps to suppress inflammation. However, it also increases production of highly pro-inflammatory cytokines such as TNFα – which is particularly implicated in the Cytokine Storm seen in people with Swine Flu. So, it is too early to tell if Black Elderberry is safe to use during an H1N1 infection. [4,5]. We are keeping a watchful eye on the current research and if it appears that Black Elderberry is safe we will notify the public via our website – through our CMA e-Newsletter Monthly Updates. (The–CMA.Org.UK).

It is vital with herbs – as with all 'medicines' – to make sure that you know which ones to take and which dosage is correct for you. It is also crucial to be absolutely certain that if you are taking herbs or any other medicines – that they come from a reputable source – so that you can be sure that they are not contaminated in any way and do indeed contain active ingredients in the right quantities. We cannot stress the importance of this enough. Many so-called herbal remedies are available in a variety of stores, but in many cases their effectiveness is limited, or almost non-existent because they have the incorrect balance of ingredients, or because they have selected herbal substances that sound correct, but which are in fact 'inert'.

In addition, herbal medicines are different to the herbs that you can go and buy from the grocery store for example. In order to make herbal medicines, it is necessary to extract the active parts of the herb and to formulate these into a "Standardised Extract" so that anyone taking the herb knows precisely what dose of the herbal medicine they are actually taking. Herbs used for cooking may have been stored for some time – or may not have enough of the active constituent in them to begin with, which would mean that they would be ineffective.

SO, WHICH HERBS DO WE RECOMMEND?

We advocate a programme of preparing your immune system so that you are as resistant to any disease as possible and this includes Swine Flu. To set up this basic underlying 'wellness' – a state of health "fitness" in all your body systems – we recommend the herbs in the following section. The herbs that we have brought together here, coupled with the nutrition programme that we propose in this book, will serve to enhance your robustness, or fitness i.e. your ability to be as unsusceptible, or immune as possible, to viruses (like Swine Flu) and other pathogens (disease causing agents). This robustness, or fitness, is not to be confused with physical fitness, like being able to run fast for example – that is totally different.

Which Herbs Should I Take?

We have exhaustively researched which herbs will help to best prepare your host immunity. In recommending which herbs you should take, we are well aware of the incredible balancing act that needs to be performed in this area – so that we do not "turn up" certain parts of your immune system – thereby possibly exposing you to the risk of Cytokine Storm. We have identified groups of herbs that can achieve this balance– but it is an incredibly delicate issue and therefore it is essential to consult a qualified herbalist, who will tell you what is right for you as an individual. It is essential to follow precise dosages of correctly sourced herbs (that you know for certain have not been tampered with or adulterated in any way). These must be taken in precisely the correct manner.

We recommend that you take the following herbs because they have been scientifically demonstrated to optimise your immune response, they have anti-oxidant properties and are also anti-viral.

Some of these herbs are also anti-pyretic (fever-reducing), anti-microbial and are anti-inflammatory and thus have specific relevance to the types of problems faced by people with severe influenza. (The anti-inflammatory component is also useful in combating the chronic inflammation seen in people throughout industrialised nations who are following a standard "Western Diet" which is discussed in much greater depth in the Nutrition section of this book.)

Of course, these have not been clinically tested on any cases of severe Swine Flu specifically so we cannot yet say for certain that these will work against Swine Flu. However, we are basing our recommendations on the best scientific research available and also upon the enormous amount of knowledge gleaned from hundreds – and in the case of herbs used in Traditional Chinese Herbal Medicine and Ayurveda – thousands of years of historical use.

We recommend that you take a balance of the following herbs:

- TURMERIC
- RESVERATROL
- GINGER
- ROSEMARY
- OLIVE LEAF EXTRACT

TURMERIC (CURCUMIN)

Due to its enormously wide range of benefits, Turmeric is probably one of the most valuable herbs available. It is used in India in food to give curries their typical yellow colour.

We include Turmeric in our herbal recommendations primarily due to its anti-viral and anti-inflammatory properties – but it does have other broad-spectrum properties that are invaluable to good health. The particular form of Turmeric that we recommend is a high-potency standardised extract of Curcuminoid complex – this Curcuminoid complex is the "active" part of Turmeric[6].

You would not be able to achieve the same health results by taking Turmeric that is sold in grocery stores, as in order to get enough of the active substance "Curcumin" you would need to eat vast amounts of Turmeric.

Scientific research supports the wide-ranging beneficial properties of the Curcuminoids, and especially Curcumin. These include powerful anti-oxidant properties, modulation of the production of inflammatory signal molecules (prostanoids and leukotrienes), and inhibition of the growth of cells which have not properly differentiated, or whose growth pattern is abnormal (either can lead to cancer).

In PubMed there are over 2,903 references to these and other facets of Curcumin activity. (PubMed is a service of the U.S. National Library of Medicine that includes over 16 million citations of published scientific papers from MEDLINE and other life science journals for biomedical articles back to the 1950s.)[7]

As we explained in the "Your Immune System and The Cytokine Storm" section of this book, one of the crucial cytokines that is implicated in the type of Cytokine Storm seen in Influenza A is TNFα.

TNFα is particularly elevated in Bird Flu and we would hypothesise this is also the case with severe Swine Flu as well. [8,9,10] Furthermore, as we have seen, scientists currently hypothesise that a particular inflammatory pathway called MAPK p38 [11,12] is predominantly implicated in the Cytokine Storm.

Curcumin is an effective TNF suppressor and the research in this area indicates that Curcumin may well reduce the lethality of Swine Flu and Bird Flu. In fact, there are currently 93 references to "MAPK Curcumin" in "PubMed". On searching PubMed for "TNF Curcumin", 196 research papers (citations) were found, which demonstrates that scientists are certain that Curcumin is a useful and promising herbal extract for potentially many illnesses. Curcuminoids act through both intervention and preventative means, thus they are accordingly considered among the most potent of the known anti-oxidants.

MORE TECHNICAL INFORMATION ABOUT CURCUMIN

Curcuma Longa is a perennial herb that belongs to the Ginger family. The rhizome is extensively used for imparting colour and flavour to food including curries, it is also used for medicinal purposes and religious ceremonies.

CHEMISTRY

Curcuma longa rhizomes yield about 8% essential oils and 10% fatty oil. Three major constituents have been identified:

(1.) Curcumin (diferuloyl methane)
(2.) Curcumin methane.
(3.) Di-hydroxy cinnamoyl methane.

The volatile oils in Curcumin contain cineol, camphor and linalool and are probably responsible for its anti-spasmodic activity. Borneol is present in the essential oil fraction and is largely responsible for the digestion-improving properties.

PHARMACOLOGICAL PROPERTIES:

The following research demonstrates that Curcumin has an important role to play in fighting Swine Flu and its complications:

1. ANTIOXIDANT PROPERTIES

Numerous studies[13] have shown that the various constituents of Curcuma longa possess potent anti-oxidant properties. The ability of cucuminoids to reduce hydroxyl and peroxyl free-radicals is well documented.

As long ago as 1976, respected researcher, Dr Sharma[14] reported Curcumin to be an effective agent against lipid peroxidation, which if uncontrolled can lead to high cholesterol levels. Antioxidants are very useful when combating any viral illness as many free-radicals are produced as a result of our body's infection-fighting activities.

2. ANTI-INFLAMMATORY PROPERTIES

The Central Drug Research Institute in India found Curcumin to be the major constituent responsible for the anti-inflammatory activity of Turmeric. The classical model for studying acute effects of anti-inflammatory agents, is to test their inhibitory action on the development of rat paw oedema – the exudative phase of inflammation – induced, for instance, by the local injection of carrageenins – which are a substance that causes inflammation.

Inflammation is thought to be in part due to the action of prostaglandins derived from arachidonic acid metabolism (see our Nutrition section for more information about this). A detailed evaluation of Curcumin as a potential non-steroidal anti-inflammatory agent by the scientists Srimal and Dhawan[15] found Curcumin to be highly effective after oral administration.

Scientists do not yet know why Curcumin has strong anti-inflammatory properties. The results of scientific trials are conflicting, some researchers found Curcumin to be less effective in adrenalectomised rats (rats whose adrenal glands had been removed so that they could not produce the "stress hormone" Cortisol), suggesting a participation of corticoidal steroids, while others did not observe any effect of Curcumin salts on steroid release from the adrenal cortex.

Ultimately, the conclusion that we can draw is that it certainly appears that Curcumin is a useful anti-inflammatory, but its exact mechanism of action is as yet, unknown. Scientists continue to test Curcumin to find out how it actually works. Currently, there are 568 research papers displayed on PubMed which explore the role of Curcumin as an anti-inflammatory substance.[16]

3. ANTI-VIRAL PROPERTIES

A 2000 study[17] showed Curcumin is an effective ally in the fight against HIV. Curcumin was effective in inhibiting the replication of HIV [18,19,20,21] in both acutely infected and chronically infected cells. Given the anti-viral properties of Curcumin this may well mean that it can inhibit the replication of other viruses such as the H1N1 virus.

4. ANTI-BACTERIAL/ANTI-FUNGAL PROPERTIES

Curcumin has been shown to inhibit the growth of most organisms [22,23,24] including: Staph aureus, Streptococci, Lactobacilli, Corynebacterium, Baccilus aureus, and Micrococcus pyogenes. The crude ether and chloroform extracts of Curcuma Longa showed anti-fungal activity[25] against several dermatophytes as well as anti-amoebic activity against Entamoeba histolytica. It also has anti-parasitic properties. [26,27,28]

As discussed earlier, one of the serious problems that can arise after a severe bout of flu is the issue of "opportunistic infection", such as bacterial or fungal infection. These pathogens can easily infect a body that is already weakened by having to cope with a bout of virulent flu. In 1918, a major contributor to the enormous numbers of fatalities was a post-flu pneumonia. If Curcumin can help to combat bacteria and fungus then there is a good case for its use during and after a Swine Flu infection too.

The following research is included here to demonstrate the vast sphere of activity of Curcumin, although this research doesn't have as direct a relationship with fighting Swine Flu as the research findings outlined above:

5. GASTRO-INTESTINAL EFFECTS

Curcumin increases mucin content (large, heavily glycosylated proteins that are secreted to make the slimy mucus we need in various places in our bodies to protect, or 'oil' them), thereby protecting our gastric mucosa (stomach lining) against irritants. This may have some relevance to protecting us from Swine Flu as it may prevent viruses from gaining entry to our bodies via stomach mucosa – although this is just a hypothesis and not proven.

Controversial data also exist regarding the ability of Curcumin to prevent the formation of stomach ulcers. Some researchers found a protective effect for Curcumin against histamine-induced gastric ulceration [29,30,31] while others reported an ulcerogenic effect for Curcumin.[32]

6. ANTI-SPASMODIC EFFECTS
Curcumin also possesses anti-spasmodic properties (to prevent spasms). Curcumin showed liver protective effects against carbon tetrachloride, D-Galactosamine and peroxide induced cytotoxicity. Curcumin increased bile acid production in dogs and rats.

7. CARDIOVASCULAR EFFECTS
A sharp and transient hypotensive effect (lower blood pressure) of Curcumin was reported in dogs. Curcumin also inhibited collagen and adrenaline-induced aggregation of platelets but did not affect prostacyclin (PGI2) synthesis. [33,34,35]

8. LIPID METABOLISM
The scientists, Rao and co-workers [36,37] reported that rats fed with Curcumin and cholesterol in their diet had only half to one-third of the serum and liver cholesterol levels compared to the controlled groups receiving cholesterol alone. [38,39,40,41]

9. ANTI-TUMOUR ACTIVITY
The anti-tumour activity of various extracts of Curcuma longa has been noted by several researchers. Topical application (i.e. the Curcumin was applied directly onto the tumour) of Curcumin inhibited the number of TPA-induced tumours by as much as 98%. Curcumin was found to be a selective and non-competitive inhibitor of phosphorylase kinase. There are many indications that Curcumin will be very useful in the fight against cancer and much work is being undertaken by Dr Sharma [42] and colleagues at the University of Leicester to advance the understanding of its anti-cancer properties.

NOT ALL TURMERIC (CURCUMIN) IS EQUAL:

We realise that with so many types of Turmeric available in the shops and on the internet it can be difficult for you as a consumer to select which type you need in order to deliver enough of the bioavailable, physiologically active quantities of the Curcumin that your body can absorb and actually utilise. This is especially important as some types of Turmeric, even those sold as health supplements, are basically almost useless for your system. [43] When purchasing any herbal product it is vital to ensure that it contains a Standardised Extract of the active ingredients.

RED GRAPE EXTRACT – RESVERATROL

A potent COX-2 inhibitor, [44,45] (this is a substance that selectively inhibits the actions of COX-2, an enzyme involved in the inflammation pathway), known as Resveratrol is produced in the skin of red grapes, where it protects the grapes against oxidation and fungal infections. Resveratrol is found in grape juice and red wine; red Bordeaux and French and Chilean Cabernets contain a particularly high concentration of the compound.

Note: as tempting as it is for some people to think that the best way to get sufficient quantities of Resveratrol is from drinking lots of red wine, it is best to take Resveratrol as a supplement to get the most benefit from it as you would need to drink quite a lot of wine in order to get enough Resveratrol.

Although red wine is considered to be good for us in moderation, [46,47] drinking too much of any form of alcohol has deleterious effects upon your immune system and is particularly dangerous and must be avoided completely if you actually contract Swine Flu. In addition, pregnant women should avoid alcohol. For more information about the way that alcohol affects your immune system please see the section in this book on alcohol and your immune system in our Nutrition section.

RESVERATROL IN MORE DEPTH

Of particular interest when thinking about ways to combat Swine Flu is that a cell culture study has found that Resveratrol compromises the ability of the influenza virus from carrying viral proteins to the viral building site and this restricts the ability of the virus to self-replicate.

The effect is both marked and long lasting. The self-replication restrictive effect was 90% when Resveratrol was added to cells six hours after infection and continued for 24 hours thereafter! This was reported in the respected publication; The Journal of Infectious Diseases in May 2005.[48]

The scientists reported:

"That RV (Resveratrol) acts by inhibiting a cellular, rather than a viral function, suggests that it could be a particularly valuable anti-influenza drug."

In addition, Resveratrol is a neuraminidase inhibitor [49] – like Tamiflu – but a 'natural' one – but, unlike Tamiflu, it is one where it has not yet been demonstrated that Influenza A viruses have become resistant to it.[50]

As we know, one of the serious problems seen in Swine Flu is inflammation. Scientists have recently discovered that up-regulation of a cytokine, fractalkine, is involved in vascular and tissue damage in inflammatory conditions and the inflammatory cytokine that is particularly elevated in Bird Flu (and we would hypothesize that the same will be true for Swine Flu) - and TNFα has a role to play in this. [51]

Resveratrol has been shown to combat TNFα. In addition, Resveratrol has anti-oxidant, and anti-tumour activities.[52] Although not of direct relevance to Swine Flu, we include the following information to demonstrate the other enormous health benefits of Resveratrol:

Resveratrol appears to help protect against cancer in at least three ways:

- It has anti-inflammatory effects,
- It's a powerful anti-oxidant,
- It may prevent cancer cells from progressing to the next stage. Resveratrol interferes with initiation, promotion and progression of cancers.

Experiments using Resveratrol show that there are a multitude of factors responsible for its pharmacological activities. At the time of writing there are currently 900 scientific papers on PubMed that are exploring the ways in which Resveratrol can be used to treat cancers. The anti-cancer properties of Resveratrol include various factors such as the inhibition of the transcription factor NF-kappa B, cytochrome P450 isoenzyme CYP1A1, androgenic actions and expression and activity of cyclooxygenase (COX) enzymes.[53] For more information about these please see this book's section on Nutrition.

Resveratrol has been shown to be involved with Fas/Fas ligand mediated apoptosis (cell death), p53 (tumour protein 53) and cyclins (a family of proteins involved in the progression of cells through the cell cycle) A, B1 and cyclin-dependent kinases (protein kinases originally discovered as being involved in the regulation of the cell cycle) cdk 1 and 2. [54,55,56,57,58,59,60,61,62,63]

Furthermore, it possesses anti-oxidant and anti-angiogenic properties. Angiogenesis means *"the growth of blood vessels"* and is a normal process in our growth and development, as well as in wound healing. However, angiogenesis – if it gets out of control – is also a fundamental step in the transition of tumours from a dormant state to a malignant state. Due to the discovery of the anti-angiogenic properties of Resveratrol, it is currently being investigated extensively by scientists as a cancer chemo-preventive agent.

Diseases such as Huntington's disease and Alzheimer's may both benefit from Resveratrol's ability to be effective against neuronal cell dysfunction and cell death. [64,65,66,67,68,69] Recent research at Ohio State University indicated that Resveratrol inhibits the development of cardiac fibrosis (the formation or development of excess fibrous connective tissue in the heart). [70]

NOT ALL RESVERATROL SUPPLEMENTS ARE EQUAL

As with Turmeric – it can be very confusing for consumers who wish to buy Resveratrol as there are so many options on the market. However, there are different types of Resveratrol available – some of which are more bioavailable and better for you than others.

We particularly recommend Trans-Resveratrol as opposed to the Cis-Resveratrol that is also commonly available.[71] This is because the "Trans" version of Resveratrol is more potent and has performed better in studies. When purchasing any herbal product it is vital to ensure that it contains a Standardised Extract of the active ingredients.

ROSEMARY

This common herb is of particular interest when considering Swine Flu as it is another strong anti-inflammatory,[72] COX-2 inhibitor,[73] anti-oxidant,[74,75] and it also increases the activity of detoxification enzymes. Given that Rosemary contains these extremely useful and health-protective qualities in abundance, these factors may be of help in combating the types of problems seen in those with Swine Flu.

Apart from its anti-oxidant,[76] anti-inflammatory and detoxification properties, an extract of Rosemary, named carnosol, has anti-cancer properties[77,78] and has inhibited the development of both breast and skin tumours in animals.[79] It is also a potent aid in the fight against lipid peroxidisation – which can lead to high LDL ("bad") cholesterol levels.[80]

Evidence suggests that Rosemary can support the action of Vitamin D3 to combat some forms of leukaemia.[81] Rosemary also has strong anti-viral properties against the HIV virus – in test tube studies.[82] Mesangial Cell Proliferation is a feature of some types of disease that affect the kidneys. It is caused by a variety of cytokines of which one is TNFα – which is, as we have seen, also implicated in the type of Cytokine Storm produced by Swine Flu (H1N1). Rosemary has been shown to inhibit the cytokines responsible for Mesangial Cell Proliferation.[83]

MORE ABOUT ROSEMARY

Rosemary is a small evergreen shrub that has a distinctive fragrance. It can be grown in most locations although it is native to the Mediterranean area. It is commonly used to flavour food and in aromatherapy. The name Rosemary means "sea dew". The leaves are needle-like and dark green and its flowers produce a pale blue volatile oil.

Herbalists traditionally use Rosemary to treat digestive and circulatory problems, pain, neuralgia, mild spasms, wounds, eczema, sciatica, rheumatism and depression as well as parasites. Rosemary has excellent anti-microbial properties.[84] Research has shown that it may improve memory, relieve muscle pain, and stimulate the circulatory and nervous systems. Used topically, Rosemary can assist in healing wounds.

Researchers are looking at Rosemary carefully as it has so many potential benefits for health – in fact – there are 802 studies on PubMed which have investigated the effects of this herb.

Rosemary also shows promise as an additive to cosmetic products[85] as it has such powerful anti-oxidant capabilities which are very beneficial to skin, which is susceptible to damage from exposure to sunlight (solar radiation), and of course oxygen – which leads to oxidization. In addition – the food industry is attempting to harness the powers of Rosemary for its anti-oxidant effects which help food preservation and of course it is non-toxic.

It is used as an antispasmodic[86] and diuretic for increasing urine production and can stimulate menstrual blood flow. Herbalists prescribe Rosemary in conjunction with St. John's Wort and Ginkgo Biloba to improve cognitive function and some visual and speech difficulties associated with brain inflammation.

NOT ALL ROSEMARY HERBAL SUPPLEMENTS ARE EQUAL

You can't just go to the grocery store and buy Rosemary herbs and hope that they will "do the job" and protect you from Swine Flu.

As with all herbal medicines, it is absolutely essential to make sure that you are getting enough of the bioavailable, physiologically active quantities of the Rosemary that your body can absorb and actually utilise. This is especially important as some types of Rosemary, even those sold as health supplements, are almost useless therapeutically.[87]

When purchasing any herbal product it is vital to ensure that it contains a Standardised Extract of the active ingredients.

GINGER

Ginger has been used as a medicine and a condiment since ancient times. It has been cultivated for so long that its origin is unclear. It was imported to Alexandria via the Red Sea over two thousand years ago. It is still one of the most popular hot-tasting spices today. The plant stands 15-150 cm tall. References to the medicinal use of Ginger root are found in early Chinese, Greek, Roman and Arabic texts.

The Asians used it for thousands of years to treat stomach aches, diarrhoea and nausea and it was used in Africa as much as it was used in Asia.

Today, it is found in the national pharmacopoeia of Austria, China, Egypt, Germany, Great Britain, Japan and Switzerland. Yearly production of Ginger is estimated at 100,000 tons. Ginger is sometimes referred to as "hands" because of the rhizome's resemblance to human hands.

Ginger has anti-viral, anti-emetic and anti-diarrhoeal properties – it kills viruses, it reduces vomiting and diarrhoea [88,89,90,91,92,93] – and in addition it has anti-pyretic (fever-reducing) and analgesic (pain-reducing) properties – all of which have been a feature of Swine Flu (H1N1).[94,95]

Ginger has many other extremely beneficial health-giving properties – such as being a rich source of anti-oxidants. There are over 1,089 research studies into the immunological and anti-oxidant capacity of Ginger on PubMed and we highlight just a few of these in our references below. [96,97,98,99,100,101]

The immune-modulating and anti-oxidant effect of Ginger will be of great value in fighting viral disease – because your body produces enormous amounts of free radicals when under the stress of a virulent infection – such as we would see with Swine Flu, for example.

TECHNICAL DETAILS FOR GINGER

PHARMACOLOGY:
• The odour and flavour of Ginger are highly dependent on the content in its volatile acids, roughly 1-3%: zingerone, shoagoles and Gingerols.
• The Gingerols are responsible for the pungency and are also thought to be some of the most pharmacologically active ingredients of the plant.
• The anti-pyretic (fever-reducing) and analgesic (pain-relieving) effects of the plant are due to Gingerol and shogaol, two compounds that produce an inhibition of spontaneous motor activity. Both ingredients also suppress gastric contractions.[102]
• The plant contains several anti-oxidants.
• Ginger's platelet aggregation-lowering effect (it stops red blood cells from clumping together)

was shown to be superior to that produced by Garlic and Onions. [103]
- Ginger stimulates the conversion of cholesterol into bile acids and impairs cholesterol absorption. [104,105,106,107,108,109,110,111,112,113,114]
- Ginger is a potent cardiotonic. [115,116,117]
- Shogaol found in Ginger inhibits the release of "Substance P", reducing pain.
- Ginger is a potent anti-inflammatory and suppresses both prostaglandins and arachidonic acid [118,119,120,121,122,123,124,125,126,127,128,129,130,131,132] – both of which are implicated in inflammatory cascades – which of course has relevance to Swine Flu. First by reducing generalised chronic inflammation that most of us who eat a standard Western Diet are hostage to, we improve our health and this can render us more resistant to viral infection. Secondly, as we know, inflammatory cascades are part of the Cytokine Storm phenomenon as seen in Swine Flu, so Ginger could well be helpful in combating this too.
- Ginger's nausea reducing action is probably linked to its ability to increase digestive fluid secretion.
- The pungent compounds found in Ginger also appear to have significant anti-ulcer properties. The root was shown to prevent ulcer formation which is due to a variety of chemicals such as ethanol, aspirin and indomethacin. [133,134,135,136,137,138]

INDICATIONS:

As we have seen above, Ginger has effects on many body systems such as on the digestive, central nervous and cardiovascular systems.
- Some of Ginger's main applications include the treatment and prevention of motion and sea-sickness, post-surgical nausea and vomiting, to relieve joint pain and to improve mobility for rheumatoid arthritis patients.
- Ginger is a carminative (produces an anti-spasmodic activity that can be used against cramps of the digestive tract in combination with flatulence) anti-emetic (stops vomiting), spasmolytic (stops spasms/cramps), anti-inflammatory and peripheral circulatory stimulant (increases circulation to your extremities).
- Ginger modulates the production of certain prostaglandins and this effect is thought to be responsible for the root's anti-inflammatory activity – very important in fighting a virus as devastating as H1N1.
- As the history of the plant suggests, Ginger is an excellent treatment for dyspepsia (a constant pain in the stomach). The plant also shows hypoglycemic effects (blood sugar lowering), promotes the secretion of saliva, bile and gastric juices and increases tonus (muscular tone) and peristalsis (movement of muscles) in the intestines.
- Ginger has been used for the treatment and prevention of migraine headaches.
- Ginger has been shown to inhibit diarrhea – this is useful as severe diarrhoea has been a feature in some people who have contracted Swine Flu.

RESEARCH SUMMARY

- Several studies have confirmed Ginger's effectiveness in the treatment of motion sickness; Naval cadets using the herb to fend off sea-sickness had fewer reported incidences of vomiting and cold sweats.[139] In another study, 940 mg of dried Ginger was given to 36 volunteers who were blindfolded and placed in a rotating chair. The group receiving the Ginger lasted 5.5 minutes while the group receiving dimenhydrinate, an anti-histamine used in over-the-counter motion sickness products lasted 3.5 minutes. This shows that Ginger is more effective at reducing nausea and vomiting than pharmaceutical drugs!
- Research demonstrates that Ginger can inhibit Prostaglandins, increase the strength of contraction of the heart, and reduce gastric lesions.
- Recent studies on the use of Ginger for morning sickness during pregnancy concluded that low doses of the herb appeared to be fairly low risk and effective for such treatment.
- Ginger has thermogenic properties (being able to increase the body's metabolism through the generation of heat) and in animal experiments Ginger helped to maintain body temperature and inhibit serotonin induced hypothermia (low body temperature). Gingerol is the most thermogenic compound found in Ginger.[140,141]

GINGER – IN CONCLUSION

Ginger is an extraordinary herbal medicine and it is not surprising that it has been used for thousands of years. Its health benefits extend to a wide variety of body systems. As outlined above, Ginger can help a number of conditions such as abdominal discomfort or nausea, poor digestion and loss of appetite, heart disease, inflammation – something that most of us suffer from if we eat a Western Diet. In addition, Ginger has been shown to be of great use to those who suffer from rheumatoid pain and joint stiffness. Its use is supported by thousands of years of tradition and by modern science and clinical research.

NOT ALL MEDICAL QUALITY GINGER IS EQUAL

As with the other commonly available herbs above, it is essential that you realise that you cannot just go into a supermarket and buy Ginger off the shelf and assume that it has enough of the right quantities of active substances that will be bioavailable and that your body can properly utilise. One of the problems is that herbs and spices can hang around on shop shelves for weeks and during this time they can slowly lose their active, medicinal qualities. As with all of the other herbs discussed in this section, we realise that you may have a problem in selecting the ones that actually work. As with the other herbs, some types of Ginger, even some of those sold as health supplements, can be a waste of money and are almost useless from a health point of view.[142]

Olive Leaf Extract, as the name suggests is a substance that is extracted from the leaves of the olive tree. This extract has a wide number of constituents, including oleuropein and several types of flavonoids (e.g., rutin, apigenin, luteolin). Research is showing that these constituents play a very important and broad spectrum role in health and well-being. One of the reasons for the inclusion of Olive Leaf Extract in this section is the very marked ability of Olive Leaf Extract to prevent viruses from replicating.[143,144]

Another reason for its inclusion is that Olive Leaf Extract has excellent anti-oxidant capabilities.[145,146,147,148,149,150] All of these factors are likely to be of great relevance in preventing and treating Swine Flu although Olive Leaf Extract has not been tested on the H1N1 virus as yet.

One of the most important elements in Olive Leaf Extract is oleuropein. When enzymes in your body process oleuropein it promotes several substantial wellness benefits, which include helping the body battle viruses, bacteria, and fungi. In addition, it supports healthy cell growth and replication, provides anti-oxidant protection to support cardiovascular health and has been shown to improve energy levels.

MORE ABOUT OLIVE LEAF EXTRACT

Olive trees are strongly resistant to damage from insects, bacteria, viruses and fungi and they are not eaten by animals.[151] This is because the tree, its roots, fruit and leaves contain oleuropein, known as an iridoid, which is a polyphenolic fraction – or a plant chemical that is located everywhere in the plant, it is also found in olive oil. There is a chemical called elenolic acid which is found in oleuropein, and it is this that has been found to promote your body's immune defence.

Research studies have found that elenolic acid helps the body to balance levels of "friendly" bacteria and support the immune system. Furthermore, the energy-boosting benefits of Olive Leaf Extract are believed to be the result of its ability to combat fungi, which can sometimes overburden the immune system.

These fungi include Candida Albicans – the yeast that causes infections such as thrush and is implicated in many diverse conditions such as chronic fatigue syndrome. Olive Leaf Extract helps us with the essential process of detoxification at the cellular level, and this is especially important when the body is under stress.

It has also been shown to protect RNA structure – which could be relevant if it becomes important to stop viral RNA (like H1N1) from mutating. This anti-viral activity has been recognised since 1969, when researchers at the Upjohn Company discovered that elenolic acid was the main anti-viral ingredient in Olive Leaf Extract.

Which Herbs Should I Take?

They discovered that the calcium salt of elenolic acid acts as a broad spectrum anti-viral agent and that it was active against every virus they tested.

Elenolic acid basically seems to inhibit the multiplication of potentially any virus. Upjohn scientists also confirmed the exceptional safety of elenolic acid by feeding it to animals in very large amounts – many times greater than needed for anti-viral effects.

As with Resveratrol, the polyphenolic constituent of red wine, oleuropein has some important anti-oxidant benefits that may help prevent the oxidation of LDL – also commonly called "bad cholesterol" which can severely damage the walls of arteries and so oleuropein helps support healthy heart function.

Both Resveratrol and oleuropein are important factors in the acclaimed Mediterranean Diet (which includes olive oil), which research shows to be responsible for the reduced incidence of heart disease in those who follow this diet.[152] (See our Nutrition section for more information about the Mediterranean Diet.)

NOT ALL OLIVE LEAF EXTRACT IS EQUAL

The same caveats apply to Olive Leaf Extract as to the other herbs discussed. We realise that it can be difficult for purchasers to select the best Olive Leaf Extract product – which will deliver enough of the bioavailable, physiologically active quantities of the Olive Leaf Extract that your body can absorb and actually utilise. As with the other herbs, some types of Olive Leaf Extract can be pharmacologically inactive.[153] When purchasing any herbal product it is vital to ensure that it contains a Standardised Extract of the active ingredients.

ADAPTOGENS

In addition, another class of herbs called "adaptogens" may be of great use in a post-viral situation – where people may well be vulnerable to infection from bacteria and other pathogens. Russian Scientist Dr. Nicolai Lazarev invented the word "adaptogen", which refers to a natural herb which has the ability to increase your body's resistance to stresses such as trauma, anxiety and bodily fatigue.

WELL-KNOWN ADAPTOGENS ARE:

- Ginseng
- Rhodiola rosea
- Liquorice
- Ashwagandha

OTHERS ARE:

- Noni
- Suma (Pfaffia paniculata)
- Ginkgo biloba
- Tulsi (Ocimum tenuiflorum)
- Jiaogulan
- Siberian Chag.

Instructions on how to use any of these will be included on their packaging.

Our research into adaptogens continues and we will report any new discoveries that could be helpful in optimising immune health or that are relevant in the fight against Swine Flu in our CMA Monthly Ezine Updates – available through The Complementary Medical Association's website, The-CMA.Org.UK

LAZAREV CREATED THE FOLLOWING GUIDELINES WHICH DICTATE WHETHER AN HERB CAN BE CONSIDERED ADAPTOGENIC:

1. It must cause negligible disruption to your body's physiological functions;

2. It must increase your body's resistance to adverse influences i.e. disease, stress, trauma etc. not by a specific action but by a wide range of physical, chemical, and biochemical factors;

3. It must have an overall "normalising" effect, which improves all kinds of conditions and aggravating none.

WHICH HERBS SHOULD I AVOID?

As we outlined at the beginning of this section, one of our biggest concerns is that ill-informed individuals and organisations are telling people that they need to "boost" their immune systems if they suspect that they have been exposed to Swine Flu. At the risk of repeating ourselves, we reiterate that, in our considered opinion, it is essential that you do not do this!

Any boost to your immune system may well cause the overproduction of cytokines – which, as we know, are involved in the Cytokine Storm phenomenon which is a vicious circle of the production and reproduction of the inflammatory response that can totally overwhelm us.

Our current advice is to avoid Echinacea and Black Elderberry Extract until we have more evidence that the anti-viral activities of both of these outweigh the risks posed by their up-regulation of inflammatory cytokines.[154,155,156,157,158]

We will keep you informed via our CMA Monthly Ezine Updates, available from The Complementary Medical Association's website: The-CMA.Org.UK

AFTER YOU CATCH THE FLU – AND SURVIVE – THAT'S THE TIME TO USE THE IMMUNE BOOSTERS

If people do catch Swine Flu and survive – as most people will, there is a possibility that they may go on to develop an opportunistic infection such as bacterial pneumonia which is also highly lethal – it is at this stage that the so called "immune boosters" may well be of great value.

As we have seen above, herbs that can boost your immune system include Echinacea and Elderberry extract. Another formula that is likely to be of great use in combating post-viral opportunistic infections is a combination of Echinacea and Goldenseal – the Echinacea helps us to produce more of the stem cells that go on to become immune system cells and the Goldenseal is a very effective anti-bacterial herb. [159,160,161,162]

REFERENCES

1 Ugeskr Laeger. 2003 Apr 28;165(18):1868-71.
Effect of Coenzyme Q10 and Ginkgo biloba on warfarin dosage in patients on long-term warfarin treatment. A randomized, double-blind, placebo-controlled cross-over trial; (Article in Danish).
Engelsen J, Nielsen JD, Hansen KF. Klinisk Biokemisk Afdeling, Koagulationslaboratoriet, Amtssygehuset i Gentofte, Niels Andersens Vej 165, DK-2900 Hellerup. jeng@dadlnet.dk

2 FEBS Lett. 2004 Nov 19;577(3):563-9.
Echinacea alkylamides modulate TNF-alpha gene expression via cannabinoid receptor CB2 and multiple signal transduction pathways. Gertsch J, Schoop R, Kuenzle U, Suter A. Swiss Federal Institute of Technology, Institute of Pharmaceutical Sciences, Wolfgang-Pauli-Str. 10 CH-8093 Zurich, Switzerland. juerg.gertsch@pharma.ethz.ch

3 J Virol. 2005 Aug;79(16):10147-54.
p38 mitogen-activated protein kinase-dependent hyperinduction of tumor necrosis factor alpha expression in response to Avian Influenza virus H5N1.Lee DC, Cheung CY, Law AH, Mok CK, Peiris M, Lau AS. Department of Paediatrics and Adolescent Medicine, The University of Hong Kong, Queen Mary Hospital, Pokfulam, Hong Kong Special Administrative Region, People's Republic of China.

4 Isr Med Assoc J. 2002 Nov;4(11 Suppl):919-22.

Comment in: Isr Med Assoc J. 2002 Nov;4(11 Suppl):944-6. The effect of herbal remedies on the production of human inflammatory and anti-inflammatory cytokines. Barak V, Birkenfeld S, Halperin T, Kalickman I. Immunology Laboratory for Tumor Diagnosis, Department of Oncology, Hadassah University Hospital, Jerusalem, Israel. barak845@yahoo.com

5 Eur Cytokine Netw. 2001 Apr-Jun;12(2):290-6.

The effect of Sambucol, a black elderberry based, natural product, on the production of human cytokines: I. Inflammatory cytokines. Barak V, Halperin T, Kalickman I. Immunology Laboratory for Tumor Diagnosis, Department of Oncology, Hadassah University Hospital, Jerusalem, Israel.

6 Please see individual herb sections in this chapter for references to supporting research

7 A service of the National Library of Medicine and the National Institutes of Health and may be accessed at www.ncbi.nlm.nih.gov/entrez

8 Zhou J, Law HK, Cheung CY, Ng IH, Peiris JS, Lau YL. Functional tumor necrosis factor-related apoptosis-inducing ligand production by Avian Influenza virus-infected macrophages. J Infect Dis. 2006 Apr 1;193(7):945-53. Epub 2006 Feb 27.

9 Lee DC, Cheung CY, Law AH, Mok CK, Peiris M, Lau AS. p38 mitogen-activated protein kinase-dependent hyperinduction of tumor necrosis factor alpha expression in response to Avian Influenza virus H5N1. J Virol. 2005 Aug;79(16):10147-54.

10 Cheung CY, Poon LL, Lau AS, Luk W, Lau YL, Shortridge KF, Gordon S, Guan Y,

Peiris JS. Induction of proinflammatory cytokines in human macrophages by Influenza A (H5N1) viruses: a mechanism for the unusual severity of human disease? Lancet. 2002 Dec 7;360(9348):1831-7.

11 Lee DC, Cheung CY, Law AH, Mok CK, Peiris M, Lau AS. p38 mitogen-activated protein kinase-dependent hyperinduction of tumor necrosis factor alpha expression in response to Avian Influenza virus H5N1. J Virol. 2005 Aug;79(16):10147-54.

12 Cheung CY, Poon LL, Lau AS, Luk W, Lau YL, Shortridge KF, Gordon S, Guan Y, Peiris JS. Induction of proinflammatory cytokines in human macrophages by Influenza A (H5N1) viruses: a mechanism for the unusual severity of human disease? Lancet. 2002 Dec 7;360(9348):1831-9.

13 105 studies in PubMed using "Curcumin" and "Lipid Peroxidation" as keywords

14 Sharma OP.

Antioxidant activity of Curcumin and related compounds. Biochem Pharmacol. 1976 Aug 1;25(15):1811-2.

15 Srimal R.C. and Shawan, B.N, (1973). "Pharmacology of Curcumin, a non-steroidal anti-inflammatory agent". J. Clin Pharmacol Ther Toxicol; 24:651-654.

16 Search term used was "Curcumin" and "antiinflammatory"

17 Med Res Rev. 2000 Sep;20(5):323-49.

Current lead natural products for the chemotherapy of human immunodeficiency virus (HIV) infection. De Clercq E. Rega Institute for Medical Research, Katholieke Universiteit Leuven, Belgium. erik.declerq@rega.kuleven.ac.be

18 Mazumder A, Wang S, Neamati N, Nicklaus M, Sunder S, Chen J, Milne GW, Rice WG, Burke TR Jr, Pommier Y. Antiretroviral agents as inhibitors of both human immunodeficiency virus type 1 integrase and protease. J Med Chem. 1996 Jun 21;39(13):2472-81.

19 Jordan WC, Drew CR.

Curcumin--a natural herb with anti-HIV activity J Natl Med Assoc. 1996 Jun;88(6):333.

20 Mazumder A, Raghavan K, Weinstein J, Kohn KW, Pommier Y. Inhibition of human immunodeficiency virus type-1 integrase by Curcumin. Biochem Pharmacol. 1995 Apr 18;49(8):1165-70.

21 Li CJ, Zhang LJ, Dezube BJ, Crumpacker CS, Pardee AB. Three inhibitors of type 1 human immunodeficiency virus long terminal repeat-directed gene expression and virus replication.

Proc Natl Acad Sci U S A. 1993 Mar 1;90(5):1839-42.

22 Park BS, Kim JG, Kim MR, Lee SE, Takeoka GR, Oh KB, Kim JH. Curcuma longa L. constituents inhibit sortase A and Staphylococcus aureus cell adhesion to fibronectin. J Agric Food Chem. 2005 Nov 16;53(23):9005-9.

23 Negi PS, Jayaprakasha GK, Jagan Mohan Rao L, Sakariah KK. Antibacterial activity of Turmeric oil: a byproduct from Curcumin manufacture.J Agric Food Chem. 1999 Oct;47(10):4297-300.

24 Dahl TA, McGowan WM, Shand MA, Srinivasan VS. Photokilling of bacteria by the natural dye Curcumin. Arch Microbiol. 1989;151(2):183-5.

25 Wuthi-udomlert M, Grisanapan W, Luanratana O, Caichompoo W. Antifungal activity of Curcuma longa grown in Thailand. Southeast Asian J Trop Med Public Health. 2000;31 Suppl 1:178-82.

26 Chan MM, Adapala NS, Fong D. Curcumin overcomes the inhibitory effect of nitric oxide on Leishmania. Parasitol Res. 2005 Apr;96(1):49-56.

Epub 2005 Mar 17.

27 Reddy RC, Vatsala PG, Keshamouni VG, Padmanaban G, Rangarajan PN. Curcumin for malaria therapy. Biochem Biophys Res Commun. 2005 Jan 14;326(2):472-4.

28 Araujo CA, Alegrio LV, Gomes DC, Lima ME, Gomes-Cardoso L, Leon LL. Studies on the effectiveness of diarylheptanoids derivatives against Leishmania amazonensis. Mem Inst Oswaldo Cruz. 1999 Nov-Dec;94(6):791-4.

29 Chattopadhyay I, Bandyopadhyay U, Biswas K, Maity P, Banerjee RK. Indomethacin inactivates gastric peroxidase to induce reactive-oxygen-mediated gastric mucosal injury and Curcumin protects it by preventing peroxidase inactivation and scavenging reactive oxygen. Free Radic Biol Med. 2006 Apr 15;40(8):1397-408. Epub 2006 Jan 17.

30 Kim DC, Kim SH, Choi BH, Baek NI, Kim D, Kim MJ, Kim KT. Curcuma longa extract protects against gastric ulcers by blocking H2 histamine receptors. Biol Pharm Bull. 2005 Dec;28(12):2220-4.

31 Swarnakar S, Ganguly K, Kundu P, Banerjee A, Maity P, Sharma AV. Curcumin regulates expression and activity of matrix metalloproteinases 9 and 2 during prevention and healing of indomethacin-induced gastric ulcer. J Biol Chem. 2005 Mar 11;280(10):9409-15. Epub 2004 Dec 22. Erratum in: J Biol Chem. 2005 Aug 19;280(33):29988.

32 Gupta B, Kulshrestha VK, Srivastava RK, Prasad DN. Mechanisms of Curcumin induced gastric ulcer in rats. Indian J Med Res. 1980

Which Herbs Should I Take?

May;71:806-14. No abstract available.
33 Shah BH, Nawaz Z, Pertani SA, Roomi A, Mahmood H, Saeed SA, Gilani AH. Inhibitory effect of Curcumin, a food spice from Turmeric, on platelet-activating factor- and arachidonic acid-mediated platelet aggregation through inhibition of thromboxane formation and Ca^{2+} signaling.
Biochem Pharmacol. 1999 Oct 1;58(7):1167-72.
34 Srivastava KC, Bordia A, Verma SK. Curcumin, a major component of food spice Turmeric (Curcuma longa) inhibits aggregation and alters eicosanoid metabolism in human blood platelets. Prostaglandins Leukot Essent Fatty Acids. 1995 Apr;52(4):223-7.
35 Srivastava R, Puri V, Srimal RC, Dhawan BN. Effect of Curcumin on platelet aggregation and vascular prostacyclin synthesis. Arzneimittelforschung. 1986 Apr;36(4):715-7.
36 Rao DS, Sekhara NC, Satyanarayana MN, Srinivasan M. Effect of Curcumin on serum and liver cholesterol levels in the rat. J Nutr. 1970 Nov;100(11):1307-15. No abstract available.
37 Sreejayan, Rao MN. Curcuminoids as potent inhibitors of lipid peroxidation.J Pharm Pharmacol. 1994 Dec;46(12):1013-6.
38 Kempaiah RK, Srinivasan K. Integrity of erythrocytes of hypercholesterolemic rats during spices treatment. Mol Cell Biochem. 2002 Jul;236(1-2):155-61.
39 Asai A, Miyazawa T. Dietary Curcuminoids prevent high-fat diet-induced lipid accumulation in rat liver and epididymal adipose tissue. J Nutr. 2001 Nov;131(11):2932-5.
40 Babu PS, Srinivasan K. Hypolipidemic action of Curcumin, the active principle of Turmeric (Curcuma longa) in streptozotocin induced diabetic rats. Mol Cell Biochem. 1997 Jan;166(1-2):169-75.
41 Yasni S, Imaizumi K, Nakamura M, Aimoto J, Sugano M. Effects of Curcuma xanthorrhiza Roxb. and Curcuminoids on the level of serum and liver lipids, serum apolipoprotein A-I and lipogenic enzymes in rats. Food Chem Toxicol. 1993 Mar;31(3):213-8.
42 Eur J Cancer. 2005 Sep;41(13):1955-68. Curcumin: the story so far Sharma RA, Gescher AJ, Steward WP. Cancer Biomarkers and Prevention Group, Department of Cancer Studies and Molecular Medicine, University of Leicester, Leicester Royal Infirmary, Leicester LE2 7LX, UK. ras20@le.ac.uk
43 Garrard J, Harms S, Eberly LE, Matiak A. Variations in product choices of frequently purchased herbs: caveat emptor. Arch Intern Med. 2003 Oct 27;163(19):2290-5.
44 Life Sci. 2001 Feb 2;68(11):1317-21. Resveratrol decreases hyperalgesia induced by carrageenan in the rat hind paw. Gentilli M, Mazoit JX, Bouaziz H, Fletcher D, Casper RF, Benhamou D, Savouret JF. Universite de Paris-Sud: Laboratoire d'Anesthesie, UPRES EA392 Faculte de Medecine du Kremlin-Bicetre, Le Kremlin-Bicetre, France.
45 Biochem Pharmacol. 2000 Apr 1;59(7):865-70. Effect of Resveratrol, a natural polyphenolic compound, on reactive oxygen species and prostaglandin production.Martinez J, Moreno JJ.
Department of Physiology, Faculty of Pharmacy, Barcelona University, Spain.
46 Curr Med Chem. 2006;13(9):989-96. Vascular dysfunction in aging: potential effects of Resveratrol, an anti-inflammatory phytoestrogen. Labinskyy N, Csiszar A, Veress G, Stef G, Pacher P, Oroszi G, Wu J, Ungvari Z. Department of Physiology, New York Medical College, Valhalla, New York 10595,
USA. zoltan_ungvari@nymc.edu.
47 Mol Interv. 2006 Feb;6(1):36-47. Resveratrol in cardioprotection: a therapeutic promise of alternative medicine. Das DK, Maulik N. Cardiovascular Research Center, University of Connecticut School of Medicine, Farmington, CT 06030-1110, USA.
48 J Infect Dis. 2005 May 15;191(10):1719-29. Epub 2005 Apr 13. Inhibition of Influenza A virus replication by Resveratrol. Palamara AT, Nencioni L, Aquilano K, De Chiara G, Hernandez L, Cozzolino F, Ciriolo MR, Garaci E. Institute of Microbiology, University of Rome La Sapienza, Rome, Italy.
annateresa.palamara@uniroma1.it
49 Arch Pharm Res. 2003 May;26(5):367-74. Neuraminidase inhibitors from Reynoutria elliptica. Lee CH, Kim SI, Lee KB, Yoo YC, Ryu SY, Song KS. Division of Applied Biology & Chemistry, College of Agriculture & Life Sciences, Kyungpook National University, 1370, Sankyuk-Dong, Daegu 702-701, Korea.
50 N Engl J Med. 2005 Sep 29;353(13):1363-73. Neuraminidase inhibitors for influenza. Moscona A Department of Pediatrics, Weill Medical College of Cornell University, New York, NY 10021, USA. anm2047@med.cornell.edu
51 Mol Pharmacol. 2006 Apr 13; [Epub ahead of print] Resveratrol Suppresses TNF-{alpha}-Induced Fractalkine Expression in Endothelial Cells. Moon SO, Kim W, Sung MJ, Lee S, Kang KP, Kim DH, Lee SY, So JN, Park SK. Chonbuk National University Medical School.
52 Anticancer Res. 2004 Sep-Oct;24(5A):2783-840.
Role of Resveratrol in prevention and therapy of cancer: preclinical and clinical studies. Aggarwal BB, Bhardwaj A, Aggarwal RS, Seeram NP, Shishodia S, Takada Y. Cytokine Research Laboratory, Department of Bioimmunotherapy, The University of Texas M. D. Anderson Cancer Center, Box 143, 1515 Holcombe Boulevard, Houston, Texas 77030, USA. aggarwal@mdanderson.org
53 Biochem Pharmacol. 2000 Apr 1;59(7):865-70. Effect of Resveratrol, a natural polyphenolic compound, on reactive oxygen species and prostaglandin production. Martinez J, Moreno JJ. Department of Physiology, Faculty of Pharmacy, Barcelona University, Spain.
54 Tolomeo M, Grimaudo S, Di Cristina A, Roberti M, Pizzirani D, Meli M, Dusonchet L, Gebbia N, Abbadessa V, Crosta L, Barucchello R, Grisolia G,
Invidiata F, Simoni D. Pterostilbene and 3'-hydroxypterostilbene are effective apoptosis-inducing agents in MDR and BCR-ABL-expressing leukemia cells. Int J Biochem Cell Biol. 2005 Aug;37(8):1709-26. Epub 2005 Apr 26.
55 Atten MJ, Godoy-Romero E, Attar BM, Milson T, Zopel M, Holian O. Resveratrol regulates cellular PKC alpha and delta to inhibit growth and induce apoptosis in gastric cancer cells. Invest New Drugs. 2005 Mar;23(2):111-9. Review.
56 Su JL, Lin MT, Hong CC, Chang CC, Shiah SG, Wu CW, Chen ST, Chau YP, Kuo ML. Resveratrol induces FasL-related apoptosis through Cdc42 activation of ASK1/JNK-dependent signaling pathway in human leukemia HL-60 cells.
Carcinogenesis. 2005 Jan;26(1):1-10. Epub 2004 Jun 24.
57 Wang Q, Li H, Wang XW, Wu DC, Chen XY, Liu J. Resveratrol promotes differentiation and induces Fas-independent apoptosis of human

medulloblastoma cells. Neurosci Lett. 2003 Nov 13;351(2):83-6.

58 Delmas D, Rebe C, Lacour S, Filomenko R, Athias A, Gambert P, Cherkaoui-Malki M, Jannin B, Dubrez-Daloz L, Latruffe N, Solary E. Resveratrol-induced apoptosis is associated with Fas redistribution in the rafts and the formation of a death-inducing signaling complex in colon cancer cells. J Biol Chem. 2003 Oct 17;278(42):41482-90. Epub 2003 Aug 5.

59 Pervaiz S. Resveratrol--from the bottle to the bedside? Leuk Lymphoma. 2001 Feb;40(5-6):491-8. Review.

60 Dorrie J, Gerauer H, Wachter Y, Zunino SJ. Resveratrol induces extensive apoptosis by depolarizing mitochondrial membranes and activating caspase-9 in acute lymphoblastic leukemia cells.Cancer Res. 2001 Jun 15;61(12):4731-9.

61 Bernhard D, Tinhofer I, Tonko M, Hubl H, Ausserlechner MJ, Greil R, Kofler R, Csordas A. Resveratrol causes arrest in the S-phase prior to Fas-independent apoptosis in CEM-C7H2 acute leukemia cells.Cell Death Differ. 2000 Sep;7(9):834-42.

62 Tsan MF, White JE, Maheshwari JG, Bremner TA, Sacco J. Resveratrol induces Fas signalling-independent apoptosis in THP-1 human monocytic leukaemia cells. Br J Haematol. 2000 May;109(2):405-12.

63 Clement MV, Hirpara JL, Chawdhury SH, Pervaiz S. Chemopreventive agent Resveratrol, a natural product derived from grapes, triggers CD95 signaling-dependent apoptosis in human tumor cells. Blood. 1998 Aug 1;92(3):996-1002.

64 Frank B, Gupta S. A review of anti-oxidants and Alzheimer's disease. Ann Clin Psychiatry. 2005 Oct-Dec;17(4):269-86. Review.

65 Anekonda TS, Reddy PH. Neuronal protection by sirtuins in Alzheimer's disease. J Neurochem. 2006 Jan;96(2):305-13. Epub 2005 Oct 7. Review.

66 Chen J, Zhou Y, Mueller-Steiner S, Chen LF, Kwon H, Yi S, Mucke L, Gan L. SIRT1 protects against microglia-dependent amyloid-beta toxicity through inhibiting NF-kappaB signaling. J Biol Chem. 2005 Dec 2;280(48):40364-74. Epub 2005 Sep 23.

67 Marambaud P, Zhao H, Davies P. Resveratrol promotes clearance of Alzheimer's disease amyloid-beta peptides. J Biol Chem. 2005 Nov 11;280(45):37377-82. Epub 2005 Sep 14.

68 Savaskan E, Olivieri G, Meier F, Seifritz E, Wirz-Justice A, Muller-Spahn F. Red wine ingredient Resveratrol protects from beta-amyloid neurotoxicity. Gerontology. 2003 Nov-Dec;49(6):380-3.

69 Draczynska-Lusiak B, Doung A, Sun AY. Oxidized lipoproteins may play a role in neuronal cell death in Alzheimer disease. Mol Chem Neuropathol. 1998 Feb;33(2):139-48.

70 Am J Physiol Heart Circ Physiol. 2005 Mar;288(3):H1131-8. Epub 2004 Oct 21. Inhibition of cardiac fibroblast proliferation and myofibroblast differentiation by Resveratrol. Olson ER, Naugle JE, Zhang X, Bomser JA, Meszaros JG. Department of Physiology and Pharmacology, Northeastern Ohio Universities College of Medicine, Rootstown 44272-0095, USA.

71 Garrard J, Harms S, Eberly LE, Matiak A. Variations in product choices of frequently purchased herbs: caveat emptor. Arch Intern Med. 2003 Oct 27;163(19):2290-5.

72 Lo AH, Liang YC, Lin-Shiau SY, Ho CT, Lin JK. Carnosol, an antioxidant in Rosemary, suppresses inducible nitric oxide synthase through down-regulating nuclear factor-kappaB in mouse macrophages. Carcinogenesis. 2002 Jun;23(6):983-91.

73 Cancer Res. 2002 May 1;62(9):2522-30. Retinoids and carnosol suppress cyclooxygenase-2 transcription by CREB-binding protein/p300-dependent and -independent mechanisms. Subbaramaiah K, Cole PA, Dannenberg AJ. Department of Medicine, New York Presbyterian Hospital-Cornell and Strang Cancer Prevention Center, New York, New York 10021, USA. ksubba@med.cornell.edu

74 Food Chem Toxicol. 1996 May;34(5):449-56. An evaluation of the antioxidant and antiviral action of extracts of Rosemary and Provencal herbs. Aruoma OI, Spencer JP, Rossi R, Aeschbach R, Khan A, Mahmood N, Munoz A, Murcia A, Butler J, Halliwell B. Pharmacology Group, University of London King's College, UK.

75 Valenzuela A, Sanhueza J, Nieto S. Cholesterol oxidation: health hazard and the role of anti-oxidants in prevention. Biol Res. 2003;36(3-4):291-302. Review.

76 Free Radic Res. 2006 Feb;40(2):223-31. Antioxidant and antimicrobial activities of Rosemary extracts linked to their polyphenol composition. Moreno S, Scheyer T, Romano CS, Vojnov AA. Instituto de Investigaciones Bioquimicas, Buenos Aires I.I.B.B.A.-CONICET, Universidad de Buenos Aires, Fundacion Instituto Leloir, Facultad de Ciencias Exactas y Naturales, Patricias Argentinas 435, Buenos Aires, 1405, Argentina. smoreno@leloir.org.ar

77 Cancer Lett. 1995 Sep 4;96(1):23-9. Effects of three dietary phytochemicals from tea, Rosemary and Turmeric on inflammation-induced nitrite production. Chan MM, Ho CT, Huang HI. Department of Biological Sciences, Rutgers, State University of New Jersey, Piscataway 08855-1059, USA.

78 Del Bano MJ, Castillo J, Benavente-Garcia O, Lorente J, Martin-Gil R, Acevedo C, Alcaraz M. Radioprotective-antimutagenic effects of Rosemary phenolics against chromosomal damage induced in human lymphocytes by gamma-rays. J Agric Food Chem. 2006 Mar 22;54(6):2064-8.

79 Cancer Res. 1994 Feb 1;54(3):701-8. Inhibition of skin tumorigenesis by Rosemary and its constituents carnosol and ursolic acid. Huang MT, Ho CT, Wang ZY, Ferraro T, Lou YR, Stauber K, Ma W, Georgiadis C, Laskin JD, Conney AH. Department of Chemical Biology and Pharmacognosy, College of Pharmacy, Rutgers, State University of New Jersey, Piscataway 08855-0789.

80 Asai A, Nakagawa K, Miyazawa T. Antioxidative effects of Turmeric, Rosemary and capsicum extracts on membrane phospholipid peroxidation and liver lipid metabolism in mice. Biosci Biotechnol Biochem. 1999 Dec;63(12):2118-22.

81 Int J Cancer. 2006 Jun 15;118(12):3012-21. Cooperative antitumor effects of Vitamin D(3) derivatives and Rosemary preparations in a mouse model of myeloid leukemia. Sharabani H, Izumchenko E, Wang Q, Kreinin R, Steiner M, Barvish Z, Kafka M, Sharoni Y, Levy J, Uskokovic M, Studzinski GP, Danilenko M. Department of Clinical Biochemistry, Ben-Gurion University of the Negev, Beer-Sheva, Israel.

82 Food Chem Toxicol. 1996 May;34(5):449-56. An evaluation of the antioxidant and antiviral action of extracts of Rosemary and Provencal herbs. Aruoma OI, Spencer JP, Rossi R, Aeschbach R, Khan A, Mahmood N, Munoz A, Murcia A, Butler J, Halliwell B. Pharmacology Group, University of London King's College, UK.

83 Nephrol Dial Transplant. 2000 Aug;15(8):1140-5. Inhibitory effects of rosmarinic acid on the proliferation of cultured murine mesangial cells. Makino T, Ono T, Muso E, Yoshida H, Honda G, Sasayama S. Department of Pharmacognosy, Graduate School of Pharmaceutical

Sciences, Kyoto University, Kyoto, Japan.

84 Free Radic Res. 2006 Feb;40(2):223-31. Antioxidant and antimicrobial activities of Rosemary extracts linked to their polyphenol composition. Moreno S, Scheyer T, Romano CS, Vojnov AA.

Instituto de Investigaciones Bioquimicas, Buenos Aires I.I.B.B.A.-CONICET, Universidad de Buenos Aires, Fundacion Instituto Leloir, Facultad de Ciencias Exactas y Naturales, Patricias Argentinas 435, Buenos Aires, 1405, Argentina. smoreno@leloir.org.ar

85 Int J Tissue React. 2000;22(1):5-13. Biochemical studies of a natural antioxidant isolated from Rosemary and its application in cosmetic dermatology. Calabrese V, Scapagnini G, Catalano C, Dinotta F, Geraci D, Morganti P. Department of Biochemistry, Faculty of Medicine, University of Catania, Italy. Calabrese@mbox.Unict.it

86 al-Sereiti MR, Abu-Amer KM, Sen P. Pharmacology of Rosemary (Rosmarinus officinalis Linn.) and its therapeutic potentials.Indian J Exp Biol. 1999 Feb;37(2):124-30. Review.

87 Garrard J, Harms S, Eberly LE, Matiak A. Variations in product choices of frequently purchased herbs: caveat emptor. Arch Intern Med. 2003 Oct 27;163(19):2290-5.

88 Obstet Gynecol. 2005 Apr;105(4):849-56. Comment in: Obstet Gynecol. 2005 Sep;106(3):640; author reply 640-1. Effectiveness and safety of Ginger in the treatment of pregnancy-induced nausea and vomiting. Borrelli F, Capasso R, Aviello G, Pittler MH, Izzo AA. Department of Experimental Pharmacology, University of Naples Federico II, Naples, Italy. franborr@unina.it

89 Ghayur MN, Gilani AH. Pharmacological basis for the medicinal use of Ginger in gastrointestinal disorders. Dig Dis Sci. 2005 Oct;50(10):1889-97.

90 Koretz RL, Rotblatt M. Complementary and alternative medicine in gastroenterology: the good, the bad, and the ugly. Clin Gastroenterol Hepatol. 2004 Nov;2(11):957-67.

91 Borrelli F, Capasso R, Pinto A, Izzo AA. Inhibitory effect of Ginger (Zingiber officinale) on rat ileal motility in vitro. Life Sci. 2004 Apr 23;74(23):2889-96.

92 Langmead L, Rampton DS. Review article: herbal treatment in gastrointestinal and liver disease--benefits and dangers. Aliment Pharmacol Ther. 2001 Sep;15(9):1239-52. Review.

93 Huang Q, Matsuda H, Sakai K, Yamahara J, Tamai Y. The effect of Ginger on serotonin induced hypothermia and diarrhea. Yakugaku Zasshi. 1990 Dec;110(12):936-42. Japanese.

94 Chrubasik S, Pittler MH, Roufogalis BD. Zingiberis rhizoma: a comprehensive review on the Ginger effect and efficacy profiles. Phytomedicine. 2005 Sep;12(9):684-701. Review.

95 Mascolo N, Jain R, Jain SC, Capasso F. Ethnopharmacologic investigation of Ginger (Zingiber officinale). J Ethnopharmacol. 1989 Nov;27(1-2):129-40.

96 Rababah TM, Hettiarachchy NS, Horax R. Total phenolics and antioxidant activities of fenugreek, green tea, black tea, grape seed, Ginger, Rosemary, gotu kola, and ginkgo extracts, Vitamin E, and tert-butylhydroquinone. J Agric Food Chem. 2004 Aug 11;52(16):5183-6.

97 Blomhoff R. Antioxidants and oxidative stress. Tidsskr Nor Laegeforen. 2004 Jun 17;124(12):1643-5. Review. Norwegian.

98 Murcia MA, Egea I, Romojaro F, Parras P, Jimenez AM, Martinez-Tome M. Antioxidant evaluation in dessert spices compared with common food additives. Influence of irradiation procedure.

J Agric Food Chem. 2004 Apr 7;52(7):1872-81.

99 Lu P, Lai BS, Liang P, Chen ZT, Shun SQ. Antioxidation activity and protective effection of Ginger oil on DNA damage in vitro] Zhongguo Zhong Yao Za Zhi. 2003 Sep;28(9):873-5. Chinese.

100 Park EJ, Pezzuto JM. Botanicals in cancer chemoprevention. Cancer Metastasis Rev. 2002;21(3-4):231-55. Review.

101 Surh YJ. Anti-tumor promoting potential of selected spice ingredients with antioxidative and anti-inflammatory activities: a short review. Food Chem Toxicol. 2002 Aug;40(8):1091-7. Review.

102 Mascolo N, Jain R, Jain SC, Capasso F. Ethnopharmacologic investigation of Ginger (Zingiber officinale).J Ethnopharmacol. 1989 Nov;27(1-2):129-40.

103 Thromb Res. 2003;111(4-5):259-65. Effective anti-platelet and COX-1 enzyme inhibitors from pungent constituents of Ginger. Nurtjahja-Tjendraputra E, Ammit AJ, Roufogalis BD, Tran VH, Duke CC. Herbal Medicines Research and Education Center, Faculty of Pharmacy, University of Sydney, NSW 2006, Australia.

104 Kadnur SV, Goyal RK. Beneficial effects of Zingiber officinale Roscoe on fructose induced hyperlipidemia and hyperinsulinemia in rats. Indian J Exp Biol. 2005 Dec;43(12):1161-4.

105 Sivakumar V, Sivakumar S. Effect of an indigenous herbal compound preparation 'Trikatu' on the lipid profiles of atherogenic diet and standard diet fed Rattus norvegicus. Phytother Res. 2004 Dec;18(12):976-81.

106 Bhandari U, Kanojia R, Pillai KK. Effect of ethanolic extract of Zingiber officinale on dyslipidaemia in diabetic rats. J Ethnopharmacol. 2005 Feb 28;97(2):227-30.

107 Verma SK, Singh M, Jain P, Bordia A. Protective effect of Ginger, Zingiber officinale Rosc on experimental atherosclerosis in rabbits. Indian J Exp Biol. 2004 Jul;42(7):736-8.

108 Akhani SP, Vishwakarma SL, Goyal RK. Anti-diabetic activity of Zingiber officinale in streptozotocin-induced type I diabetic rats.J Pharm Pharmacol. 2004 Jan;56(1):101-5.

109 Fuhrman B, Rosenblat M, Hayek T, Coleman R, Aviram M. Ginger extract consumption reduces plasma cholesterol, inhibits LDL oxidation and attenuates development of atherosclerosis in atherosclerotic, apolipoprotein E-deficient mice. J Nutr. 2000 May;130(5):1124-31.

110 Bhandari U, Sharma JN, Zafar R. The protective action of ethanolic Ginger (Zingiber officinale) extract in cholesterol fed rabbits.J Ethnopharmacol. 1998 Jun;61(2):167-71.

111 Bordia A, Verma SK, Srivastava KC. Effect of Ginger (Zingiber officinale Rosc.) and fenugreek (Trigonella foenumgraecum L.) on blood lipids, blood sugar and platelet aggregation in patients with coronary artery disease. Prostaglandins Leukot Essent Fatty Acids. 1997 May;56(5):379-84.

112 Tanabe M, Chen YD, Saito K, Kano Y. Cholesterol biosynthesis inhibitory component from Zingiber officinale Roscoe. Chem Pharm Bull (Tokyo). 1993 Apr;41(4):710-3.

113 Sambaiah K, Srinivasan K. Effect of cumin, cinnamon, Ginger, mustard and tamarind in induced hypercholesterolemic rats.Nahrung. 1991;35(1):47-51.

114 Srinivasan K, Sambaiah K. The effect of spices on cholesterol 7 alpha-hydroxylase activity and on serum and hepatic cholesterol levels in the rat. Int J Vitam Nutr Res. 1991;61(4):364-9.

115 Kobayashi M, Ishida Y, Shoji N, Ohizumi Y. Cardiotonic action of [8]-Gingerol, an activator of the Ca++-pumping adenosine triphosphatase of sarcoplasmic reticulum, in guinea pig atrial muscle.
J Pharmacol Exp Ther. 1988 Aug;246(2):667-73.

116 Kobayashi M, Shoji N, Ohizumi Y. Gingerol, a novel cardiotonic agent, activates the Ca2+-pumping ATPase in skeletal and cardiac sarcoplasmic reticulum. Biochim Biophys Acta. 1987 Sep 18;903(1):96-102.

117 Shoji N, Iwasa A, Takemoto T, Ishida Y, Ohizumi Y. Cardiotonic principles of Ginger (Zingiber officinale Roscoe).J Pharm Sci. 1982 Oct;71(10):1174-5.

118 Han AR, Kim MS, Jeong YH, Lee SK, Seo EK. Cyclooxygenase-2 inhibitory phenylbutenoids from the rhizomes of Zingiber cassumunar. Chem Pharm Bull (Tokyo). 2005 Nov;53(11):1466-8.

119 Shen CL, Hong KJ, Kim SW. Comparative effects of Ginger root (Zingiber officinale Rosc.) on the production of inflammatory mediators in normal and osteoarthrotic sow chondrocytes. J Med Food. 2005 Summer;8(2):149-53.

120 Grzanna R, Lindmark L, Frondoza CG. Ginger-an herbal medicinal product with broad anti-inflammatory actions.J Med Food. 2005 Summer; 8(2):125-32. Review.

121 Jolad SD, Lantz RC, Chen GJ, Bates RB, Timmermann BN. Commercially processed dry Ginger (Zingiber officinale): composition and effects on LPS-stimulated PGE2 production. Phytochemistry. 2005 Jul;66(13):1614-35.

122 Kim SO, Kundu JK, Shin YK, Park JH, Cho MH, Kim TY, Surh YJ. [6]-Gingerol inhibits COX-2 expression by blocking the activation of p38 MAP kinase and NF-kappaB in phorbol ester-stimulated mouse skin.Oncogene. 2005 Apr 7;24(15):2558-67.

123 Kim SO, Chun KS, Kundu JK, Surh YJ. Inhibitory effects of [6]-Gingerol on PMA-induced COX-2 expression and activation of NF-kappaB and p38 MAPK in mouse skin. Biofactors. 2004;21(1-4):27-31.

124 Frondoza CG, Sohrabi A, Polotsky A, Phan PV, Hungerford DS, Lindmark L. An in vitro screening assay for inhibitors of proinflammatory mediators in herbal extracts using human synoviocyte cultures. In Vitro Cell Dev Biol Anim. 2004 Mar-Apr;40(3-4):95-101.

125 Jolad SD, Lantz RC, Solyom AM, Chen GJ, Bates RB, Timmermann BN. Fresh organically grown Ginger (Zingiber officinale): composition and effects on LPS-induced PGE2 production.
Phytochemistry. 2004 Jul;65(13):1937-54.

126 Thomson M, Al-Qattan KK, Al-Sawan SM, Alnaqeeb MA, Khan I, Ali M. The use of Ginger (Zingiber officinale Rosc.) as a potential antiinflammatory and antithrombotic agent. Prostaglandins Leukot Essent Fatty Acids. 2002 Dec;67(6):475-8.

127 Koo KL, Ammit AJ, Tran VH, Duke CC, Roufogalis BD. Gingerols and related analogues inhibit arachidonic acid-induced human platelet serotonin release and aggregation. Thromb Res. 2001 Sep 1;103(5):387-97.

128 Tjendraputra E, Tran VH, Liu-Brennan D, Roufogalis BD, Duke CC. Effect of Ginger constituents and synthetic analogues on cyclooxygenase-2 enzyme in intact cells.
Bioorg Chem. 2001 Jun;29(3):156-63.

129 Kiuchi F, Iwakami S, Shibuya M, Hanaoka F, Sankawa U. Inhibition of prostaglandin and leukotriene biosynthesis by Gingerols and diarylheptanoids. Chem Pharm Bull (Tokyo). 1992 Feb;40(2):387-91.

130 Suekawa M, Yuasa K, Isono M, Sone H, Ikeya Y, Sakakibara I, Aburada M, Hosoya E. Pharmacological studies on Ginger. IV. Effect of (6)-shogaol on the arachidonic cascade. Nippon Yakurigaku Zasshi. 1986 Oct;88(4):263-9. Japanese.

131 Srivas KC. Effects of aqueous extracts of onion, garlic and Ginger on platelet aggregation and metabolism of arachidonic acid in the blood vascular system: in vitro study. Prostaglandins Leukot Med. 1984 Feb;13(2):227-35.

132 Kiuchi F, Shibuya M, Sankawa U. Inhibitors of prostaglandin biosynthesis from Ginger. Chem Pharm Bull (Tokyo). 1982 Feb;30(2):754-7.

133 Mahady GB, Pendland SL, Stoia A, Hamill FA, Fabricant D, Dietz BM, Chadwick LR. In vitro susceptibility of Helicobacter pylori to botanical extracts used traditionally for the treatment of gastrointestinal disorders. Phytother Res. 2005 Nov;19(11):988-91.

134 Koretz RL, Rotblatt M. Complementary and alternative medicine in gastroenterology: the good, the bad, and the ugly.Clin Gastroenterol Hepatol. 2004 Nov;2(11):957-67.

135 Mahady GB, Pendland SL, Yun GS, Lu ZZ, Stoia A. Ginger (Zingiber officinale Roscoe) and the Gingerols inhibit the growth of Cag A+ strains of Helicobacter pylori. Anticancer Res. 2003 Sep-Oct;23(5A):3699-702.

136 Yoshikawa M, Yamaguchi S, Kunimi K, Matsuda H, Okuno Y, Yamahara J, Murakami N. Stomachic principles in Ginger. III. An anti-ulcer principle, 6-gingesulfonic acid, and three monoacyldigalactosyl-glycerols, Gingerglycolipids A, B, and C, from Zingiberis Rhizoma originating in Taiwan.Chem Pharm Bull (Tokyo). 1994 Jun;42(6):1226-30.

137 al-Yahya MA, Rafatullah S, Mossa JS, Ageel AM, Parmar NS, Tariq M. Gastroprotective activity of Ginger zingiber officinale rosc., in albino rats. Am J Chin Med. 1989;17(1-2):51-6.

138 Yamahara J, Mochizuki M, Rong HQ, Matsuda H, Fujimura H. The anti-ulcer effect in rats of Ginger constituents. J Ethnopharmacol. 1988 Jul-Aug;23(2-3):299-304.

139 Acta Otolaryngol. 1988 Jan-Feb;105(1-2):45-9.
Ginger root against seasickness. A controlled trial on the open sea Grontved A, Brask T, Kambskard J, Hentzer E. Department of Oto-Rhino-Laryngology, Svendborg Hospital, Denmark.

140 Westerterp-Plantenga M, Diepvens K, Joosen AM, Berube-Parent S, Tremblay A. Metabolic effects of spices, teas, and caffeine. Physiol Behav. 2006 Mar 28; [Epub ahead of print]

141 Eldershaw TP, Colquhoun EQ, Dora KA, Peng ZC, Clark MG. Pungent principles of Ginger (Zingiber officinale) are thermogenic in the perfused rat hindlimb. Int J Obes Relat Metab Disord. 1992 Oct;16(10):755-63.

142 Garrard J, Harms S, Eberly LE, Matiak A. Variations in product choices of frequently purchased herbs: caveat emptor. Arch Intern Med.

Which Herbs Should I Take?

2003 Oct 27;163(19):2290-5.

143 Micol V, Caturla N, Perez-Fons L, Mas V, Perez L, Estepa A. The Olive Leaf Extract exhibits antiviral activity against viral haemorrhagic septicaemia rhabdovirus (VHSV). Antiviral Res. 2005 Jun;66(2-3):129-36. Epub 2005 Apr 18.

144 Lee-Huang S, Zhang L, Huang PL, Chang YT, Huang PL. Anti-HIV activity of Olive Leaf Extract (OLE) and modulation of host cell gene expression by HIV-1 infection and OLE treatment. Biochem Biophys Res Commun. 2003 Aug 8;307(4):1029-37.

145 Zaslaver M, Offer S, Kerem Z, Stark AH, Weller JI, Eliraz A, Madar Z. Natural compounds derived from foods modulate nitric oxide production and oxidative status in epithelial lung cells. J Agric Food Chem. 2005 Dec 28;53(26):9934-9.

146 Al-Azzawie HF, Alhamdani MS. Hypoglycemic and antioxidant effect of oleuropein in alloxan-diabetic rabbits. Life Sci. 2006 Feb 16;78(12):1371-7. Epub 2005 Oct 19.

147 Madar Z, Maayan N, Sarit O, Eliraz A. Antioxidants modulate the nitric oxide system and SOD activity and expression in rat epithelial lung cells. Asia Pac J Clin Nutr. 2004;13(Suppl):S101.

148 Farag RS, El-Baroty GS, Basuny AM. Safety evaluation of olive phenolic compounds as natural anti-oxidants. Int J Food Sci Nutr. 2003 May;54(3):159-74.

149 Benavente-Garcia O, Castillo J, Lorente J, Alcaraz M. Radioprotective effects in vivo of phenolics extracted from Olea europaea L.leaves against X-ray-induced chromosomal damage: comparative study versus several flavonoids and sulfur-containing compounds.J Med Food. 2002 Fall;5(3):125-35.

150 Paiva-Martins F, Gordon MH. Isolation and characterization of the antioxidant component 3,4-dihydroxyphenylethyl 4-formyl-3-formylmethyl- 4-hexenoate from olive (Olea europaea) leaves. J Agric Food Chem. 2001 Sep;49(9):4214-9.

151 J AOAC Int. 2004 Jan-Feb;87(1):146-50. A gas chromatographic determination of residues of eleven insecticides and two metabolites on olive tree leaves. Aplada-Sarlis P, Miliadis GE, Liapis K, Tsiropoulos NG. Benaki Phytopathological Institute, Pesticide Residues Laboratory, 7 Ekalis St, 145 61, Kifissia, Greece.

152 Arterioscler Thromb Vasc Biol. 2003 Apr 1;23(4):622-9. Epub 2003 Feb 20. Olive oil and red wine antioxidant polyphenols inhibit endothelial activation: antiatherogenic properties of Mediterranean diet phytochemicals. Carluccio MA, Siculella L, Ancora MA, Massaro M, Scoditti E, Storelli C, Visioli F, Distante A, De Caterina R. C.N.R. Institute of Clinical Physiology, Lecce, Italy.

153 Garrard J, Harms S, Eberly LE, Matiak A. Variations in product choices of frequently purchased herbs: caveat emptor. Arch Intern Med. 2003 Oct 27;163(19):2290-5.

154 Barak V, Birkenfeld S, Halperin T, Kalickman I. The effect of herbal remedies on the production of human inflammatory and anti-inflammatory cytokines. Isr Med Assoc J. 2002 Nov;4(11 Suppl):919-22.

155 Jefferson T. Advances in the Diagnosis and Management of Influenza. Curr Infect Dis Rep. 2002 Jun;4(3):206-210.

156 Lindenmuth GF, Lindenmuth EB. The efficacy of echinacea compound herbal tea preparation on the severity and duration of upper respiratory and flu symptoms: a randomized, double-blind placebocontrolled study. J Altern Complement Med. 2000 Aug;6(4):327-34.

157 Sun LZ, Currier NL, Miller SC. The American coneflower: a prophylactic role involving nonspecific immunity. J Altern Complement Med. 1999 Oct;5(5):437-46.

158 Barak V, Halperin T, Kalickman I. The effect of Sambucol, a black elderberry-based, natural product, on the production of human cytokines: I. Inflammatory cytokines. Eur Cytokine Netw. 2001Apr-Jun;12(2):290-6.

159 Yu HH, Kim KJ, Cha JD, Kim HK, Lee YE, Choi NY, You YO. Antimicrobial activity of berberine alone and in combination with ampicillin or oxacillin against methicillin-resistant
Staphylococcus aureus. J Med Food. 2005 Winter;8(4):454-61.

160 Freile ML, Giannini F, Pucci G, Sturniolo A, Rodero L, Pucci O, Balzareti V, Enriz RD. Antimicrobial activity of aqueous extracts and of berberine isolated from Berberis heterophylla.
Fitoterapia. 2003 Dec;74(7-8):702-5.

161 Hwang BY, Roberts SK, Chadwick LR, Wu CD, Kinghorn AD. Antimicrobial constituents from goldenseal (the Rhizomes of Hydrastis canadensis) against selected oral pathogens.Planta Med. 2003 Jul;69(7):623-7.

162 Cernakova M, Kostalova D. Antimicrobial activity of berberine--a constituent of Mahonia aquifolium. Folia Microbiol (Praha). 2002;47(4):375-8.

163 http://jech.bmj.com/cgi/content/abstract/jech.2008.082198v1

143 Liu S, Song Y, Ford ES, Manson JE, Buring JE, Ridker PM. Dietary calcium, vitamin D, and the prevalence of metabolic syndrome in middle-aged and older U.S. women. Diabetes Care. 2005 Dec;28(12):2926-32.

144 Gloth FM 3rd, Alam W, Hollis B. Vitamin D vs broad spectrum phototherapy in the treatment of seasonal affective disorder. J Nutr Health Aging.1999;3(1):5-7.

145 Lansdowne AT, Provost SC. Vitamin D3 enhances mood in healthy subjects during winter. Psychopharmacology (Berl). 1998 Feb;135(4):319-23.

146 Imazeki I, Matsuzaki J, Tsuji K, Nishimura T. Immunomodulating effect of vitamin D3 derivatives on type-1 cellular immunity. Biomed Res. 2006 Feb;27(1):1-9.

147 Staud R. Vitamin D: more than just affecting calcium and bone. Curr Rheumatol Rep. 2005 Oct;7(5):356-64.

148 Matsuzaki J, Tsuji T, Zhang Y, Wakita D, Imazeki I, Sakai T, Ikeda H, Nishimura T. 1alpha,25-Dihydroxyvitamin D3 downmodulates the functional differentiation of Th1 cytokine-conditioned bone marrow-derived dendritic cells beneficial for cytotoxic T lymphocyte generation. Cancer Sci. 2006 Feb;97(2):139-47.

149 Life Sci. 2006 Mar 27;78(18):2088-98. Epub 2006 Feb 3. Tocotrienols: Vitamin E beyond tocopherols. Sen CK, Khanna S, Roy S. Department of Surgery, Davis Heart and Lung Research Institute, The Ohio State University Medical Center, Columbus, Ohio 43210, USA. chandan.sen@osumc.edu

150 Thevenot T, Di Martino V, Lunel-Fabiani F, Vanlemmens C, Becker MC, Bronowicki JP, Bresson- Hadni S, Miguet JP. [Complementary treatments of chronic viral hepatitis C] Gastroenterol Clin Biol. 2006 Feb;30(2):197-214. French.

151 Thevenot T, Di Martino V, Lunel-Fabiani F, Vanlemmens C, Becker MC, Bronowicki JP, Bresson- Hadni S, Miguet JP. [Complementary

treatments of chronic viral hepatitis C] Gastroenterol Clin Biol. 2006 Feb;30(2):197-214. French.

152 Sprengers D, Janssen HL. Immunomodulatory therapy for chronic hepatitis B virus infection. Fundam Clin Pharmacol. 2005 Feb;19(1):17-26. Review.

153 Med Hypotheses. 2006 Apr 16; [Epub ahead of print] A nutritional supplement formula for Influenza A (H5N1) infection in humans. Friel H, Lederman H. 32 Paradise Road, Northampton, MA 01060, USA.

154 Trends Microbiol. 2004 Sep;12(9):417-23. Host nutritional status: the neglected virulence factor. Beck MA, Handy J, Levander OA. Department of Pediatrics and Nutrition, University of North Carolina at Chapel Hill, Chapel Hill, North Carolina, NC 27599, USA. melinda_beck@unc.edu

155 Jiang Q, Wong J, Fyrst H, Saba JD, Ames BN. gamma-Tocopherol or combinations of vitamin E forms induce cell death in human prostate cancer cells by interrupting sphingolipid synthesis. Proc Natl Acad Sci U S A. 2004 Dec 21;101(51):17825-30. Epub 2004 Dec 13.

156 Min J, Guo J, Zhao F, Cai D. [Effect of apoptosis induced by different vitamin E homologous analogues in human hepatoma cells(HepG2)] Wei Sheng Yan Jiu. 2003 Jul;32(4):343-5. Chinese.

157 McIntyre BS, Briski KP, Gapor A, Sylvester PW. Antiproliferative and apoptotic effects of tocopherols and tocotrienols on preneoplastic and neoplastic mouse mammary epithelial cells. Proc Soc Exp Biol Med. 2000 Sep;224(4):292-301.

158 Galli F, Piroddi M, Iannone A, Pagliarani S, Tomasi A, Floridi A. A comparison between the antioxidant and peroxynitrite-scavenging functions of the vitamin E metabolites alpha- and gammacarboxyethyl-6-hydroxychromans. Int J Vitam Nutr Res. 2004 Sep;74(5):362-73.

159 Baliarsingh S, Beg ZH, Ahmad J. The therapeutic impacts of tocotrienols in type 2 diabetic patients with hyperlipidemia. Atherosclerosis. 2005 Oct;182(2):367-74. Epub 2005 Apr 20.

160 Tomeo AC, Geller M, Watkins TR, Gapor A, Bierenbaum ML. Antioxidant effects of tocotrienols in patients with hyperlipidemia and carotid stenosis. Lipids. 1995 Dec;30(12):1179-83.

161 Qureshi AA, Bradlow BA, Brace L, Manganello J, Peterson DM, Pearce BC, Wright JJ, Gapor A, Elson CE. Response of hypercholesterolemic subjects to administration of tocotrienols. Lipids. 1995 Dec;30(12):1171-7.

162 Lipids. 1995 Dec;30(12):1179-83. Antioxidant effects of tocotrienols in patients with hyperlipidemia and carotid stenosis. Tomeo AC, Geller M, Watkins TR, Gapor A, Bierenbaum ML. Kenneth L. Jordan Research Group, Montclair, New Jersey 07042, USA.

163 Jiang Q, Elson-Schwab I, Courtemanche C, Ames BN. gamma-tocopherol and its major metabolite, in contrast to alpha-tocopherol, inhibit cyclooxygenase activity in macrophages and epithelial cells. Proc Natl Acad Sci U S A. 2000 Oct 10;97(21):11494-9.

164 Vraka PS, Drouza C, Rikkou MP, Odysseos AD, Keramidas AD. Synthesis and study of the cancer cell growth inhibitory properties of alpha-, gammatocopheryl and gamma-tocotrienyl 2-phenylselenyl succinates. Bioorg Med Chem. 2006 Apr 15;14(8):2684-96. Epub 2005 Dec 27.

165 Jiang Q, Wong J, Ames BN. Gamma-tocopherol induces apoptosis in androgen-responsive LNCaP prostate cancer cells via caspase-dependent and independent mechanisms. Ann N Y Acad Sci. 2004 Dec;1031:399-400.

166 Galli F, Stabile AM, Betti M, Conte C, Pistilli A, Rende M, Floridi A, Azzi A. The effect of alpha- and gamma-tocopherol and their carboxyethyl hydroxychroman metabolites on prostate cancer cell proliferation. Arch Biochem Biophys. 2004 Mar 1;423(1):97-102.

167 Khanna S, Roy S, Slivka A, Craft TK, Chaki S,Rink C, Notestine MA, DeVries AC, Parinandi NL, Sen CK. Neuroprotective properties of the natural vitamin E alpha-tocotrienol. Stroke. 2005 Oct;36(10):2258-64. Epub 2005 Sep 15.

168 Sen CK, Khanna S, Roy S. Tocotrienol: the natural vitamin E to defend the nervous system? Ann N Y Acad Sci. 2004 Dec;1031:127-42. Review.

169 Khanna S, Roy S, Ryu H, Bahadduri P, Swaan PW, Ratan RR, Sen CK. Molecular basis of vitamin E action: tocotrienol modulates 12-lipoxygenase, a key mediator of glutamate-induced neurodegeneration. J Biol Chem.2003 Oct 31;278(44):43508-15. Epub 2003 Aug 13.

170 Sen CK, Khanna S, Roy S, Packer L. Molecular basis of vitamin E action. Tocotrienol potently inhibits glutamate-induced pp60(c-Src) kinase activation and death of HT4 neuronal cells J Biol Chem. 2000 Apr 28;275(17):13049-55.

171 Chao JT, Gapor A, Theriault A. Inhibitory effect of delta-tocotrienol, a HMG CoA reductase inhibitor, on monocyte-endothelial cell adhesion. J Nutr Sci Vitaminol (Tokyo). 2002 Oct;48(5):332-7.

172 Theriault A, Chao JT, Gapor A. Tocotrienol is the most effective vitamin E for reducing endothelial expression of adhesion molecules and adhesion to monocytes. Atherosclerosis. 2002 Jan;160(1):21-30.

173 J Gerontol A Biol Sci Med Sci. 2000 Jun;55(6):B280-5. Effects of tocotrienols on life span and Protein carbonylation in Caenorhabditis elegans. Adachi H, Ishii N. Life Science Research Center, Lion Corporation, Kanagawa, Japan. hadachi@lion.co.jp

174 Morris MC, Evans DA, Tangney CC, Bienias JL, Wilson RS, Aggarwal NT, Scherr PA. Relation of the tocopherol forms to incident Alzheimer disease and to cognitive change. Am J Clin Nutr. 2005 Feb;81(2):508-14.

175 Williamson KS, Gabbita SP, Mou S, West M, Pye QN, Markesbery WR, Cooney RV, Grammas P, Reimann-Philipp U, Floyd RA, Hensley K. The nitration product 5-nitro-gamma-tocopherol is increased in the Alzheimer brain. Nitric Oxide. 2002 Mar;6(2):221-7.

176 Nitric Oxide. 2002 Mar;6(2):221-7. The nitration product 5-nitro-gamma-tocopherol is increased in the Alzheimer brain. Williamson KS, Gabbita SP, Mou S, West M, Pye QN, Markesbery WR, Cooney RV, Grammas P, Reimann-Philipp U, Floyd RA, Hensley K. Free-Radical Biology and Aging Research Program, Oklahoma Medical Research Foundation, 825 NE 13th Street, Oklahoma City, OK 73104, USA.

177 Kishimoto C, Tomioka N, Nakayama Y, Miyamoto M. Anti-oxidant effects of coenzyme Q10 on experimental viral myocarditis in mice. J Cardiovasc Pharmacol. 2003 Nov;42(5):588-92.

178 Folkers K, Brown R, Judy WV, Morita M. Survival of cancer patients on therapy with coenzyme Q10. Biochem Biophys Res Commun. 1993 Apr 15;192(1):241-5.

179 Folkers K, Langsjoen P, Nara Y, Muratsu K, Komorowski J, Richardson PC, Smith TH. Biochemical deficiencies of coenzyme Q10 in HIVinfection and exploratory treatment. Biochem Biophys Res Commun. 1988 Jun 16;153(2):888-96.

180 Planta Med. 1992 Oct;58(5):417-23. In vitro virucidal effects of Allium sativum (Garlic) extract and compounds. Weber ND, Andersen DO, North JA, Murray BK, Lawson LD, Hughes BG. Department of Microbiology, Brigham Young University, Provo, Utah 84602.

181 Zhen H, Fang F, Liu ZF, Nie XC, Cui W, Li G. [Effects of allitridin on the expression of human cytomegalovirus immediate early antigens-IE72 and IE86 in human embryonic lung cells] Zhongguo Zhong Yao Za Zhi. 2005 Jan;30(1):47-9.

Which Herbs Should I Take?

182 Liu ZF, Fang F, Dong YS, Li G, Zhen H.Experimental study on the prevention and treatment of murine cytomegalovirus hepatitis by using allitridin. Antiviral Res. 2004 Feb;61(2):125-8.

183 Silverberg N. Pediatric molluscum contagiosum: optimal treatment strategies. Paediatr Drugs. 2003;5(8):505-12.

184 Harris JC, Cottrell SL, Plummer S, Lloyd D. Antimicrobial properties of Allium sativum (Garlic). Appl Microbiol Biotechnol. 2001 Oct;57(3):282-6. Review.

185 Luo R, Dong Y, Fang F. [The experimental study of the anti-enterovirus effects of drugs in vitro] Zhonghua Shi Yan He Lin Chuang Bing Du Xue Za Zhi. 2001 Jun;15(2):135-8.

186 Ankri S, Mirelman D. Antimicrobial properties of allicin from Garlic. Microbes Infect. 1999 Feb;1(2):125-9.

187 Weber ND, Andersen DO, North JA, Murray BK, Lawson LD, Hughes BG. In vitro virucidal effects of Allium sativum (Garlic) extract and compounds. Planta Med. 1992 Oct;58(5):417-23.

188 Esanu V. Research in the field of antiviral chemotherapy performed in the "Stefan S. Nicolau" Institute of Virology. Virologie. 1984 Oct-Dec;35(4):281-93.

189 Esanu V. Recent advances in the chemotherapy of herpes virus infections. Virologie. 1981 Jan-Mar;32(1):57-77.

190 J Nutr. 2001 Mar;131(3s):1054S-7S. The influence of heating on the anticancer properties of Garlic. Song K, Milner JA. Graduate Program in Nutrition and Nutrition Department, The Pennsylvania State University, University Park, PA 16802, USA.

191 Life Sci. 2006 Jan 11;78(7):761-70. Epub 2005 Aug 16. Reactive oxygen species scavenging capacity of different cooked Garlic preparations. Pedraza-Chaverri J, Medina-Campos ON, Avila-Lombardo R, Berenice Zuniga-Bustos A, Orozco-Ibarra M. Facultad de Quimica, Edificio B, Segundo Piso, Laboratorio 209, Departamento de Biologia, Universidad Nacional Autonoma de Mexico (UNAM), Ciudad Universitaria, 04510, Mexico, D.F., Mexico. pedraza@servidor.unam.mx

192 Allison GL, Lowe GM, Rahman K. Aged Garlic extract may inhibit aggregation in human platelets by suppressing calcium mobilization. J Nutr. 2006 Mar;136(3 Suppl):789S-792S.

193 Allison GL, Lowe GM, Rahman K. Aged Garlic extract and its constituents inhibit platelet aggregation through multiple mechanisms. J Nutr. 2006 Mar;136(3 Suppl):782S-788S.

194 Teranishi K, Apitz-Castro R, Robson SC, Romano E, Cooper DK. Inhibition of baboon platelet aggregation in vitro and in vivo by the Garlic derivative, ajoene. Xenotransplantation. 2003 Jul;10(4):374-9.

195 Lanzotti V. The analysis of onion and Garlic.J Chromatogr A. 2006 Apr 21;1112(1-2):3-22. Epub 2006 Jan 18

196 Augusti KT, Narayanan A, Pillai LS, Ebrahim RS, Sivadasan R, Sindhu KR, Subha I, Abdeen S, Nair SS. Beneficial effects of Garlic (Allium sativum Linn) on rats fed with diets containing cholesterol and either of the oil seeds, coconuts or groundnuts. Indian J Exp Biol. 2001 Jul;39(7):660-7.

197 Fugh-Berman A. Herbs and dietary supplements in the prevention and treatment of cardiovascular disease. Prev Cardiol. 2000 Winter;3(1):24-32.

198 Neil A, Silagy C. Garlic: its cardio-protective properties. Curr Opin Lipidol. 1994 Feb;5(1):6-10. Review.

199 Neil A, Silagy C. Garlic: its cardio-protective properties. Curr Opin Lipidol. 1994 Feb;5(1):6-10. Review.

200 Isensee H, Rietz B, Jacob R. Cardioprotective actions of Garlic (Allium sativum). Arzneimittelforschung. 1993 Feb;43(2):94-8.

201 Penner R, Fedorak RN, Madsen KL. Probiotics and nutraceuticals: non-medicinal treatments of gastrointestinal diseases. Curr Opin Pharmacol. 2005 Dec;5(6):596-603. Epub 2005 Oct 7.

202 Katz S. Update in medical therapy of ulcerative colitis: newer concepts and therapies. J Clin Gastroenterol. 2005 Aug;39(7):557-69. Review. Erratum in: J Clin Gastroenterol. 2005 Oct;39(9):843.

203 Pool-Zobel BL. Inulin-type fructans and reduction in colon cancer risk: review of experimental and human data. Br J Nutr. 2005 Apr;93 Suppl 1:S73-90.

204 Le Leu RK, Brown IL, Hu Y, Bird AR, Jackson M, Esterman A, Young GP. A synbiotic combination of resistant starch and Bifidobacterium lactis facilitates apoptotic deletion of carcinogen-damaged cells in rat colon. J Nutr. 2005 May;135(5):996-1001.

205 Lim CC, Ferguson LR, Tannock GW. Dietary fibres as "prebiotics": implications for colorectal cancer. Mol Nutr Food Res. 2005 Jun;49(6):609-19.

206 Ishikawa H, Akedo I, Otani T, Suzuki T, Nakamura T, Takeyama I, Ishiguro S, Miyaoka E, Sobue T, Kakizoe T. Randomized trial of dietary fiber and Lactobacillus casei administration for prevention of colorectal tumors. Int J Cancer. 2005 Sep 20;116(5):762-7.

207 Roller M, Pietro Femia A, Caderni G, Rechkemmer G, Watzl B. Intestinal immunity of rats with colon cancer is modulated by oligofructoseenriched inulin combined with Lactobacillus rhamnosus and Bifidobacterium lactis. Br J Nutr. 2004 Dec;92(6):931-8. Nutrition And Supplements References 281

208 Lewis SJ, Burmeister S. A double-blind placebocontrolled study of the effects of Lactobacillus acidophilus on plasma lipids. Eur J Clin Nutr. 2005 Jun;59(6):776-80.

209 Liong MT, Shah NP. Acid and bile tolerance and cholesterol removal ability of lactobacilli strains. J Dairy Sci. 2005 Jan;88(1):55-66.

210 Brown AC, Valiere A. Probiotics and medical nutrition therapy. Nutr Clin Care. 2004 Apr-Jun;7(2):56-68.

211 Pereira DI, Gibson GR. Effects of consumption of probiotics and prebiotics on serum lipid levels in humans. Crit Rev Biochem Mol Biol. 2002;37(4):259-81.

212 Kiessling G, Schneider J, Jahreis G. Long-term consumption of fermented dairy products over 6 months increases HDL cholesterol. Eur J Clin Nutr. 2002 Sep;56(9):843-9. 213 Nasser M, Wolosker N, Uint L, Rosoky RA, Lobato M, Wajngarten M, Puech-Leao P. Relationship between soluble thrombomodulin in patients with intermittent claudication and critical ischemia. Thromb Res. 2006;117(3):271-7.

214 Thomas SR, Stocker R. Molecular action of vitamin E in lipoProtein oxidation: implications for atherosclerosis. Free Radic Biol Med. 2000 Jun 15;28(12):1795-805.

215 Conri C, Seigneur M, Constans J, Mercier J, Baste JC, Dufourcq P, Boisseau MR. [Evidence of elevated soluble plasma thrombomodulin in atherosclerosis] J Mal Vasc. 1993;18(2):112-8.

216 Tsuda H, Sekine K. Milk Components as Cancer Chemopreventive Agents. Asian Pac J Cancer Prev. 2000;1(4):277-282.

217 Sternhagen LG, Allen JC. Growth rates of a human colon adenocarcinoma cell line are regulated by the milk protein alpha-lactalbumin.

Adv Exp Med Biol. 2001;501:115-20.

218 Hakkak R, Korourian S, Ronis MJ, Johnston JM,Badger TM. Dietary Whey Protein protects against azoxymethane-induced colon tumors in male rats. Cancer Epidemiol Biomarkers Prev. 2001 May;10(5):555-8.

219 Tsuda H, Sekine K, Ushida Y, Kuhara T, Takasuka N, Iigo M, Han BS, Moore MA. Milk and dairy products in cancer prevention: focus on bovine lactoferrin. Mutat Res. 2000 Apr;462(2-3):227-33.

220 McIntosh GH. Colon cancer: dietary modifications required for a balanced protective diet. Prev Med. 1993 Sep;22(5):767-74.

221 Anticancer Res. 1995 Nov-Dec;15(6B):2643-9. The use of a Whey Protein concentrate in the treatment of patients with metastatic carcinoma: a phase I-II clinical study. Kennedy RS, Konok GP, Bounous G,Baruchel S, Lee TD. Department of Surgery, Dalhousie University, Halifax, Nova Scotia, Canada.

222 Eason RR, Velarde MC, Chatman L Jr, Till SR, Geng Y, Ferguson M, Badger TM, Simmen RC. Dietary exposure to Whey Proteins alters rat mammary gland proliferation, apoptosis, and gene expression during postnatal development. J Nutr. 2004 Dec;134(12):3370-7.

223 Sternhagen LG, Allen JC. Growth rates of a human colon adenocarcinoma cell line are regulated by the milk protein alpha-lactalbumin. Adv Exp Med Biol. 2001;501:115-20.

224 Markus CR, Olivier B, Panhuysen GE, Van Der Gugten J, Alles MS, Tuiten A, Westenberg HG, Fekkes D, Koppeschaar HF, de Haan EE. The bovine protein alpha-lactalbumin increases the plasma ratio of tryptophanto the other large neutral amino acids, and in vulnerable subjects raises brain serotonin activity, reduces cortisol concentration, and improves mood under stress. Am J Clin Nutr. 2000 Jun;71(6):1536-44.

225 Matsumoto H, Shimokawa Y, Ushida Y, Toida T, Hayasawa H. New biological function of bovine alpha-lactalbumin: protective effect against ethanoland stress-induced gastric mucosal injury in rats.Biosci Biotechnol Biochem. 2001 May;65(5):1104-11.

226 Ishikado A, Imanaka H, Takeuchi T, Harada E, Makino T. Liposomalization of lactoferrin enhanced it's anti-inflammatory effects via oral administration. Biol Pharm Bull. 2005 Sep;28(9):1717-21.

227 Hayashida K, Kaneko T, Takeuchi T, Shimizu H, Ando K, Harada E. Oral administration of lactoferrin inhibits inflammation and nociception in rat adjuvant-induced arthritis. J Vet Med Sci. 2004 Feb;66(2):149-54.

228 Haversen L, Ohlsson BG, Hahn-Zoric M, Hanson LA, Mattsby-Baltzer I. Lactoferrin down-regulates the LPS-induced cytokine production in monocytic cells via NF-kappa B. Cell Immunol. 2002 Dec;220(2):83-95.

229 Ward PP, Uribe-Luna S, Conneely OM. Lactoferrin and host defense. Biochem Cell Biol. 2002;80(1):95-102.

230 Caccavo D, Pellegrino NM, Altamura M, Rigon A, Amati L, Amoroso A, Jirillo E. Antimicrobial and immunoregulatory functions of lactoferrin and its potential therapeutic application. J Endotoxin Res. 2002;8(6):403-17.

231 Am J Respir Crit Care Med. 2001 Jun;163(7):1591-8. Comment in: Am J Respir Crit Care Med. 2001 Jun;163(7):1516-7. Local inflammatory responses following bronchial endotoxin instillation in humans. O'Grady NP, Preas HL, Pugin J, Fiuza C, Tropea M, Reda D, Banks SM, Suffredini AF. Critical Care Medicine Department, Warren G. Magnuson Clinical Center, National Institutes of Health, Bethesda, Maryland, USA.

232 J Am Coll Nutr. 2001 Oct;20(5 Suppl):389S-395S; discussion 396S-397S. Antiinflammatory activitiesof lactoferrin.Conneely OM.Department of Molecular and Cellular Biology, Baylor College of Medicine, Houston, Texas 77030, USA.orlac@bcm.tmc.edu

233 Biochem Cell Biol. 2002;80(1):95-102. Lactoferrin and host defense. Ward PP, Uribe-Luna S, Conneely OM. Department of Molecular and Cellular Biology, Baylor College of Medicine,Houston, TX 77030, USA.

234 Biochim Biophys Acta. 1994 Jun 23;1213(1):82-90. Lactoferrin inhibits cholesterol accumulation in macrophages mediated by acetylated or oxidized low-density lipoproteins. Kajikawa M, Ohta T, Takase M, Kawase K, Shimamura S, Matsuda I. Nutritional Science Laboratory, Morinaga Milk Industry Company Limited, Kanagawa, Japan.

235 Neurol Neurochir Pol. 2005 Nov-Dec;39(6):482-9. [Lactoferrin in the central nervous system] [Article in Polish] Sacharczuk M, Zagulski T, Sadowski B, Barcikowska M, Pluta R. Zaklad Cytogenetyki Molekularnej, Instytut Genetyki i Hodowli Zwierzat, Polska Akademia Nauk, ul. Postepu 1, 05-552 Jastrzebiec. M.Sacharczuk@ighz.pl

236 Glycoconj J. 2006 Feb;23(1-2):27-37. Role of Sialic Acids in rotavirus infection.Isa P, Arias CF, Lopez S. Departamento de Genetica del Desarrollo y Fisiologia Molecular, Instituto de Biotecnologia, Universidad Nacional Autonoma de Mexico, Cuernavaca, Morelos, 62210, Mexico, pavel@ibt.unam.mx.

237 Wolska K, Rudas P, Jakubczak A. Reduction in the adherence of Pseudomonas aeruginosa to human buccal epithelial cells with neuraminidase inhibition. Pol J Microbiol. 005;54(1):73-6.

238 Wolska K, Rudas P, Jakubczak A. Reduction in the adherence of Pseudomonas aeruginosa to human buccal epithelial cells with neuraminidase inhibition. Pol J Microbiol. 2005;54(1):73-6.

239 Unemo M, Aspholm-Hurtig M, Ilver D, Bergstrom J, Boren T, Danielsson D, Teneberg S. The Sialic Acid binding SabA adhesin of Helicobacter pylori is essential for nonopsonic activation of human neutrophils. J Biol Chem. 2005 Apr 15;280(15):15390-7. Epub 2005 Feb 2.

240 Castaneda-Roldan EI, Avelino-Flores F, Dall'Agnol M, Freer E, Cedillo L, Dornand J, Giron JA. Adherence of Brucella to human epithelial cells and macrophages is mediated by Sialic Acid residues. Cell Microbiol. 2004 May;6(5):435-45.

241 Curr Drug Targets Infect Disord. 2005 Dec;5(4):401-9. Neuraminidase inhibitors as antiviral agents. Alymova IV, Taylor G, Portner A. Department of Infectious Diseases, St Jude Children's Research Hospital, Memphis, TN 38105- 2794, USA.

242 N Engl J Med. 1997 Sep 25;337(13):874-80. Comment in: N Engl J Med. 1997 Sep 25;337(13):927- 8. Efficacy and safety of the neuraminidase inhibitor zanamivir in the treatment of influenza virus infections. GG167 Influenza Study Group. Hayden FG, Osterhaus AD, Treanor JJ, Fleming DM, Aoki FY, Nicholson KG, Bohnen AM, Hirst HM, Keene O, Wightman K. University of Virginia, Charlottesville 22908, USA.

CHAPTER 21

NUTRITION AND SUPPLEMENTS

WHAT FOODS AND SUPPLEMENTS WILL BEST PREPARE ME TO FACE SWINE FLU?

START A HEALTHY DIET – NOW

One of the most important things to do to prepare yourself to be best placed to face a medical threat like Swine Flu is to eat a diet that will help you to become as healthy as possible. This diet needs to incorporate special features that ensure that you are:

> 1) Preparing your immune system to cope at its optimum level with the threat and
> 2) That also, "sets you up", so that you are not as predisposed to 'inflammatory responses' as normal.

This approach is based upon the extensive research we have undertaken in this field and the reason that this is important is because when your body is under attack, as we have seen, your immune system produces an inflammatory response as a way to get lots of white blood cells to wherever they are needed in order to protect your cells. In normal instances this is a vital and helpful response to problems such infection.

However, as we have seen, H1N1 is believed to cause a huge surge of TNFα and other inflammatory cytokines and in certain circumstances, the effect on your body can be overpowering. This incites your body's white blood cells to 'attack' everything – rather than just potentially harmful viruses. Your immune system fails to recognise "Self" i.e. your healthy cells from "Non-Self" i.e. pathogens and infected cells that have already been penetrated by the virus. So, understanding what we can do to calm these responses down in a crisis – or keep them in balance – is crucial to helping you survive a threat like Swine Flu.

The research papers we have analysed indicate that a reduction in pro-inflammatory (inflammation-causing) foods leads to a reduction in your body's production of this inflammatory response – and evidence suggests that establishing this kind of regime in your body may be helpful if you are ever faced with a potentially highly virulent virus such as H1N1, given that part of the potential lethality of H1N1 is due to the Cytokine Storm that your immune system deliberately creates to fight the invader – and which, as we know can, in a worst–case scenario, overwhelm your body, leading to viral pneumonia causing other very dangerous, life-threatening problems such as multiple-organ failure.

"WHY IS MY CURRENT DIET A PROBLEM?"

If you are already eating a healthy, balanced diet you could already be optimally healthy. However, it is worth considering what foods you do eat, to see if there is any room for improvement – and also taking a look at the foods you need to avoid. In many cases, most of us eat what is known as the Western Diet.

The typical Western Diet (as opposed to the Mediterranean Diet for example) is heavily reliant on fat and simple sugars and is 'pro-inflammatory' or inflammation-causing. Scientists now have conclusive proof that this pro-inflammatory diet contributes directly to the initiation and worsening of chronic (long term) inflammation [1,2,3,4,5.] This leads to disorders that are directly related to inflammation and these include joint destruction, diabetes mellitus (i.e. Type 2 diabetes and it can exacerbate the complications of both Type 1 and 2), cardiovascular disease, neuropsychiatric disease (e.g. Alzheimer's and Parkinson's diseases) and some cancers.

In Western society, we are seeing a huge increase in these degenerative diseases and this is due, to a large extent, to the foods and drinks we consume. In fact, medical scientists – and even the UK and US Governments now tell us that 50% of cancers are totally preventable and this is one of the key reasons why we are all told to eat "at least 5 portions of fruit and vegetables each day". In the USA some doctors recommend a higher amount; 9+ portions each day!

One of the problems with Western society is that there is a reliance on convenience foods, which are nutritionally depleted and which do not give us enough of the kinds of vitamins, minerals and other molecules that are essential to our health – but they do provide us with too many of the kinds of chemicals that our bodies don't need, such as pesticides, preservatives, "improvers", flavourings, colorants, "E" numbers, insecticides, fungicides and in fact almost all of these are injurious to our health.

Recently, it has come to light that some additives, while fairly innocuous by themselves, are highly dangerous, even carcinogenic, in combination. In the UK, foods and drinks that contained a combination of Benzoates – a preservative – and Ascorbic Acid (Vitamin C) were found to link together to form Benzines – which are highly carcinogenic substances. The highest levels of Benzines were found in a selection of fruit drinks and these were removed from the market. The FDA in the USA has also been investigating this problem, but has yet to remove any products from the market.

TOO MUCH OF A GOOD THING?

In the Western Diet, there is also an over-abundance of the essential fatty acid, Omega 6 – which is good for us when we take it in the right dosage and when it is mixed in the correct balance with other relevant foods but we tend to get too much of this – and not enough Omega 3 – which is crucial in the fight against inflammation.

This over-representation of Omega 6 can, in fact, actually cause inflammation. In addition, trans fats, simple sugars and starches all contribute to inflammation and are implicated in other health problems. To read more about the effects that trans fats and simple sugars have on our immune system, see the sections on Eating Too Much Sugar and Eating Too Much Fat, in this book.

A particularly deleterious aspect of the typical Western Diet is that it lacks Omega 3 Essential Fatty Acids, vitamins, minerals and phytonutrients – complex nutrients which are derived directly from plants, in their natural state. Omega 3 has vast numbers of health promoting properties and is crucial to our well-being.

The problems posed by the Western Diet were outlined by Dr David Seaman (renowned chiropractic doctor and noted writer on the links between food and inflammation) in 2002 and since then there has been a lot of scientific research about his assertion that the Western Diet is bad for us.[6] Of course it has long been documented that the intake of refined carbohydrates is responsible for many of the major diseases of Western civilisation but we are only just learning exactly why this is so and which dietary components influence which parts of our physiology and health.

1. TOO MUCH SUGAR

Eating too much sugar is one of the very worst things you can do for your immune system. Did you know that the amount of sugar in an ordinary glass of cola is equivalent to TEN teaspoons' worth?

The weakening effects of excessive sugar intake that suppress your immune system, can last for anything up to 5 hours after drinking it?

Sugar consumption is on the rise everywhere. In the USA, for example, official research into the "Standard American Diet" – also known as "S.A.D.", has shown that the average American consumes twice as much as the 'maximum' recommended levels, by taking in 20 teaspoons of added sugar each day. (After all – that is only 2 cans of cola. Many people take in much more than this).

The over-consumption of sugar is becoming standard throughout most industrialised nations. "Added sugar" does not include sugar naturally found in milk and fruit. This over-consumption is on top of the levels of sugar we take in from 'normal' foods.

Underneath all the statistics is the fact that certain sugars, such as polysaccharides and glyconutrients, found in plants such as Aloe Vera etc, are good for you – but only at particular levels. They form a vital part of a healthy diet – but only if you take them in moderation. It's a bit like alcohol consumption. Most doctors now accept that some alcohol – in moderation – can be good for you, but as with alcohol, the problems start when you take in vast amounts, or start "bingeing".

You might look at these consumption levels and think they are really excessive and that they can't possibly apply to you – but just look at how it all adds up. Just 1 can of 'fizzy drink' e.g. cola gives you your daily maximum "recommended allowance!"

- A 12 ounce Pepsi or Coke contains 10 teaspoons of sugar
- A 2 ounce package of sweets/candy contains 11 teaspoons of sugar
- A small bowl of Frosted Flakes cereal provides more than 4 teaspoons of sugar.

While moderate amounts of sugar in your diet are acceptable, there's a problem when high-sugar, low-nutrient food, such as soft drinks, or sweets/candy, replaces more nutritious food such as fruit. These are called "empty calories". These are calorie-dense foods that do not offer much in the way of nutrition, e.g. vitamins/minerals etc. It is surprising how fast all the empty calories add up!

Here are some of the conditions that are linked to high levels of sugar intake:

- Atherosclerosis (hardening of the arteries)
- Panic Attacks/Stress/Anxiety
- Obesity and problems related to obesity
- Adult acne
- Type 2 diabetes

WHAT ARE THE WORST SUGAR OFFENDERS?

SOFT DRINKS

Soft drinks e.g. cola and other fizzy drinks, isotonic "sports" drinks, and to our minds the worst offenders of all are the "Fruit Drinks", that look as if they are "healthy" fruit juice, but are actually diluted fruit juice, with high levels of sugar. Look for the term "Fruit Drink" on the label and avoid these. These generally represent the single largest source of added sweeteners to our diet. They account for one-third of all calories we consume from added sweeteners, which for the average person equals over 23 pounds of sugar from 47.4 gallons of Soft Drinks annually.

SWEETS/CANDY/BISCUITS/COOKIES

Daily and excessive eating of 'treats' like these are energy-sapping, immune-depressing, anxiety-provoking, behaviour-disrupting etc. and contribute to obesity. These are definitely not "treats" and in fact, are very unkind to your body.

HOW TO REDUCE SUGAR IN YOUR DIET

How can we modify our intake of excess 'added sugars' in order to strengthen our immune system?

A. BY DIET

If you are trying to reduce the amount of sugar that you consume, you can't just cut it out and expect everything to be OK. Sugar is a highly addictive substance and is considered by many health practitioners to be **the most insidious drug of the 20th Century** – a period when sugar consumption skyrocketed.

Professionals who deal with addictive behaviour know that you can't rely on will-power alone – you need to modify your behaviour, and find things that you can use as substitutes, to manage this.

When you have a sugar craving, try to eat something that actually provides a sweet flavour but is not just full of empty calories. Try eating dates, apples, sweet potatoes, dried fruits.

See a nutritionist who will be able to help you to figure out if you are craving sweets because your blood sugar levels are not well controlled. This is a condition called hypoglycaemia and is surprisingly common. You can find a qualified nutritionist in the UK, on The Complementary Medical Association's web site: The-CMA.Org.UK

B. EAT MORE FRUIT

Fruit has natural sugars, as well as lots of other 'goodies' your body needs, like natural Vitamin C, and it tastes great, especially if it is fresh. There is an enormous amount of sugar in fruit juices, so fresh fruit is better for you, not least because the fibre in the fruit is full to the brim with amazingly healthy substances, such as bioflavonoids and anti-oxidants. You can read more about these later in this chapter.

C. DRINK MORE WATER
Replace any high sugar drinks (Soft Drinks) with water and you will reap the benefits – see the section on "Hydration" to read about how you should correctly hydrate yourself.

D. TRY COMPLEMENTARY MEDICAL APPROACHES
Treatments like acupuncture – which have been used to control addictions for years – have been shown to be a help in getting people to eat less sugar. Certain nutritional supplements seem to be able to help balance sugar levels for some people. These include Chromium Picolinate, B Complex vitamins and the herb, Gymnema, which can put on your tongue to reduce your ability to taste sweet things – thus reducing cravings.

"WHY IS SUGAR SO BAD FOR ME?"

When you consume anything that comes into the category of a 'refined carbohydrate' e.g. sweets/candy, white bread/flour/rice and fruit juice, there is a very rapid rise in the glucose levels in your blood.

Your body immediately produces insulin to counter this rise and to metabolise the sugar. (The pancreas of the Type 1 diabetic does not produce insulin, which is why Type 1 diabetics have to inject this hormone and Type 2 diabetics are either insulin-resistant or produce very little insulin and therefore they need to take anti-diabetic medication).

It is well known that an increase in consumption of 'simple sugars' leads to an increase in 'oxidative stress'. Put simply, this is the increase of harmful oxidants (also called "free-radicals") in the blood stream that cause systemic damage. This oxidative stress is often countered by taking anti-oxidants, such as Vitamins A, C and E, bioflavonoids and minerals such as Selenium. (This is not to say that anti-oxidants can undo all the damage that excess sugar consumption causes and taking anti-oxidants is not a licence to over-indulge!)

The oxidative stress from sugar consumption has also been shown to suppress your immune system because it inhibits neutrophil-mediated phagocytosis i.e. it prevents certain key white blood cells from being able to efficiently "gobble up" harmful bacteria and viruses.

In addition, it has only recently been shown that simple sugar consumption (sugar, refined carbohydrates etc. containing 75 grammes, or 300 calories of glucose), directly promotes inflammation and that this leads to the production of chondrolytic enzymes such as MMP-2 and MMP-9. The presence of higher levels of these specific enzymes is now believed to promote the progression of joint destruction in diseases such as arthritis[7].

2. EATING TOO MUCH FAT

Our immune systems are badly affected by overeating, eating the wrong foods, obesity and rapid weight gain. There are certain elements of our diet that are particularly immune-depressing and these include the "wrong" kinds of fat. Most experts agree that we shouldn't take in more than 30% of our calories as fat and only 10% of our total caloric intake should be provided by saturated fats. Saturated fats are found in fatty meat, cooking oils and dairy foods, including milk and cream. Aside from its deleterious effects upon our immune system, saturated fat tends to increase blood cholesterol levels. Most saturated fats are solid at room temperature, with the exception of tropical oils such as coconut and palm oil.

THE REALLY "BAD" FATS – TRANS FATS (PARTIALLY HYDROGENATED OILS)

Your immune system is subjected to all kinds of onslaughts each moment of each day and many of these are unavoidable. However, there is a particular type of fat that is damaging to health and certainly should be avoided at all costs. This fat is so harmful to health, that foods that contain it – in the USA at least – must declare that fact on their labels.

As long ago as the late 19th century, scientists discovered a new product that would revolutionise the food industry. Chemists found out that they could change liquid vegetable oil into a solid or semi-solid by adding hydrogen atoms to the oil's "backbone". They achieved this by bubbling hydrogen gas through vegetable oil in the presence of a nickel catalyst. This created "partially hydrogenated fat".

This was a major breakthrough, as up until that time, food manufacturers had to use oils that had a very brief shelf life and spoiled easily. The new fats could also resist repeated heating without breaking down. These characteristics were very appealing to food manufacturers.

After a while everyone jumped on the "partially hydrogenated" bandwagon and over time, these partially hydrogenated oils became a foundation ingredient in margarines, commercially baked goods and high fat snack foods. At this time also, saturated fat, such as butter and lard was blamed for causing a range of ailments including heart disease and high cholesterol. So, many fast food companies such as McDonalds and Dunkin Donuts that previously used to fry their products in beef fat switched to the "more healthy" option – partially hydrogenated oils.

This "healthy-seeming" conversion from saturated fat to partially hydrogenated fats, appeared to be a great option and these food companies were applauded for supplying "healthier" products. So, the intake of trans fat increased dramatically. Before the invention of partial hydrogenation, humans did eat trans fats but these came from eating beef (and dairy products) and lamb - and of course those meats would have been organic at that time.

Ruminant's (e.g. cows) fore-stomachs are home to a type of bacteria that creates trans fats – but only in small quantities. So this was not a significant – or indeed – particularly worrying, source of trans fats. However, by the early 1990s, trans fat intake in the United States alone averaged 4–7% of calories from fat.

As long ago as 1981, researchers in Wales speculated that trans fats might be linked to heart disease. Then, twelve years later in 1993, a Harvard study strongly supported the hypothesis that intake of partially hydrogenated vegetable oils (trans fats) contributed to the risk of having a heart attack. In the Harvard study, the scientists proposed that substituting just 2% of energy from trans fat with healthy unsaturated fat (such as olive oil and Omega 3 rich oils) would decrease the risk of coronary heart disease by about one-third. The public finally became aware of the problem in the early nineties.

WHAT DO TRANS FATS ACTUALLY DO TO US?

Today we know that eating trans fats increases levels of low-density lipoprotein (LDL, also called "bad" cholesterol). Worryingly, it particularly increases the small, dense LDL particles that cause the most damage to arteries. In addition, trans fats also lower our levels of high-density lipoprotein (HDL or "good" cholesterol) particles, which act like scouring pads in our blood vessels. They scrub "bad cholesterol" up and transport it to our liver for safe disposal.

Trans fats also increase the risk of us getting blood clots which can block arteries and this can cause strokes. Trans fats also cause inflammation – which is an overreaction of the immune system that has been implicated in heart disease, stroke, diabetes, and other chronic conditions. As we know – the process that underlies inflammation is also implicated in our body's excessive and uncontrolled immune response – the Cytokine Storm.

3. AS IF THAT WASN'T BAD ENOUGH... CONTAMINANTS IN FOOD

It is possible that contaminants in food – which are often stored in the food's naturally occurring oil – are more responsible for causing us harm than the food itself. Beef in the UK still contains artificial hormones. Wild fish can be heavily contaminated with toxic heavy metals like mercury and farmed fish can contain anti-fungal chemicals and pesticides. Non-organic vegetables contain pesticide and insecticide residues. Some physiologists suggest that our bodies store fat-soluble toxins such as these in our own fat – it's a bit like our body's toxic dumping ground.

There are hypotheses – yet to be proven – which propose that one of the many reasons for the current obesity epidemic is that we are taking in so many toxins which are fat-soluble that our bodies have to "lay down extra fat reserves" just to keep these toxins "out of the way". The jury is out on these hypotheses but they do have a ring of possible truth about them.

If you want to know whether your fat consumption is within the guidelines, you'll have to do your sums. On food labels, the content of total fat and saturated fat (and trans fats as well – which you really should avoid!) is listed as a percentage of recommended daily intake. Keep a running tab of the percentage you consume each time you eat, so you'll know when you reach your safe limit. The total fat in your diet should average no more than 30 percent of your calories and saturated fat should be no more than 10 percent. The total fat and saturated fat grams you should eat depend on how many calories you consume each day – which will vary from person to person – according to sex, weight and activity levels.

4. DRINKING TOO MUCH ALCOHOL

Research shows that consuming excess alcohol can be a factor in causing and exacerbating health problems like chronic stress, anxiety and depression. It also weakens your immune system. Alcohol is seen as being socially acceptable to consume, but in reality, it is a toxic drug and has widespread negative effects on our biochemistry – (and therefore our well-being) – when consumed at all. This is true especially when alcohol is consumed to "excess".

Any alcohol consumption has a direct effect on the chemistry of your body. When we speak of the deleterious effects of alcohol on your body, we are not talking about people who are 'alcoholics' – people who can't get through a day without resorting to alcohol. We are talking about ordinary people – who may not drink every day – but who drink at what they believe are normal levels. We are also talking about people who see no harm in the occasional resort to 'binge drinking'.

So, if you drink, it is vital that you control your intake to currently recommended levels – or give it up completely – in order to recover your optimal physical and psychological health. This is especially important in the light of what alcohol actually does to your immune system.

Both anecdotal and doctor's reports from the 1918 Spanish Flu pandemic show that people who decided "they couldn't care less" and if they were going to catch the flu, "so be it" – and carried on drinking – sometimes even more heavily than before, suffered a higher death rate than other people.

One of the problems with alcohol is that we are given very mixed information by less responsible sectors of the media who will latch onto and sometimes exaggerate the latest medical missive. In order to sell newspapers, the message can become distorted. So, it is not always clear just what the acceptable levels of alcohol actually are.

SO, HOW MUCH ALCOHOL REALLY IS "SAFE"?

The current Health Education Association alcohol safety guidelines for the UK are currently:
- 21 units per week for men
- 14 units per week for women (but no alcohol if pregnant).

WHAT IS A UNIT OF ALCOHOL?

- A half a pint (.28 litres) of ordinary beer (not strong)
- A pub measure of spirit (30ml / 1 liquid Oz US))
- A small size glass of wine (100ml / 3.31 liquid Oz US)

It is also recommended that – if you do drink – you should spread these drinks throughout the week. Some people go on a massive binge and use up the 21 units of alcohol recommended per week, over a day or two, which research has shown to be very harmful. Most doctors now agree that one glass of red wine per day can actually be beneficial due to it's antioxidant properties – not due to it's alcohol content! As discussed in our Chapter on Herbs, red wine contains a substance called "Resveratrol", which research has found to give great health benefits. So, one glass of red wine is fine for this reason but do remember that it is not actually the alcohol content of the wine that is helpful.

One word of warning about wine. Most wines contain preservatives called sulphites or sulfites. Sulphites are a commonly used preservative found in foods, alcoholic drinks (especially wines) and even in medicines. They have anti-oxidant properties and are often used to stop things from browning, e.g. salad leaves in salad bars, or on dried fruit e.g. apricots, so that they retain their colour and do not go wrinkly and stiff. About 1% to 2% of people can have an allergic reaction to sulphites, which can include nasal congestion and sneezing, skin rash, wheezing and problems with breathing. It is possible for some people to have a serious life-threatening reaction to sulphites which causes severe swelling of the throat, tongue and respiratory tract and this obstructs breathing. At least four deaths caused by reactions to sulphites have been recorded. Sulphites are found in many products, so someone who has experienced a severe reaction should carry an adrenalin injection kit – like the types used by people with any other serious allergy. If you suspect that you have problems with sulphites it is possible to ask your doctor to refer you for tests.

Anything more than one unit of alcohol can damage your immune system and lead to a depletion in your essential white blood cells. As we know, white blood cells are at the heart of our 'defence system' against disease. They are the T-cells and B-cells we discussed earlier – as well as the

NK-cells and the Macrophages that fight off pathogens like the influenza virus.

NEGATIVE EFFECTS OF ALCOHOL ON BODY AND BRAIN CHEMISTRY

Alcohol can and does have a potentially powerful and mostly negative effect on brain and body biochemistry if consumed in excessive amounts. It can cause or worsen stress, depression and anxiety. Alcohol is a chemical stressor and it causes your body to release stress hormones including adrenaline and cortisol. If you already have heightened levels of these stress hormones, the alcohol will make them higher. It does this by stimulating your sympathetic nervous system and your adrenal glands. This leads us into a vicious circle – with the end results being a cascade of increasing depression and anxiety. Another way in which alcohol can increase anxiety is by its effect on lactic acid. Alcohol increases our levels of lactic acid and research indicates that increased lactic acid levels may be an underlying factor in anxiety and panic attacks.

Although alcohol can seem to raise your mood – this is only a temporary gain. It does this by momentarily increasing the levels of your mood enhancing "feel good" chemicals such as serotonin. However there is a see-saw effect and after the temporary serotonin boost, the levels of this chemical plummet and this leads to you feeling depressed. So, you need to use alcohol in larger and larger amounts to re-create the initial high that you get after the first drink.

Certain nutrients are needed by your body in order for it to manufacture chemicals that suppress anxiety, but alcohol makes it difficult for us to utilise some of these nutrients like Vitamins B6 and Folic Acid. Your body needs these important nutrients in order to be in optimum psychological health to enable you to cope with stress.

ALCOHOL AND IMMUNITY

Because alcohol stimulates the release of the stress hormones adrenaline and cortisol, this interferes with the amino acid tryptophan, which is used to manufacture serotonin. Cortisol and adrenaline are intimately implicated in suppressing our immune system's response – this renders us far more susceptible to infection from viruses, bacteria and other pathogens. In addition, these hormones are implicated in the inflammatory response which is so deleterious to health.

ALCOHOL AND OBESITY

Many types of alcoholic drink are full of refined sugar, which is how alcohol can contribute to obesity. Obesity in itself can lead to a suppressed immune response and this makes obese people more vulnerable to viruses etc. In order to be optimally resistant to viruses you need to make sure that you are at the correct healthy weight for your height. If you are obese, or heading that way, do talk to a qualified nutritionist, who will help you to return safely to a healthy weight.

PEOPLE WITH ALCOHOL ADDICTIONS ARE AT A GREATER RISK FROM SWINE FLU

A report published by the Institute of Alcohol Research said that nearly two million people in the UK have an alcohol problem and can't get through a day without consuming alcohol. That's around one in twenty adults. Ask many people and they will say that they are concerned about the level of drug abuse in modern society, yet twice as many people are addicted to alcohol compared to other drugs. Because alcohol is socially acceptable, it is not seen as a drug. However, it is a highly addictive substance and alcohol addiction is an illness.

5. TOO MUCH WHEAT

Other parts of the typical Western Diet include high consumption of wheat, which many people report sensitivities to. These sensitivities can include migraine headaches and in recent experiments, the wheat protein, gliadin, was shown to produce a pro-inflammatory effect as it activates production of NF-KappaB, which leads to inflammation.

6. TOO MUCH ARACHIDONIC ACID: "SUPER-SIZE ME!"

Rich sources of arachidonic acid include cow's milk, beef, liver, pork and other animal products.

Research shows that **meat from grain-fed animals is one of the biggest sources of arachidonic acid** which acts as a precursor to the production of inflammatory chemicals in your body including Prostaglandins and Leukotrienes which have been shown to promote and perpetuate disease processes that end up, symptomatologically as atherosclerosis, cancer, arthritis and joint destruction.

It is important to realise that inflammation is a natural, defensive process which should, under normal healthy conditions, protect us. However, if we eat a diet that does not provide us with the nutrients that we need to be healthy, the inflammatory response can go wrong – and this process is kick-started by numerous possible factors. These factors include sugar, radiation, infection, alcohol, trans fats, injury, over-exercise, and any other factor that causes a "stress" reaction to occur. Each of these stimuli may lead to the activation of the "NF-KappaB Cascade".

This term describes the pathway that the inflammatory response follows. NF-KappaB is found in the cells of your body and from there it can promote the activation of genes that cause inflammation.

NF-KappaB is extremely important in the inflammatory process and can be thought of as an intracellular (inside your cells) "amplifier" that increases the production of the direct mediators of inflammation – such as Cytokines, Prostaglandins and Leukotrienes which are implicated in the process of inflammation (see Your Immune System and the Cytokine Storm).

The Survivor's Guide to Swine Flu

The NF-KappaB cascade is linked to both "Chronic" and "Acute" inflammatory processes.

"Chronic" inflammation is long standing and causes degenerative diseases and "Acute" inflammation is fast acting – and may be produced by your body in response to an injury or as a way of dealing with an infection i.e. viral or bacterial. In order to help prepare your immune system to be as resistant as possible to any infection – including Swine Flu – you have to reduce any chronic inflammation that you may already have so that you can become as fit and well as possible.

A fascinating experiment was reported in 2004 in the highly respected American Journal of Clinical Nutrition, where the test subjects were given a single meal of egg and sausage muffin with two hash browns. The documented increase in NF-KappaB after the meal was 150% and this enormous increase in NF-KappaB lasted for a full two hours after the meal.

The 150% increase in NF-KappaB was also associated with an increase in oxidative stress and an increase in the inflammatory marker CRP (C Reactive protein – this is a protein that is measured in blood tests to ascertain the presence of inflammation).

No doubt, anyone who has seen the film "Super-Size Me" will be able to relate to this. If you have not seen this excellent film, here's a quick recap to explain that documentary film maker Morgan Spurlock decided to try to live on three MacDonald's meals per day for thirty days – taking the "Super-Size" option whenever it was offered to him.

Spurlock started out fitter than average and by the end of the 30 day period he was in very poor health indeed. He gained 25 pounds (11 kg), suffered severe liver dysfunction and developed symptoms of depression. Spurlock's supervising doctors noted the effects caused by his high-saturated fat, high-refined carbohydrate diet and one even compared it to a case of severe binge alcoholism.

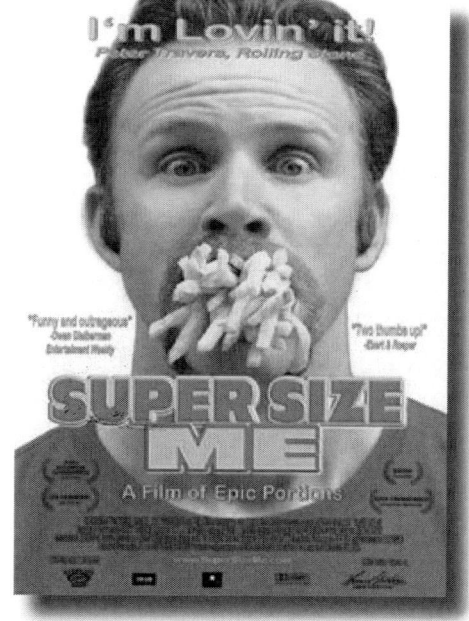

Of course, it is highly unlikely that people would actually eat fast food three times a day and nothing else – or is it? Teenage boys in the film actually said that in fact they were likely to eat fast food more than once a day.

The scientific data that we have nowadays indicates – quite compellingly – that the standard Western Diet, which is simple-carbohydrate rich (refined flour and sugars), and high in arachidonic-rich animal products, milk and wheat – will promote inflammation.

This inflammation will in turn, promote pain, free-radical damage, immune system suppression and many other diseases that are related to inflammatory processes. When taking all these factors into consideration it becomes obvious that it makes absolute sense to address these dietary factors in people who are suffering from the results of inflammatory disease, before subjecting them to medication that may have harmful side effects. Unfortunately, very few people who suffer from inflammatory based diseases are ever given sound nutritional advice that could be of enormous benefit to them.

6. TOO MUCH DAIRY FOOD?

Cow's milk is also another major part of the Western Diet and this too can cause many problems and not just for those who are lactose intolerant. These problems can include migraines, otitis media (middle ear infection) and joint inflammation.

Cow's milk is not an ideal human "food" as its actual purpose is to feed calves – not humans, or human babies. Most adults are sensitive to lactose – the type of sugar that is in milk – to a greater or lesser extent and this can cause a number of problems ranging from abdominal discomfort to bloating, diarrhoea, constipation and many other allergy-type reactions, such as eczema, and even asthma in some people.

Of course, milk does contain calcium which is good for us – but weight-for-weight - there are many comparable sources of calcium that have better overall health benefits than milk. One example of this would be sardines and other oily fish (if eaten with their bones). Also green vegetables such as broccoli contain large amounts of calcium.

On a more positive note – Scottish scientists have recently discovered that although milk does contain healthy Omega 3 Essential Fatty Acids, the levels of Omega 3 in organic milk are up to 71% higher and contain a healthier ratio of Omega 3 to Omega 6. Nevertheless, there are other, better, sources of Omega 3 available that do not come with the burden of lactose and the inflammation-causing arachidonic acid.

WHY CAN MILK CAUSE INFLAMMATION?

Milk is a rich source of emulsified arachidonic acid and as we have seen, this acts as a precursor to the production of chemicals called Prostaglandins and Leukotrienes. We do need both Prostaglandins and Leukotrienes for good health – they help to protect us by causing inflammation, which can help us to fight off pathogens – invaders, such as viruses, or bacteria, that could otherwise harm us. However, occasionally this inflammatory response is not helpful to us as it can get over produced – and even in an acute infection, lead to an overwhelming inflammatory response – the Cytokine Storm.

On the other hand there is a type of inflammation called chronic inflammation which means that the inflammation is long-lasting and causes big problems for our health as it is linked to diseases such as cancer, diabetes, cardio-vascular illnesses and arthritis and inflammation is also linked to premature ageing.

So, as we have seen above – Prostaglandins and Leukotrienes are highly pro-inflammatory and they can also cause other problems as they are 'Bronchospastic' – i.e. they cause airflow limitation and can therefore cause breathing difficulties due to the contraction of the smooth airway muscle. They are also 'vasodilatory' i.e. they can cause excessive relaxation or dilation of the blood vessel walls. The resulting low blood pressure that this causes creates an inadequate blood supply to your body's cells, which can result in shock as blood pressure becomes too low to sustain life.

As if all this was not bad enough – certain Prostaglandins (written as PG) and Leukotrienes (written as LT) also have pain enhancing and joint destroying properties via Prostaglandin-E2 (PG-E2), PG12 and PGF2a, Leukotriene-B4 and a chemical called 5HETE (5HETE is sometimes called the "cancer food" as some cancer cells feed off this).

GOOD COWS. BAD COWS?

Article taken from The CMA e-Newsletter July 2009:
(To sign up for the monthly e-Newsletter visit The CMA website; The-CMA.Org.UK)

A recent book - The Devil in the Milk - by Dr. Kevin Woodford, looks at the health-related effects of our consumption of milk, and milk-derived products, in some depth, taking evidence from more than 100 scientific papers examining population studies and research in both animals and humans as well as scientific research on various conditions.

At the heart of the findings is the fact that there are in this world, two types of cows: A1 cows (bad cows) and A2 cows (good cows).

Woodford obviously knows what he is talking about as he is the Professor of Farm Management and Agribusiness at Lincoln University (New Zealand) and he points out the key difference between A1 and A2 cows is in a protein they each express differently; beta casein.

Woolford points out - having examined all the epistemological evidence from 10 countries - that milk that comes from A1 cows has a version of this protein that is implicated in the development of a range of diseases - from Type 1 diabetes to autism, from schizophrenia to heart disease.

Milk that comes from A2 cows is "Not Guilty", as it does not have this particular adaptation to its beta casein.

So, high intake of milk (and milk products) from A1 cows is bad for your health!

Beta casein is a protein chain with 229 amino acids and branches coming off it. They have identified a specific site, at number 27 on this chain, where in A2 cows, "good cows", an amino acid called proline branches off it.

The good A2 cows, that he describes as 'old-fashioned' cows, include breeds such as Guernseys, Jerseys, Asian and African cows.

About 5,000 years ago a mutation occurred at the proline site, which converted the proline to histadine. So the 'bad cows' - the A1 cows - include more recent breeds of cows, like Holsteins and Friesians.

This is where it gets interesting! This side chain coming off of this histidine turns out to be a powerful opiate, or narcotic known as BCM7 (beta-casomorphin-7). It is also an oxidant.

BCM 7 is associated with milk intolerance and a range of auto-immune diseases including Type 1 diabetes and is linked to findings that it is implicated in autism and schizophrenia.

When BCM7 has been injected into rats it was taken into 32 different areas in the brain, including those for vision, communication and hearing, although scientists believe that the initial response to BCM7 occurs in the gut. Given that the sensory areas are so affected by BCM7, this could explain why they began to exhibit autistic spectrum phenomena such as being oblivious to external sounds.

http://articles.mercola.com/sites/articles/archive/2008/01/02/milk-linked-to-autism.aspx
http://www.naturalnews.com/026684_cows_diabetes_casein.html

THE DIETARY SOLUTION

We have extensively researched the many and varied diets that exist, in order to ascertain which of these would be most relevant in creating optimal immune wellness, and simultaneously promoting an anti-inflammatory effect in our bodies, in order to best prepare against an attack from Swine Flu (H1N1).

There is a lot of confusion surrounding all of the diets that are available and it is a complete minefield for the lay person who is not nutritionally trained, as so many commercially successful diets are aggressively hyped in the media but do not necessarily provide any real health benefits. We have discovered that one of the very best and most effective anti-inflammatory, health promoting diets is the "Paleo-Mediterranean Diet" [8,9,10,11,12,13] as proposed by Dr Alex Vasquez, a highly respected doctor and noted researcher in the field of inflammatory response.

This diet is a combination of the Palaeolithic Diet [14,15,16,17,18,19] and the Mediterranean Diet, for which there are over 1,688 cited studies in PubMed, but see References at the end of this Chapter for just a small selection of illustrative papers. [20,21,22,23,24,25,26,27]

The combination of the Palaeolithic and Mediterranean Diets have a vast number of health benefits ranging from preventing inflammation – which as we have seen – leads to degenerative diseases that include some cancers, heart disease, arthritis and diabetes – and as an added advantage is that it will help you to normalise your weight.

Many doctors and scientists who support this diet also believe that it will help you to look better too. This is because the inflammatory response that we are prone to if we eat a standard Western Diet is also a key factor in the ageing process – and the "recommendations" outlined below could also be classed as an anti-ageing programme.

In fact, it is never too late to change your diet for the better. One large study followed a group of elderly people for ten years. At the start of the study they were aged between 70 and 90. The ten year outcome of the study demonstrated that by following the Mediterranean Diet, their death rate from cardio-vascular disease, cancer, heart disease and other causes was reduced by over 50% compared to people who did not follow this diet [28].

"WHAT IS THE 'PALÆOLITHIC DIET'?"

The Palæolithic Diet (or Hunter/Gatherer Diet) is based upon a wide variety of foods that were available to our ancestors some 50,000 years ago. The justification for following this type of diet is that it would be similar to the way of eating that typified the period of time when humanity experienced its most rapid evolutionary phase. Furthermore, hunter/gatherer societies do not display any of the chronic (long-term, degenerative) diseases that are common to Western society such as heart disease, joint disease, cancers and diabetes. [29,30,31,32,33]

The most compelling argument for moving 'back' to a diet like this, is that this is the diet that our ancestors were 'bred on' for at least 100,000 generations, the diet that our bodies became 'biologically used to' for thousands of years. A diet we have only 'recently' as human beings, moved away from.

Although the Palæolithic Diet is a relatively new concept in medical circles, there have already been 14 scientific trials on it, to date.

"WHAT IS THE 'MEDITERRANEAN DIET'?"

The Mediterranean Diet – also hugely popular – is characterised by the use of mono-unsaturated fats, fruit and vegetables, olive oil, garlic and the odd glass of wine. There have been some very large-scale scientific studies on the Mediterranean Diet and the outcomes of these provide proof that this diet is extremely healthy. There are consistent reductions in cardiovascular disease [34,35,36,37,38,39,40,41,42], diabetes [43,44,45,46,47,48,49], cancer [50,51,52,53,54,55,56,57,58,59,60,61,62,63,64,65] and all other causes of death, and excellent improvements in insulin sensitivity in people who follow this diet.

SMALL AMOUNT OF WINE DAILY BOOSTS LIFE EXPECTANCY BY 5 YEARS

As we have said, heavy alcohol consumption is bad for your health. But did you know that light consumption of wine, in men, can add five years to their life expectancy?

A study in 2009, from the Netherlands, published in the Journal of Epidemiology and Community Health, looked at men (1,373) who were born between 1900 and 1920, and then looked at studies of their health taken from 1960 onwards until 2000. It suggests a positive health benefit for light alcohol consumption – but especially for light wine consumption. Some researchers think that red wine consumption in mediterranean countries may contribute to better cardio-vascular heath.

"WHY DOES THE PALÆO-MEDITERRANEAN DIET WORK?"

A scientifically sound, biochemical justification is well established for this type of diet. Doctors and scientists now know that this approach works and nutritional practitioners and functional medicine practitioners have been advocating this approach for many years.

For example, there are numerous very large trials that show that elements of this diet dramatically reduce death rates. It is well known that diets that are rich in fruit and vegetables are sources of over 5,000 phytochemicals (natural plant chemicals) that have anti-oxidant, anti-viral, anti-inflammatory and anti-cancer properties.

Olive Oil
Olive oil contains oleic acid, squalene and phenolics, all of which have health promoting properties.

Resveratrol
Resveratrol in red wine is a potent anti-oxidant, anti-inflammatory and anti-cancer agent, which also has cardio-protective qualities.[76,77]

Omega 3
The diet incorporates considerable amounts of Omega 3 Essential Fatty Acids, which have a great number of health benefits as discussed previously.

Dietary Fibre
Dietary fibre is another important aspect of the Palæo-Mediterranean Diet, as this is increased by the intake of fruit and vegetables. Increased fibre from these sources favourably affects good bacteria in the gut (gut flora) and it promotes the elimination of "bad" or "unhelpful" bacteria (xenobacteria).

This benefit comes about as a result of a modification of gut bacteria i.e. promoting the numbers of "good" bacteria, laxation (a laxative effect) and reduction in enterohepatic recirculation – i.e. it reduces the recirculation of toxins time and again through your liver, and this reduction improves the efficiency of detoxification and thus lightens the toxic burden on your body – enabling it to function more efficiently.

AMINO ACIDS

Amino acids are an important feature of the Palæo-Mediterranean diet and these are found in quantity in Omega 3-rich lean meat, oily fish and also in a nutritional supplement called "Whey Protein". They are essential building blocks used in the formation of protein – which has many roles in our body – not least of which is the formation and growth of our muscles. In addition, valuable amino acids support "phase-2 detoxification" (amino acid and sulphate conjugation – which helps with the elimination of "unfriendly bacteria").

Amino acids also provide us with precursors to neurotransmitter synthesis, e.g. Serotonin etc., which helps in the maintenance of mood, memory and cognitive performance (thinking and intellectual function). In addition, they also prevent immuno-supression thus helping us to become as resistant to pathogens as possible and they also prevent the degradation of our musculo-skeletal status.

The condition of our muscles, skeleton and connective tissues can sometimes be affected if people are eating a low-protein diet, following a vegetarian diet but not getting enough protein – or as is too often the case in the developed world – they are not absorbing protein correctly.

MORE PALÆO-MEDITERRANEAN DIET HEALTH BENEFITS

ALKALINITY VS ACIDOSIS

One of the beneficial features of the Palæo-Mediterranean Diet is that the large amount of fruit and vegetables that you eat on this programme will help to alkalinise your body. Why is this important? Increased levels of acidity in your body that are brought about by eating a standard Western Diet, can adversely affect your health in many ways. [78] The fruits and vegetables in the Palæo-Mediterranean diet increase the alkalinity of your body, thus combating high acid levels, which can compromise health.

Acidosis is a process that leads to increased levels of acidity in your blood and this can, for example, cause a range of symptoms such as osteoporosis, [79,80,81,82,83,84,85] as calcium is leached from bones in order to protect your body by buffering the excess acid in the blood. It has been shown, scientifically, that the Palæolithic Diet can lead to the alkalinisation of urine [86,87] which increases the urinary elimination of many toxins and "unfriendly" bacteria. It also, helps us to retain many valuable minerals that would otherwise be excreted in urine.

Although controversial – as scientists disagree about the relative impact that the levels of acidity within cells actually has on viral replication – there is a growing body of evidence that shows that bacteria and viruses "prefer" a more acidic environment as higher acidity is, theoretically, linked to the ability of a virus' uncoating ability [88,89] and the common cold virus is more able to thrive and is more virulent in an acidic environment [90].

We feel that, given the growing support for the hypothesis that supports the beneficial effects of alkalinity, it is as well to err on the side of caution and attempt to develop a more alkaline body environment because of the potential anti-viral and anti-bacterial effects that this may offer.

So, the Palæo-Mediterranean Diet will make you look better and feel better. It has been scientifically proven to make you healthier and will help protect you from disease. In addition, research indicates that it might well be pivotal in preparing your immune system to be more resilient to Swine Flu. Last but not least, the foods that it features are delicious and appetising!

"WHAT DO YOU EAT IF YOU WANT TO COMBINE THE BEST OF BOTH DIETS?"

Dr Vasquez recommends eating the olive oil, whole fruits, vegetables, nuts (especially almonds), seeds, olive oil, lean Omega 3 rich meats, Omega 3 rich oily fish, mono-unsaturated essential fatty acids and drinking the red wine (in moderation) – of the Mediterranean Diet - and incorporating the absence of grains from the Palæolithic Diet to give the best of both approaches.

For real food lovers, dark chocolate and garlic are also included – although not necessarily at the same time. Both of these have been proven to be tremendously health promoting.

Dark chocolate is a rich source of cardio-protective anti-oxidant and anti-inflammatory polyphenolic flavonoids and scientists are researching dark chocolate extensively [66,67,68,69,70,71,72,73,74,75]. They currently predict that dark chocolate will be able to reduce adverse cardio-vascular events, such as strokes and heart attacks by over 76%.

Garlic, is well known for its health promoting properties and is also anti-viral, antibiotic and anti-fungal. You can read more about the amazing health benefits of garlic later in this chapter.

Both the Palæolithic and Mediterranean Diets **exclude** refined carbohydrates (bread, cakes, sugar, sweets/candies, white pasta, white rice), chemicals (preservatives, E-numbers, including artificial colourings, "improvers"), sweeteners and other carbohydrate-dominant foods such as refined grains, potatoes and so on.

This list is not dissimilar to the Low Glycaemic Index (GI) diet that has recently become popular, although the Low Glycaemic Index diet is still somewhat controversial and many nutritionists consider the Low Glycaemic Load diet to be superior.

"WHAT CAN I EAT ON A 'PALÆO-MEDITERRANEAN ANTI-INFLAMMATORY DIET'?"

Lots of delicious healthy things!

You can have lots of fresh fruits and vegetables. You can enjoy fresh meat and fish, as well as a wide variety of nuts and seeds. You can also use olive oil because it is so healthy – and do use it liberally unless you have severe weight problems. Olive oil has a vast number of health benefits and was used originally as a medicine long before it was ever used as a food. Garlic is also a useful tasty and healthy addition to any meal, and, as we have seen dark chocolate can be used in moderation, as can red wine.

Aim for five servings or more each day of fruit and vegetables. Ideally, these should, where possible, be organic so as to reduce the toxic load on the body which happens as a result of the use of herbicides, fungicides and pesticides on fruit and vegetables.

Drink fruit juice in moderation only and make certain that it is organic. The reason for the moderation is that fruit juice is full of simple sugars that can suppress your immune system.

The reason that we recommend you only consume organic juices is because there is evidence that neurological diseases such as Parkinson's disease are more common in people who drink non-organic fruit juice. Scientists suspect that the pesticides, fungicides and insecticides that are sprayed on the fruit are contributory or even causative factors in the development of these diseases in people who consume non-organic juices. This is also borne out by the increased incidence of Parkinson's disease in fruit plantation workers.

Cook foods for the minimum time possible so as not to lose vital nutrients and wherever possible, try to incorporate local produce into your diet – fruit and vegetables lose nutritional value when they are transported long distances. Try steaming food lightly – not only does it retain vitamins, it tastes wonderful and has great texture.

Drink plenty of water – read this book's Chapter on Hydration for more information about ways in which you can ensure that you are properly hydrated.

"WILL I NEED ANY DIETARY SUPPLEMENTS, SUCH AS VITAMINS OR MINERALS IF I AM ON THIS DIET?"

VITAMINS

This is a highly debatable point. The UK Government currently advises that we get enough vitamins in our diet – provided we do eat the recommended "five portions" of good quality fruit and vegetables each day.

They do not have a recommended level of meat/fish, or other protein that we should eat so they may not be aware of the dangers of amino-acid depletion. In the US, the Government, supported by excellent research from various respected institutions such as Harvard Medical School, advises people to take a daily multi-vitamin/mineral supplement.

So, who is right? In this situation, we would have to side with the US Government. All respected nutritionists agree that there is such a high level of mineral depletion from intensively-farmed soil that there are not enough minerals available in fruits and vegetables grown on this soil to properly support our nutritional requirements.

"WHAT ARE VITAMINS?"

The word "vitamine" was coined by the Polish biochemist Casimir Funk in 1912. *Vita* in Latin means life and the *amine* suffix is for 'amine' because at the time it was thought that all vitamins were derived from or related to organic compounds called amines. This is now known to be incorrect.

A vitamin is, by definition, an organic substance that you don't make in your body – you have to get it directly from your food or supplements. A vitamin is absolutely necessary for carrying out the essential biochemical functions that are vital for your survival.

Most vitamins do this by forming "co-enzymes". These are molecules that activate the enzymes that catalyse key biochemical reactions –although a few of them, like vitamin C, contribute to enzyme function without forming a co-enzyme in your body.

You can think of co-enzymes as being like the PIN number on your debit card. Swiping your card (an enzyme) through a card machine (a metabolic substrate; the natural environment in which an organism lives) is an essential part of accessing your bank account (completing the biochemical "transaction"). However, unless you also punch in your PIN number (the coenzyme) to activate it, the transaction can't go through.

This makes vitamins a very distinct kind of nutrient. While there are relatively many substances that are essential to human life in both health and disease (as a group, these are the "orthomolecules"), only a few of them have all of the features that would mark them as vitamins.

OTHER VITAL NUTRIENTS

Some orthomolecules (like R(+)-lipoic acid or carnitine) are undeniably essential to the biochemistry that supports life, however, unlike vitamins they can be made by the body – if not necessarily in the amounts required for a lifetime of the best possible health, then certainly in the minimum quantities needed to keep you basically alive but not in a state of optimum health.

Other nutrients are needed for normal health – and you do have to get them from your diet or supplements – but they aren't vitamins because they are not organic molecules in the chemical sense. This category includes the essential minerals, which may be bound to organic molecules (like citrate, aspartate, or malate) but are not, themselves, chemically organic.

So calcium, magnesium and zinc – and new research suggests vanadium, silicon, lithium, and strontium – are needed for normal biochemistry and have to come from outside the body, enabling you to perform many functions including the generation of energy, optimising growth and speeding the healing process. All enzyme activities require minerals, so they are essential for you to be able to use vitamins and other nutrients correctly.

"WHEN IS A 'VITAMIN' NOT A 'VITAMIN'?"

There are the many substances that have been misidentified as vitamins.

HIGH DOSES OF VITAMINS 'WORK'; LOW 'RECOMMENDED' DOSES DON'T!

Taken from an article in With Our Complements; The Journal of The CMA (Summer 2009 edition)

In response to what they see as an 'anti-vitamin' media campaign in the US (e.g."Vitamins C and E don't prevent heart disease" AP 9/11/08) which follow the much talked about JAMA study, the Orthomolecular Medicine News Service has started to push for a greater understanding of exactly how beneficial vitamin supplementation is, when taken at the 'right' levels, and what a crucial branch of Nutrition science it accounts for.

They point out that thousands of research studies exist on this topic – all of which prove that vitamins do help prevent – and treat – a whole range of serious disease from cancer to heart disease – WHEN THEY ARE DELIVERED IN HIGH DOSES.

By the same token, they admit that vitamin supplementation at low levels (as recommended by Governments) doesn't work – and any research studies based on these low levels of vitamin supplementation are almost certainly bound to fail.

Top cardiologist Thomas Levy, M.D says;

> *"The three most important considerations in effective vitamin C therapy are dose, dose, and dose. If you don't take enough, you won't get the desired effects.*
>
> *When they talk about High Doses, they are effectively talking about levels that are "hundreds of times more than the US Recommended Dietary Allowance (RDA) or Daily Reference Intake (DRI)".*

These levels are set extremely low because various 'experts', in the US and in the UK, have been concerned about potential toxicity from higher dosage levels. The often stated view that "high doses of vitamins are not safe", is, they say, a myth.

The official statistics in the US over the last 25 years show that there has not even been a single death from vitamin supplementation, despite the fact that around 50% of the US population take vitamin supplements every day.

As opposed to 'recommended' maximum levels of 400 IU a day in the US, Dr Abram Hoffer, Ph.D., pointed out that;

> *"Drs. Wilfrid Shute and Evan Shute recommended doses from 400 IU to 8,000 IU of vitamin E daily. The usual dose range was 800 to 1600 IU but they report that they had given 8,000 IU without seeing any toxicity."*

The Shutes successfully treated over 35,000 patients by using vitamin E.

On the Orthomolecular Medicine News Service they point out what the;

> "......much touted JAMA study does is confirm what we already know: low doses do not work. The doses given were 400 IU of vitamin E every OTHER day and 500 milligrams of vitamin C/day. Try that same study with 2,000 to 4,000 IU of vitamin E every other day (1,000 to 2,000 IU/day) and 15,000-30,000 mg/day of vitamin C and the difference would be unmistakable. We know this because investigators using vitamins E and C in high doses have consistently reported success".

> "Decades of physicians' reports and controlled research studies support the use of large doses of vitamins. Yet to hear the media (and JAMA) tell it, vitamins are a Granny's folk remedy: a buggy-and barrel-stave technology that just doesn't make it". [243]

Further reading: Orthmolecular.org

Some of them really are essential but while they are orthomolecules, they aren't vitamins, because they can be made in your body. Orotic acid, once called Vitamin B13, is one example of this. Others are phytochemicals; substances found in plants that contribute to their health benefits but whose absence from our diet wouldn't lead to the total shutdown of an essential biochemical function in the body.

Still others are substances that are claimed to be vitamins that really have no clear biological purpose at all, like pangamic acid (so-called Vitamin B15, which not only has no essential biological purpose but may actually be a carcinogen) and Laetrile (which some people claim to be Vitamin B17, and use it in the treatment of certain cancers but for which there is no evidence of a role in normal human biochemistry).

WHY DO I NEED TO TAKE IN MINERALS?

Minerals are essential for health. Your body needs over 80 minerals in order to function properly, and in fact, every cell in your body relies on minerals for proper structure and function.

You need minerals for the correct formation of your blood and optimal growth of your bones, the proper composition of body fluids, a healthy nervous system and proper operation of your cardio-vascular system, among others.

Like vitamins, minerals function as coenzymes, enabling your body to perform many functions, including the generation of energy, optimising growth and speeding the healing process.

THERE ARE THREE BASIC CLASSIFICATIONS OF MINERALS.

The Metallic minerals, the Chelated minerals, and the Colloidal minerals.

Metallic minerals exist in their pure elemental form or in combinations as "Salts" such as Sodium Chloride and Zinc Sulphate. Many nutritional supplements usually feature minerals in the Salts form – especially the essential minerals – because larger amounts are needed by your body. However, this is not always a good policy as while the Salts form of minerals is inexpensive to manufacture – they are not necessarily bioavailable and are certainly less bioavailable than the more expensive Chelated or Colloidal minerals.

Chelated minerals are more bioavailable than mineral Salts. A chelated mineral is formed either in nature – or in the laboratory when a metallic mineral is Chelated with an amino acid. The role of the amino acid is to surround the metallic mineral, which helps to make it more soluble and this means that your body can more easily absorb it.
Examples of chelated minerals include Magnesium Ascorbate, which is Magnesium chelated with Natural Ascorbic Acid and Calcium Citrate which is Chromium chelated with Citric Acid. As a general rule of thumb, chelated minerals are generally about 40% better absorbed than Metallic minerals.

Colloidal minerals occur naturally in a "Colloid" state. They are infinitesimally tiny particles that have an enormous surface area when they are dispersed in a fluid – such as water. This results in improved solubility, greater bioavailability, better absorption and therefore your body can actually recognise and use them. Best of all the Colloidal minerals are those derived from plants as the most soluble and also your body recognises them as "plant substances" – and therefore is able to make the best use of them.

and other nutrients correctly. As discussed previously, in many areas of the world, the soil is so depleted of minerals – due to intensive farming – that the plants that grow in this soil do not have the optimal levels of minerals that we need. So, it is necessary to supplement our diets with extra minerals.

Mineral malnutrition shows up in a number of ways, some serious and others, less so. Conditions such as depleted energy, premature ageing, sensory acuity problems and degenerative diseases like osteoporosis, cardio-vascular disease and cancer are all linked to mineral depletion. The current thinking is that these could be prevented with proper mineral supplementation.

MINERALS ARE GROUPED INTO TWO CATEGORIES: ESSENTIAL MINERALS AND TRACE MINERALS

You need essential minerals such as calcium and magnesium, in large amounts. Trace minerals such as boron, chromium, iron, zinc, selenium and many others are needed in minute quantities but are, nevertheless, essential to health.

One mineral, for example, that is absolutely essential to health is Selenium – it is also extremely important in the fight against a number of viruses [91,92,93]. It is virtually impossible to get enough Selenium from food nowadays because, as we mentioned above, the mineral content of many soils –especially Selenium – has been depleted by intensive crop farming.

Farmers in Finland have taken steps to counter the depletion by using Selenium-rich fertilisers with good results and food scientists in the UK are recommending that UK farmers adopt this supplementation strategy too. There are also suggestions that crops could be hybridised to incorporate features of crops that have a better ability to take up Selenium from soil [94].

Interestingly, in the US, the soil in the Eastern part of the country is Selenium-deficient, but in the Western states it still contains Selenium.

Selenium is hard to get at the moment, in fact, the quantity of traditionally Selenium-rich food, such as brazil nuts, that you would have to consume, to get enough Selenium, would be so enormous that it would not be possible to do this on a daily basis. In fact, eating the amount of food that you would need to take in to get enough Selenium, would actually lead to nutritional imbalances and an excess of calories – which would then lead to obesity – another devastating health problem.

BIOAVAILABILITY

Recently, in the field of complementary medicine there has been a great revolution whereby there has been an enormous increase in the design, production and usage of bioavailable nutrients. As we have seen above bioavailability is vitally important as it means that your body recognises these nutrients and can use them – in the same way that it would use nutrients coming from real food.

This is extremely useful for supplement manufacturers since this means that for bioavailable nutrients to be delivered in the correct amounts, the physical dosage (i.e. size of the pill/physical quantity required) can be much lower. It also means that people taking supplements are far more likely to stick to a supplement programme, if they have to take fewer pills and capsules.

"CAN I TAKE JUST ANY VITAMINS, MINERALS OR OTHER SUPPLEMENTS?"

Not all vitamin and mineral supplements are equal and it really is a case of "Buyer Beware!"

In the world of nutritional supplements, you really do have to be aware of what you are actually spending money on! There are an awful lot of products on our supermarket, health food store and pharmacy shelves that are just not worth buying. Many vitamins available in supermarkets, for example, are composed of chemical versions, or analogues, of naturally occurring vitamins. While they may look similar under a microscope, your body doesn't recognise these chemical vitamins in the same way as it recognises and metabolises naturally occurring vitamins from food.

In the best-case scenario, many of the ingredients in these products will simply pass straight through you and it is akin to throwing your hard-earned money down the toilet.

Worst-case scenario? They may actually do you harm, if dosages are wrong, if the wrong types of vitamins are used and if vitamins interact unfavourably with each other.

PRECURSOR SUPPLEMENTS

In addition to the bioavailability revolution, there has recently been an increase in the numbers of "Precursor" nutritional supplements – a good example of one of these would be beta-carotene which is a precursor to Vitamin A. Many people are aware that there are some possible hepato-toxicity (liver toxicity) issues related to very high doses of Vitamin A and it is even associated, controversially, with the possibility of birth defects, if it is consumed in doses in excess of 10,000IU per day by pregnant women. However, beta-carotene, acting as a precursor, helps your body to form Vitamin A in just the right quantities that your body needs and there is no danger of toxicity.

"CAN SUPPLEMENTS ACTUALLY BE HARMFUL?"

Iron and Vitamin E have both been at the centre of a number of debates as to their safety:

IRON

Iron, in excess, is causatively linked to cardiovascular disease, cancer, diabetes mellitus, hypogonadism (small reproductive organs), infertility, thyroid disorders, infectious diseases and peripheral arthropathy (joint pain and/or destruction)[95,96,97].

Iron is essential to life but the vast majority of us get enough of this mineral from our food. Our recommendation is that you do not supplement with iron, unless there is a proven medical reason to do so.

VITAMIN E

Vitamin E has also come under fire and this is a great shame as there are many different kinds of Vitamin E available, and the recent reports that claimed that Vitamin E is harmful, were most misleading.

Like many media-driven health scares, these reports held a grain of truth, but the full story was not told. In fact, there is no such thing as 'Vitamin E', as this vitamin is, in fact, a Complex of eight different molecules – four tocopherols and four tocotrienols. These eight members of the E family work together to support each other.

So, the recent meta-analysis [98] of trials on Vitamin E which reported that Vitamin E usage was linked to a higher incidence of death in cardiac patients was flawed, since the substance used in the trials was only one part of the Vitamin E family – alpha-tocopherol [99,100,101,102].

In fact, taking the substance that is commonly sold as Vitamin E, alpha-tocopherol, actually depletes your body of other members of the E family.

Frighteningly, this depletion means that you end up worse off than if you just had a good diet and took no supplements.

Studies that look at people who are taking the full spectrum of the Vitamin E family paint a very different, much rosier picture!

Vitamin E Complex – with all eight members of its family is extremely good for you. [103]

It is an anti-oxidant, and has enormous cardio-protective properties, whilst also helping protect us from cancer. It is certainly of relevance when it comes to protecting yourself from a virus such as Swine Flu as Vitamin E Complex has anti-inflammatory properties and is a strong anti-oxidant which has the ability to "mop-up" the cellular damage caused by free-radicals that do untold damage to your cells during an influenza infection [104]. Vitamin E Complex is so important for good health that we cover it in much greater depth later in this section.

"WHICH SUPPLEMENTS SHOULD I TAKE?"

So, having covered some of the beneficial and problematic aspects of vitamin and mineral supplementation, we will take a look at supplements that you should be taking to safeguard yourself and to create the very best levels of health that we believe you can achieve.

We have, in conjunction with top scientists in the field of nutrition, spent many long years of research in the area of effective supplementation and we believe the recommendations that

PQQ IN FOODS (MCG/KG)[115]

FRUITS LEGUMES
Apple 6
Broad beans 18
Kiwifruit 27
Soybeans 9
Oranges 7
Tofu 24
Papaya 27
Tomatoes 9

FERMENTED FOODS
Natto (Fermented Soybeans) 61
Green tea 30

VEGETABLES
Cocoa powder 800
Cabbage 16
Carrot 17
Celery 6
Green pepper 28
Parsley 34

ANIMAL PRODUCTS
Human milk 140-180
Cow's milk 3.4
Egg yolk 7
Egg white 4.1

follow make for an excellent supplementation regime that will be suited to most people: (If a particular supplement is contra-indicated, i.e. not recommended in certain circumstances, we will make a note of this where relevant).

The reason that we have gone to the trouble of developing a specially designed health programme for people is because a good programme is urgently needed in the face of this current – and any potential future – Swine Flu, and, or Bird Flu – serious pandemic and its potentially devastating effects on health. This particular health programme will help you to become healthier – in general – to be less prone to inflammatory tendencies and to be "immunologically robust" and therefore as resistant to illness as possible.

In addition, we have identified a number of vitamins, minerals, herbs and other supplements that actually have anti-viral properties. So, we are taking a preventative approach to help you become more resilient to viruses, but which has the added dimension of utilising substances that have been shown – in trials – to disable viruses in a number of ways.

"WHAT ARE THE BEST MULTI-VITAMIN/MULTI-MINERAL FORMULAS?"

The best multi-vitamin/multi-mineral preparations will be formulated to deliver the most fundamental nutrients in the best forms in the fewest capsules possible. Some outstanding supplement manufacturers have recently created some excellent formulas that come as a powder that can be mixed with water, juice or other beverage, which is excellent for those who do not like to swallow capsules, or for children who may have difficulty with capsules. Of course, it is most helpful if the powdered formula tastes good on its own and can be mixed with other ingredients such as a Whey Protein powder to make a great-tasting "smoothie".

It may seem a bit facile to talk about "great tasting vitamin formulas", especially when faced with a problem of the potential enormity of a serious pandemic flu, but, the fact that a supplement tastes great, or is easy to take, is actually extremely important. If you enjoy taking a product, then you are more likely to stick with a programme. Practitioners and doctors call sticking to a recommended programme "compliance", and for our recommendations to benefit you, you do actually need to stick to the programme!

VITAMINS, MINERALS AND OTHER NUTRIENTS THAT IMPROVE IMMUNE STATUS AND ASSIST VIRAL RESISTANCE

THE MISSING VITAMIN B LINK – PQQ

On April 24, 2003, scientists with Japan's prestigious "RIKEN Brain Science Institute" made a startling announcement in the esteemed science journal Nature; they had discovered direct molecular evidence that a mysterious nutrient that they isolated, was in fact, a previously unidentified B Complex vitamin.

Interestingly, the new vitamin – Pyrroloquinoline Quinone, or PQQ – had actually been discovered decades previously and had long been known to be essential to the health of bacteria. However, despite decades of research and many tantalising hints, no one had previously been able to definitively tie PQQ into human nutritional needs. For fifty-five years since the isolation of the last B vitamin compound (Vitamin B12, isolated in 1948), nutritional science has overlooked an organic molecule whose absence from the diet is ruinous to your health.

But how do we know that PQQ is an essential factor in the human diet and not just another of the many mistakenly identified pseudo-vitamins? The first and most obvious evidence comes from studies in laboratory animals, which have found that eating a PQQ-free diet leads to a sweeping deficiency syndrome as devastating as scurvy, pellagra or beriberi.

PQQ-deficient animals suffer impaired reproductive and immune function; their growth is retarded; their skin is thin and breaks easily; and they develop abnormalities in their connective tissues known as osteolathyrism. Their offspring are less likely to survive the first few days after birth and if they do survive, do not make it to weaning. None of these signs and symptoms occur when animals eat the same diets along with supplemental PQQ. [105,106,107,108,109,110,111,112,113,114]

Because its role in human nutrition was unknown, PQQ has never previously been available in dietary supplements. Fortunately, many healthy foods contain PQQ (see table opposite), and a well-balanced diet will contain about one-tenth as much PQQ as folic acid on average.

However, now that scientists have finally established the basic biochemical need for PQQ at the gene level, leading-edge supplement companies are taking the initiative to make PQQ accessible to health-conscious people.

SELENIUM

As we have already noted, Selenium is a very important mineral when it comes to fighting viruses. In fact, some of the poorest geographical areas for Selenium in soil are China and parts of Southeast Asia. It is suspected by a number of scientists that this may be a contributory factor for the susceptibility of birds to Avian Influenza in his region.

Large amounts of Selenium are required for egg production [116,117,118] and this requirement means that Selenium levels in the hens laying eggs become even more depleted – thus rendering these hens open to infection – and this situation is exacerbated in geographical areas traditionally low in Selenium.

Furthermore – early research shows that Selenium may actually "protect" viruses and help them to be more resistant to mutations which would exacerbate virulence, if unprotected. It may seem strange to want to protect viruses, but, in fact, it is quite important, as this protection may help prevent a virus from mutating into a form that is much more infectious to humans.

Another fascinating piece of research on mice that were fed a depleted Selenium diet and then infected with human flu showed that they were more ill than the well-nourished control group and that they were ill for longer and had much greater degrees of lung inflammation [119].

According to Professor Alan Schenkin at Liverpool University, this research;

"Does imply that Selenium-deficiency is associated with more severe consequences through infections with viruses."

Along with its potent anti-viral properties[120], Selenium is now well established as a potent anti-cancer trace mineral. On PubMed there are 2,645 studies on Selenium and cancer and a handful are listed below in our references section. [121,122,123,124,125,126,127]

Areas of the world with more Selenium-rich soil have lower cancer rates and a randomised, double blind, placebo-controlled trial in the 1990s showed that men taking a daily 200mcg Selenium supplement experienced a 37% lower risk of developing new cancer and a whopping reduction on 50% in the risk of cancer-related death.

Not all forms of Selenium are equal though and it has now been shown that a particular part of Selenium, Se-methylselenocysteine or SeMC, is a form of Selenium that is directly converted into the key cancer fighting components required by the body.

It is important for you to know that there are many kinds of Selenium for sale and most of these are not bioavailable – so are a complete waste of money as they flush straight through you. Generally, it is thought that you only absorb 10% of the Selenium in most supplements – the rest is wasted.

BIOFLAVONOIDS AND VITAMIN C

Bioflavonoids, also called flavonoids, are naturally occurring plant pigments. They are a group of anti-oxidant substances that are present in most plants, concentrating in seeds, bark, flowers, and fruit skin, or peel. Your body cannot produce these phytochemicals (plant chemicals), so you have to get them through your diet, or by taking supplements.

They are essential for health. The chemical structure of bioflavonoids is made up of two benzene rings on either side of a three-carbon ring. flavonoids comprise a large and varied group and differ from one another by the addition of hydroxyl groups, sugars, methyl groups etc. The terminology used to distinguish the various classes of flavonoids includes: flavanols, flavanes, flavan-3-ols, OPCs, proanthocyanins, isoflavonoids, etc.

Flavonoids have a range of biological activities, acting as anti-oxidants and showing anti-inflammatory, anti-thrombotic (stops blood from clotting) and anti-neoplastic (stops tumours from forming) actions. Bioflavonoids also have a synergistic effect on Vitamin C activity, which is beneficial to our health.

HISTORY

In 1747, the Scottish naval surgeon, James Lind discovered that a mysterious nutrient in citrus foods prevented scurvy although it was not known at the time exactly what the nutrient actually was (now known to be Vitamin C and flavonoids).

British sailors, who were given limes to eat on their long voyages, did not succumb to scurvy like their counterparts who did not eat limes, hence the old American usage of the term "Limey" to describe a British sailor, and now any British person.

Vitamin C was rediscovered by Norwegians, A. Hoist and T.Froelich in 1912 and it was later artificially synthesised in 1935, and was the first synthetic vitamin.

Szent-Gyorgyi, the first person to actually isolate Vitamin C, also later discovered flavonoids accidentally in the late '30s. His friend, who had bleeding gums, was given a crude, basic version of Vitamin C – extracted from lemon and his condition improved. However, later his gums started bleeding again.

Szent-Gyorgyi gave his friend a purer form of Vitamin C thinking he would see better results. Instead, his friend's gums worsened. So Szent-Gyorgyi gave his friend an isolated flavonoid extract and Vitamin C and his friend's gums healed completely. So Szent-Gyorgyi deduced and later demonstrated that scurvy symptoms were due to a combined deficiency of Vitamin C and flavonoids. Without the 'flavonoids' – from the pith and the segments of the limes – Vitamin C would not have worked on its own. **It needs to be taken with flavonoids!**

Flavonoids were originally termed "Vitamin P", because they reduced the permeability of blood vessels. But flavonoids are so chemically diverse that they cannot be categorised as a single nutrient.

The following are some plants, fruits and herbs whose active ingredients are classified as flavonoids:

- Bilberry – anthocyanins;
- Strawberries – ellagic acids;
- Ginkgo – ginkgoflavone glycosides;
- Turmeric – curcuminoids;
- Green tea – catechins;
- Hawthorn berry – proanthocyanidins;
- Onions – quercetin;
- Grape seeds / skin – OPCs (oligomeric proanthocyanidins).

An interesting observation was made by some Indian researchers from the prestigious All India Institute of Medical Sciences: The Vitamin C in the extract of the fruit amla, which has the highest concentration of ascorbate (Vitamin C) in any plant, had over ten times the bioavailabilty of synthetic Vitamin C. Careful analysis also revealed that the tannins present in the amla fruit protected and enhanced the Vitamin C activity.

Other studies have found that the cancer cell growth inhibitory action of the flavonoid quercetin was considerably enhanced by Vitamin C. The effect on the vitamin may be due to the ability of Quercetin to recycle oxidized Vitamin C. This is because when anti-oxidants neutralise free-radicals, they become weak pro-oxidants. Flavonoids display an anti-oxidant boosting effect, returning ascorbate (Vitamin C) to its active anti-oxidant form.

Vitamin C and flavonoids are probably the most extensively researched nutritional supplements of all. A PubMed search for the term "Vitamin C" returns 32,010 results and a search for flavonoids returns 46532. [33,743]. This illustrates that scientists re keen to discover much more about the effects that Vitamin C and bioflavonoids have an enormous role to play in all aspects of human health.

VITAMIN D

The term "vitamin" as applied to Vitamin D, is somewhat inaccurate because it is synthesised by your skin after you have been exposed to sunlight.

This creation of Vitamin D depends upon a number of factors including the type and intensity of ultraviolet light, duration of exposure, skin pigmentation, age, altitude, latitude, hour of day and season.

VITAMIN D DEFICIENCY IS WIDESPREAD ACROSS ALL POPULATION GROUPS

Most doctors and practitioners recognise that the elderly population is at risk of Vitamin D deficiency, however few people realise that children, young adults and middle-age groups are also at risk. Studies have shown that children in areas as diverse as Madrid in Spain, to Maine in the US, have approximately a 50% deficit in Vitamin D in the winter months. Apart from equatorial areas, where people make enough Vitamin D, everywhere else – particularly above or below latitudes of 40°N and 40°S respectively – people make little Vitamin D.

In Edmonton, Canada, which is 52°N, Vitamin D synthesis is impaired from October through to March. This problem is further exacerbated because people are given incorrect or misleading information about sun exposure. There is of course, no doubt that over-exposure to the sun is associated strongly with skin cancer but too little Vitamin D synthesis also has its own unique health problems.

Vitamin D deficiency is becoming a problem elsewhere in the world too, as people who live in sunny climates are likely to be very aware of the need to avoid over-exposure to the sun and cover themselves with sunscreen, prior to any sun exposure [128]. In Hawaii, for example, doctors are actually being advised to screen their patients to make sure that they are not Vitamin D deficient [129].

"HOW IS VITAMIN D FORMED?"

UVB exposure to your epidermis (surface of your skin), produces Vitamin D which then undergoes hydroxylation (addition of OH or hydroxyl group), first in your liver, and then in your kidneys, to produce the active hormone 1, 25-dihydroxy Vitamin D3 – also called "D3" for short (and also called Cholecalciferol – just to confuse matters!) and this is the form of Vitamin D that we will be referring to throughout the rest of this section, as this form of Vitamin D is the most active and has the most health benefits – some of which have special relevance to protecting us from serious pandemic flu.

Vitamin D is responsible for bone development and growth in children and maintenance of bone in adults. It is also important for the prevention of osteoporosis and fractures in the elderly. Deficiency in children results in rickets and osteomalacia (a form of rickets) in adults. Both conditions are characterised by inadequate bone mineralisation.

Vitamin D is also essential for the efficient utilisation of dietary calcium.

VITAMIN D HELPS US REGULATE LEVELS OF CALCIUM

In order for us to be healthy, it is essential that calcium levels in our blood are tightly regulated. In a Vitamin D deficient state, the amount of calcium absorbed is inadequate to satisfy your body's requirements and this causes your body to release a hormone – PTH (parathyroid hormone). This hormone activates certain bone cells (osteoclasts) to break down the bone, so

The optimum formulation of Vitamin E complex contains a balance of the following eight members of the Vitamin E family:

> d-alpha-tocopherol
> d-beta-tocopherol
> d-gamma-tocopherol
> d-delta-tocopherol
> d-alpha-tocotrienol
> d-beta-tocotrienol
> d-gamma-tocotrienol
> d-delta-tocotrienol

that your body can get the much needed calcium.

This weakens your bone and results in osteopenia, which results in a decrease in your bone's mineral density, that is a precursor to the development of osteoporosis and PTH release is also linked to osteoporosis itself.

Additionally, PTH causes your kidneys to excrete phosphate and the overall net result is a decrease in calcium phosphate, which is the major mineral required for mineralising bone. The bone-building cells, osteoblasts, continue to deposit collagen matrix. This results in a rubbery matrix which expands upon hydration and causes pressure and a low grade unrelenting pain often misdiagnosed as fibromyalgia.

MUSCLE FUNCTION

Vitamin D is also important in the function of your muscles. Muscle weakness, pain and changes in gait have been described in Vitamin D insufficiency. This may be the reason that the elderly have more falls. And given that they may also be suffering from reduced bone strength, due to the Vitamin D deficiency outlined above, this may consequently lead to increased fracture rates.

OTHER PROBLEMS ASSOCIATED WITH A LACK OF VITAMIN D

Vitamin D deficiency has been associated with increased hypertension (high blood pressure) [130,131,132], increased auto-immune disease and various forms of cancer [133] including breast, prostate and ironically, skin cancer [134]. Low Vitamin D is also associated with premenstrual syndrome (PMS)[135,136], poor immune system function [137,138,139], diabetes [140,141,142,143] and the so-called 'syndrome X' and seasonally affective disorders (SAD).[144,145]

Of particular relevance to Swine Flu is the fact that Vitamin D3 can modulate your immune system, and in doing so, potentially suppress the production of various cytokines including TNF-α, which as we have previously discussed is implicated in the Cytokine Storm seen in H1N1. [146,147,148]

VITAMIN E COMPLEX

As we read earlier in this section – Vitamin E is not really one vitamin, as such, but it is, in fact, a "Complex" of eight closely related Vitamin E molecules (or "vitamers"): four tocopherols and four tocotrienols.

Each member of the Vitamin E Complex has its own unique strengths, and even unique properties not shared with other E vitamers. If your Vitamin E contains only alpha-tocopherol – or alpha-tocopherol with token quantities of mixed tocopherols, you're missing out on the benefits of the other Vitamin E molecules.

But more than that: studies show that unbalanced alpha-tocopherol supplementation actually depletes your body of the other members of the family, and can negate many of their benefits!

"SO JUST WHAT CAN THESE OTHER VITAMIN E MOLECULES DO THAT ALPHA-TOCOPHEROL CAN'T?

Tocotrienols specifically, have a unique chemical structure which allows them to move around more freely in cell membranes. As a result, the tocotrienols are forty to sixty times more potent anti-oxidants, than the tocopherols. [149]

PANDEMIC FLU

Various members of the Vitamin E family have anti-viral activities, [150,151,152] and at least one paper recommends Vitamin E as a specific treatment for the H5N1 strain of Bird Flu that is still of concern. [153]

Other research papers remind us that Host Nutritional Status (i.e. how healthily-nourished you are), is of enormous relevance when considering ways of being optimally resistant to all forms of illness, especially viral disease. [154]

CARDIO-PROTECTIVE

Extra-cellular fluid pressure (the fluid surrounding our cells) plays a key role in the regulation of blood pressure, and high extracellular fluid pressure puts you at risk of congestive heart failure, cardiac fibrosis, and liver cirrhosis. It was recently found that gamma-tocopherol and gamma-tocotrienol, but not alpha-tocopherol, help to contribute to the control of your extracellular fluid pressure.

ANTI-CANCER STUDIES

Five studies have found that that delta-tocopherol, as well as all four tocotrienols, but not alpha-tocopherol, can cause apoptosis (cellular "suicide") in breast and other cancer cells in in-vitro (test tube) tests. [155, 156,157]

ANTI-OXIDANT STUDIES

We do know that alpha-tocopherol is a good anti-oxidant against many kinds of free-radicals, but gamma-tocopherol is much more effective in detoxifying "reactive nitrogen species," which are the types of free-radicals found in things like smog. In fact, alpha-tocopherol cannot effectively remove peroxynitrite (a highly toxic, key reactive nitrogen species) without gamma-tocopherol as a partner. [158]

CHOLESTEROL STUDIES

Double-blind, placebo-controlled trials which many (but not all) scientists consider to be the gold standard of conventional scientific trials, have shown that high-dose tocotrienol complex can help correct cholesterol balance in people whose levels are too high. [159,160,161]

In one such trial, tocotrienols actually reversed the thickening of the arteries leading into the brain in patients with advanced carotid stenosis [162] (a blocking of the carotid artery leading to the brain, by fatty deposits which can cause strokes or Transient Ischemic Attacks (TIA; mini-stroke).

COX-2, GAMMA-TOCOPHEROL AND INFLAMMATION

COX-2 is a key enzyme in the inflammatory process. It is targeted by the controversial and dangerous COX-2 inhibitor drugs such as Celebrex® and Vioxx®. Researchers have recently reported that gamma- tocopherol – as found in the E complex – but not alpha-tocopherol, is an effective COX-2 inhibitor [163].

A recent study found that men who had the most gamma-tocopherol in their blood were an astounding five times less likely to develop prostate cancer than men whose blood gamma-tocopherol levels were lowest. In the same study, alpha-tocopherol and Selenium levels were only found to be protective in men whose gamma-tocopherol levels were also high [164,165,166].

BRAIN PROTECTION

When scientists tested members of the E complex to see what effect they would have on brain cells exposed to glutamate (a substance known to kill brain cells) in a test tube, they found that alpha-tocotrienol, but not alpha-tocopherol, could block brain cell death caused by glutamate [167,168,169,170].

ATHEROSCLEROSIS

A key step in the development of atherosclerosis (hardening of the arteries) is the invasion of injured blood vessel walls by immune cells, called monocytes. A recent study found that alpha-tocotrienol actually inhibited the sticking of monocytes to the endothelial cells on the blood vessel walls. Alpha-tocotrienol was much more effective than alpha-tocopherol [171,172].

WHICH "E" FOR THE HEART? CUTTING THROUGH THE VITAMIN E MYTHS

As touched on earlier, the news that "Vitamin E does not protect the heart – and in fact may increase the risk of death from cardiovascular disease!" was greeted with enormous surprise in many quarters.

This, initially, was a great blow to the general vitamin industry, as many studies (the HOPE, GISSI, CHAOS, Primary Prevention Project (PPP)) found that, despite all expectations, alpha-tocopherol does not give any protection against death from a heart attack, or other heart hazards in people at high risk. It seems however that, in fact, the researchers were using the "wrong" kind of Vitamin E.

Scientists do however know about all the heart-protective properties of the other E vitamins – cholesterol-lowering, anti-inflammatory, blood-pressure reduction, inhibition of adhesion molecules etc, – so you might expect that alpha-tocopherol, alone, is not going to be the cardiac "cure-all" that many people expect it to be. However, it has come to light that several studies have found that low plasma levels of gamma-tocopherol – but not alpha-tocopherol – exist in patients with atherosclerosis. Three such studies have actually discovered an unbalanced ratio of alpha-tocopherol to gamma-tocopherol in these patients.

Similarly, in two large epidemiological studies (one involving American women, and the other amongst Finnish people of both sexes), it has been found that Vitamin E from food, but not from supplements, was protective against death from heart disease. Why would this be?

The fact is that most of the Vitamin E in the food we eat is gamma-tocopherol, while most "Vitamin E" supplements contain an abundance of alpha-tocopherol.

LIFE EXTENSION

Researchers recently reported that tocotrienols, but not alpha-tocopherol, extend the average lifespan of flatworms, and protected them against carbonylation [173], a kind of free-radical-damage to the body's proteins. This raises interesting questions as to what tocotrienols may do for human lifespan.

ALZHEIMER'S DISEASE AND THE 'E FAMILY'

Scientists have known for a long time now that free-radicals are important in the degenerative process of Alzheimer's disease. But until recently, it hasn't been clear which kinds of free-radicals are causing such devastating neurological destruction. Furthermore, if you don't know which free-radicals are doing the damage, you can't know which anti-oxidants are likely to be most effective in combating this disease.

Recent research has begun to provide evidence that nitrogen-based free-radicals, such as peroxynitrite, are especially powerful in the brains of people with Alzheimer's disease. As discussed above, gamma-tocopherol, but not alpha-tocopherol can detoxify nitrogen-based free-radicals such as peroxynitrite.

So, scientists looked at levels of gamma-tocopherol and alpha-tocopherol in the brains of people who had died from Alzheimer's disease. They found that areas of the brain which were affected by the disease, had a particularly low level of gamma-tocopherol. Interestingly, alpha-tocopherol levels were the same in the brains of the Alzheimer's casualties as in people without the disease, but gamma-tocopherol levels were found to be lower overall throughout the brains of people with the Alzheimer's disease compared to the brains of those without it [174,175].

These depleted levels of gamma-tocopherol corresponded with increased levels of a waste product left over when gamma-tocopherol is used up in fighting nitrogen-based free-radicals. Crucially, the region-by-region pattern of used-up gamma-tocopherol followed the pattern of nitrogen-based, free-radical damage, already established in earlier studies.

Finally, the same research team showed that gamma-tocopherol but not alpha-tocopherol could significantly protect the enzyme "alpha-ketoglutarate dehydrogenase" from damage by peroxynitrite [176]. Levels of this enzyme have been found to be reduced by 50 to 75% in the brains of people with Alzheimer's compared to the brains of people not suffering from the disease. The researchers confirmed their suspicions: As much as 55% of the peroxynitrite damage to this Alzheimer's- sensitive enzyme was prevented by gamma-tocopherol, while alpha- tocopherol offered only a 15% reduction at the optimal concentration.

One large, double-blind, placebo-controlled study has already shown that alpha-tocopherol supplements can provide some limited support for people with Alzheimer's, slowing the progression of the disease. This new research suggests that gamma-tocopherol may provide far greater protection.

In fact, the scientists who carried out the study suggest that, since;

> "Dietary supplementation with alpha-tocopherol will decrease plasma levels of gamma-tocopherol . . . it is conceivable that the beneficial effects of alpha-tocopherol supplementation are confounded by a diminution of gamma-tocopherol pools in [Alzheimer's disease]. . . A better clinical paradigm might entail co-supplementation with gamma-tocopherol."

So, when it comes to Vitamin E, we recommend that you do take it, but only if it contains all eight elements in its complex form.

Please also note: any Vitamin E complex formula should also contain Co-enzyme Q10 (CoQ10), because this nutrient plays a vital role in "recharging" E vitamins to their active anti-oxidant form when they are deactivated in the battle against free-radicals.

CoQ10

CoQ10 is a fat-soluble yellow crystalline compound with a molecular weight of 338.44 Daltons. It functions as a co-enzyme in the energy-producing metabolic pathways of every cell of the body, with a powerful anti-oxidant activity. CoQ10, or Ubiquinone, is a vitamin-like substance that is found in virtually all cells of your body. In 1957, Dr. Fred L Carne noticed a frothy substance that consistently rose to the top of the test tubes of liquidised beef heart.

This yellow crystalline substance was identified by Karl Folkers (the "father" of Co-enzyme Q10) at the Merck, Sharp & Dohme laboratories in New Jersey in 1958. Dr. R.A. Morten called this Q10 compound Ubiquinone because of its widespread or "ubiquitous" appearance in living organisms – it's everywhere! Unlike vitamins, which by definition are not synthesised by the body, CoQ10 is synthesised in all of your body's tissues.

Of particular relevance to Swine Flu, CoQ10 has anti-viral properties [177,178,179] and is a strong anti-oxidant with over 2,033 research studies listed on PubMed. Research suggests that CoQ10 has the ability to inhibit the arachidonic acid metabolic pathway which, as we have discussed previously in other chapters, inhibits the formation of various prostaglandins, including those responsible for inflammation.

BIOLOGICAL PROPERTIES OF CoQ10:

ANTI-OXIDANT ACTIVITY

Biological oxidation is an event that occurs everywhere, continually in your body, causing havoc among your cells and numerous illnesses. Oxidation happens as a result of the breakdown of oxygen molecules as they combine with other molecules in your body. We see examples of oxidisation all around us – if you cut an apple in half and leave it for a while, it turns brown as the oxygen in the atmosphere reacts with the chemicals in the apple. Rust – where metals react with oxygen – is another example of oxidisation.

Oxidation can be the result of your body's normal metabolism of the foods you eat, or it can occur in your body as a result of external factors which place your body under stress, such as exercise, radiation, pollution, alcohol or heavy metal intoxication, infections etc.

The resulting free-radicals are highly reactive molecules, which interfere with enzymatic reactions and cause disturbance of cell membranes and can even adversely affect your DNA. Free-radicals are needed for a number of important cellular functions – but they are highly reactive as they contain an "unpaired electron" that needs to find another electron to pair with, in order to become stable – and this process begins an oxidisation "cascade" that can wreak havoc upon our cells.

The reason that we don't keel over and die is because we always have some endogenous anti-oxidants in our bodies naturally – the most powerful of which is called Glutathione. In addition, if we eat a healthy diet (Paleo-Mediterranean Diet, for example), which contains lots of fruit, vegetables and lean meats and oily fish, we are able to get the exogenous (coming from outside your body) anti-oxidants that we need.

CoQ10 has a marked ability to "give up" electrons quickly and it therefore acts as a powerful anti-oxidant which acts against free-radicals and this gives you protection against LDL oxidation (the oxidisation of "bad" cholesterol) and it is this oxidisation that is a pivotal step in the cause of atherosclerosis (hardening of your arteries).

CoQ10 ACTS AS A REDOX AGENT

CoQ10 keeps other anti-oxidants (e.g. Vitamins E and C) in their "reduced active" states. For example, as Vitamins C and E perform their functions as anti-oxidants, they themselves become used up or "oxidised" – it is as if they sacrifice themselves by giving up an extra electron from an oxidised molecule, to protect us. Since these vitamins are active in their "reduced" forms, CoQ10 recharges them (reduces them) to their active states, by taking the burden of their extra electron away, so that they can go back to work.

MEMBRANE STABILISATION

CoQ10 stabilises your cell membranes – including those of your red blood cells. This means that they can let the nutrients in that they need and let the used-up, waste molecules out.

ENERGY PRODUCTION

CoQ10 is critical in generating the synthesis of Adenosine Triphosphate (ATP), which is the energy "currency" of all cells. This process takes place in your mitochondria (your cells' power source) and involves an intricate and complex cascade of enzymatic reactions called the "electron transfer chain".

CHEMISTRY

Co-enzyme Q10 has a quinone-like group (hence the Q) with 10 isoprenoid units as the side-chain (hence 10). The quinone ring is synthesised from the amino acid tyrosine whilst the isoprenoid side chains are formed from acetyl CoA (of which pantethine - a form of Vitamin B5 - is also a precursor).

CONTRAINDICATIONS?

None reported. CoQ10 has been shown to be useful with beta-blockers, psychotropic drugs including phenothiazines and tricyclic anti-depressants. A 1994 Lancet study reported 3 cases

PROPER PREPARATION

- When preparing garlic to eat, it is important to chop it finely or ideally, to crush it.
- The action of crushing or chopping garlic releases an enzyme called alliinase that catalyses the formation of allicin – the active component of garlic that is so supportive to good health.
- This rapidly breaks down to form a variety of useful organosulphur compounds.
- Since cooking can inhibit the action of alliinase, scientists recommend letting garlic stand for 10 minutes after chopping or crushing before cooking it.
- Furthermore, alliinase can be inactivated by heat. In one study, microwave cooking of unpeeled, uncrushed garlic totally destroyed alliinase enzyme activity.

where CoQ10 reduced the effect of coumadin – a blood-thinning drug. No other cases have been reported. It may be wise to monitor prothrombin (blood clotting factors) in people who are taking anti-coagulant medication when supplementing with CoQ10, although clotting factors in anyone on drugs such as Warfarin or Heparin should be under observation, regardless of their supplementation status.

CoQ10, like many other supplements can be variable in its quality and bioavailability. It is therefore vital to ensure that you are taking a form of CoQ10 that is actually going to give you the health benefits that make this supplement so uniquely powerful.

GARLIC

Although not actually a vitamin, Garlic is such a valuable supplement that it earns its place in our supplements section. It can of course be eaten raw – which is the ideal way to get most of its enormous numbers of benefits and it can also be taken as a tablet. Many people prefer this method as they are concerned about the garlicky smell that lingers after eating Garlic. However, one way of combating this problem is to eat parsley at the same time – or after eating Garlic – as this is a natural deodoriser – plus it is full of Vitamin C and healthy bioflavoniods.

Garlic (Allium sativum) is a particularly rich source of organosulphur compounds, which are currently being researched in great depth as they appear to have the ability to treat a number of diseases – both acute and chronic.

One of the primary areas of interest for many scientists is the role of Garlic in inhibiting inflammation, as this appears to play an important role in the pathology of many chronic degenerative diseases including diabetes, cardiovascular disease, arthropathies and cancer.

Part of the reason for this anti-inflammatory activity is that the organosulphur compounds in garlic have been found to inhibit the activity of the inflammatory enzymes, cyclooxygenase (COX) and lipoxygenase (LOX) in tests and to decrease the expression of inducible nitric oxide synthase (iNOS) in inflammatory white blood cells (macrophages).

Also, organosulphur compounds have been found to decrease the production of inflammatory signalling molecules – such as the NFKappaB that we discussed earlier. These anti-inflammatory properties may be valuable in combating inflammation that is linked to the Cytokine Storm phenomenon.

Garlic is also a powerful anti-viral agent, which can combat a number of viruses [180,181,182,183,184, 185,186,187,188,189] and this too may be useful in combating a powerful virus such as H1N1.

A study published in the Journal of Nutrition, a respected, peer-reviewed journal, showed that when raw Garlic was administered to rats that were exposed to a chemical carcinogen, the Garlic significantly decreased the amount of DNA damage. However, heating uncrushed Garlic cloves for 60 seconds in a microwave oven or 45 minutes in a convection oven prior to feeding it to the rats blocked the protective effect of Garlic. [190,191]

The study found that the action of crushing the Garlic and allowing it to stand for 10 minutes prior to microwave heating for 60 seconds, or alternatively, cutting the tops off Garlic cloves and allowing them to stand for 10 minutes, before heating in a convection oven, partially restored the protective effect of Garlic against DNA damage.

The results of randomised controlled trials suggest that Garlic supplementation inhibits platelet aggregation [192,193,194] (the "clumping together" of red blood cells) and can improve serum lipid (cholesterol) profiles for up to three months and it is thought that garlic supplementation may prevent cardiovascular disease from developing [195,196,197,198,199,200]

PROBIOTICS

Probiotics are dietary supplements that contain so called "good bacteria". The name comes from the Greek; pro = for and bios = life. We are becoming increasingly familiar with these as many food manufacturers now sell products that are said to contain probiotic bacteria in therapeutic amounts, for example yogurt with live cultures added to them. In addition, many probiotics are present in natural sources such as lactobacillus in yogurt and sauerkraut.

The rationale for including probiotic bacterial cultures in foods is that they support and help your body's naturally-occurring flora (bacteria). Probiotics are often prescribed by nutritionists, and sometimes by doctors, for supplementation after a course of anti-biotics, or to treat candida (an overgrowth of the yeast – candida albicans).

Some of the most effective probiotic supplements will include the following bacteria :

- Bifidobacterium bifidum
- Bifidobacterium breve
- Bifidobacterium infantis
- Bifidobacterium longum
- Lactobacillus acidophilus
- Lactobacillus bulgaricus
- Lactobacillus casei
- Lactobacillus plantarum
- Lactobacillus rhamnosus
- Lactobacillus GG
- Streptococcus thermophilus

Evidence exists to suggest that probiotics strengthen your immune system and they have a number of other important functions that are extremely beneficial to your health.

Your intestines contain a miniature "ecology" of microbes, collectively known as your gut flora or "good bacteria". The number and concentration of various bacterial types can be thrown out of balance by a wide range of circumstances, including the use of anti-biotics or other drugs, excess alcohol, stress, disease, exposure to toxic substances and even the use of antibacterial soap. These circumstances can cause the bacteria that normally work well with our bodies to decrease in quantity and this may allow harmful bacterial and fungal competitors to thrive, to the detriment of your health.

The maintenance of a healthy balance of intestinal flora (bacteria) by using probiotics is very important as it aids digestion and boosts your immune system. It also prevents constipation and helps you sleep better by reducing insomnia. It is also believed to have beneficial impacts on stress-related illnesses. Research suggests that the improvement in normal gut function may also help to reduce the risks of colorectal cancer. [201,202,203,204,205,206,207]

Some strains of Lactobacillus acidophilus are documented to reduce cholesterol and improve the LDL/HDL("bad" cholesterol/"good" cholesterol) ratio. [208,209,210,211,212] Additionally, the benefits of the Lactobacillus casei and Rhamnosus strains found in popular products like Yakult and Actimel in the UK, and Activia in the USA, for example, are well documented.

The problem with some of these products is that they do contain a large amount of added sugar which may be counterproductive, especially in people with candida, or with weakened immune systems.

As we have seen, it is important to remember that sugar dramatically suppresses your immune system – which is not helpful when trying to prepare your immune system to be as optimally resistant to viruses as possible. It is possible to buy probiotics that come in capsules and do not have the extra burden of sugars found in the products above.

PREBIOTICS

It is vital to keep our good bacteria "well fed" and there are many formulations available that achieve this. These are known as "prebiotics". It is better though if you can create your own prebiotic food source by eating foods such as raw oats and unrefined wheat – providing you are not sensitive or allergic to these. The provision of a prebiotic food source in your gut is a good idea, since without the necessary food sources, your probiotics will die off.

ANTI-OXIDANTS

Although we have spoken extensively about the enormous benefits of anti-oxidants, above, we can recap with the following:

When free-radicals rampage through the body, the molecules they damage themselves become free-radicals. The same is true of anti-oxidants. After quenching a free-radical, an anti-oxidant molecule doesn't just disappear. Instead, used-up anti-oxidants are transformed into mild free-radicals. However, because the "radicalised" anti-oxidants are less immediately toxic to your body than the free-radicals they neutralise, the overall effect of anti-oxidants is positive.

Common anti-oxidants are Vitamins A, C, E, and CoQ10 and minerals such as Selenium. The bioflavonoids found in fruits and vegetables are strong anti-oxidants and other anti-oxidant families include substances such as melatonin, glutathione, anthocyanadins, super oxide dismutase (SOD) etc.

There is a great deal of scientific evidence to demonstrate that anti-oxidants are extremely valuable to health, as they have such an enormous sphere of action.

One of the best ways to ensure your anti-oxidant status is optimal is to eat the universally recommended five or more portions of fruit and vegetables each day and to supplement your diet with a good multi-vitamin/multi-mineral supplement and a well designed anti-oxidant.

THE ANTI-OXIDANT NETWORK

It is not enough to just make sure that you are taking your anti-oxidants regularly – you also need to ensure that your anti-oxidants are working to support each other and not "fighting". We recommend that you take an anti-oxidant supplement that ensures that the anti-oxidants that it contains are totally supportive and work together to give you the most benefit possible.

As we have seen above – "radicalised" anti-oxidants can do long-term harm, if they aren't properly dealt with. The most well-studied example of this phenomenon is "tocopherol-mediated peroxidation" (tocopherol as you know, is a member of the Vitamin E family), or "TMP", in which Vitamin E family members stop an incoming free-radical from attacking a particle of LDL ("bad") cholesterol.

The "radicalised" anti-oxidant then initiates a slower, more insidious pattern of lipid peroxidation. Several studies suggest that TMP may play a devastating role in the long-term development of atherosclerosis – hardening of your arteries – which eventually leads to heart disease. [213,214,215]

The potential for chronic illnesses such as heart disease developing as a result of exposure to "radicalised" anti-oxidants can be prevented through taking advantage of the unique synergistic interactions of an elite anti-oxidant strike force: the 'Networking Anti-Oxidants'.

When taken together, these specific, biologically, essential nutrients form a dynamic team of synergistic "co-anti-oxidants." Networking anti-oxidants can "recycle" one another from their "radicalised" forms back into their active, anti-oxidant forms.

By this process of mutual regeneration, Networking Anti-Oxidants enhance and extend one another's capacities and they are fuelled by the fires of life in the body's cellular power plants (mitochondria).

THE 5 NETWORKING ANTI-OXIDANTS

There are five Networking Anti-Oxidants: R (+)-lipoic acid, the Vitamin E complex (including the four tocopherols and four tocotrienols), Vitamin C, CoQ10, and glutathione (GSH).

This mutual regeneration cycle is ultimately kept going thanks to the role played by R (+)-lipoic acid in your body's energy-production cycle. As food energy is converted into cellular energy by your cellular "power plants" (the mitochondria), R (+)-lipoic acid that you take as a supplement is "charged up" into its more potent anti-oxidant form, dihydrolipoic acid (DHLA). It is DHLA, rather than R (+)-lipoic acid itself, that "recycles" other Networking Anti-Oxidants.

Therefore, because the "charging-up" of R (+)-lipoic acid to DHLA piggybacks onto the on-going process of energy production, the mitochondria fuel a renewing cycle of co-regeneration amongst the Networking Anti-Oxidants.

AN OVERVIEW OF THE ANTI-OXIDANT NETWORK RECYCLING PROCESS LOOKS LIKE THIS:

First, the original free-radical attacker is neutralised by a Networking Anti-Oxidant. Unfortunately, the result is that the networking anti-oxidant is degraded into its free-radical form. To save your body from disaster, the networking anti-oxidant is rejuvenated by a co anti-oxidant from the Anti-Oxidant Network team. A game of electron donating "pass the parcel" begins, which ultimately results in rejuvenation by DHLA of the networking anti-oxidant free-radical. And at this point, the "pass the parcel" game is stopped when DHLA is restored through R (+)-lipoic acid's cycling through the mitochondrial energy-production process. For the Anti-Oxidant Network to work optimally, it's crucial to ensure that your lipoic acid supplement is in the form of R (+)-lipoic acid.

ANOTHER CASE OF "BUYER BEWARE"...

Supplements labelled "alpha-lipoic acid", or simply "lipoic acid", contain up to 50% S (-)-lipoic acid, which is an unnatural molecule that hinders the ability of mitochondria to "charge up" R (+)-lipoic acid into DHLA. As a result, the S (-)-lipoic acid in conventional lipoic acid supplements actually interferes with the recycling activity of the Networking Anti-Oxidants.

The Networking Anti-Oxidants have a genuine synergy with one another. The effects of each Networking Anti-Oxidant support greater and better functionality of the Anti-Oxidant Network as a whole. No other anti-oxidants participate in the interlocking cycles of the Anti-Oxidant Network. In fact, the ability of other anti-oxidants, such as melatonin and glutathione, to play a protective role in your body depends on having a well functioning Anti-Oxidant Network – but not vice-versa.

However, a few anti-oxidants do play a supporting role to Networking Anti-Oxidants, without fully participating in the Anti-Oxidant Network recycling system. The best understood of these Network "boosters" are bioflavonoids and the mineral Selenium.

Among bioflavonoids, Carnosic Acid – which is found in the herb Rosemary – is especially interesting because of its ability to repeatedly rearrange itself into a "cascade" of new anti-oxidant "booster" forms before being exhausted.

Selenium supports the network by maintaining your body's supply of two key enzymes: glutathione peroxidase (GSH-Px) and thioredoxin reductase (TrxR) both of which are essential for your health. Only very low doses of Selenium are needed to maximise the levels and activity of these enzymes.

You can purchase the various members of the Networking Anti-Oxidant "team" individually but you need to be cautious and ensure you heed the advice given above regarding which ones work and which ones do not work. As we have indicated there are large discrepancies between products that you can buy that may hinder or enhance their effectiveness – due to their bioavailability, their composition and even the amount of active substance they contain.

WHEY PROTEIN

We all need high quality protein and the more active we are the more of this we need.

This is especially the case when preparing your body to be optimally resistant to viral infections such as Swine Flu. There is much data to suggest that while many good sources of quality proteins are available, e.g. lean meat, poultry, oily fish etc. the form of protein that reigns supreme is Whey Protein.

Research indicates that Whey Protein may be useful in the treatment of:

- Certain cancers
- High cholesterol levels
- Catabolism (muscle wasting)
- Impaired immune function

You can't support, maintain, repair, or grow muscle tissue without protein (which the body breaks down into vitally important amino acids). Which means you can't build muscle unless you consume protein. Due to the fact that many of us in Western society are deficient in our amino acid profiles, this indicates that there may well be a lack of high enough quality protein being eaten, or actually absorbed, in such a way that it can be used by your body (metabolised).
This can be as a result of general poor diet or an imbalance of the correct combinations of nutrients that are required for proper protein digestion and metabolism.

Whey Protein, one of several forms of protein derived from milk, is regarded by many nutritionists and also sports and peak performance experts as the highest quality protein available. It does not contain lactose and is therefore not a problem for people with lactose intolerance.

It is considered to be the foundation for building and maintaining muscle mass and the reason that Whey has gained its solid reputation as the supreme protein supplement is due to these important factors:

- It is highly bioavailable (i.e. readily absorbed and utilised by the body) and this means that it provides you with a faster and better uptake of amino acids into your muscle cells than other forms of protein.
- Whey Protein has an extremely rich amino acid content, including the two vitally important amino acids; Glutamine and Cysteine and these are direct precursors to the most powerful free-radical fighting amino acid; Glutathione. Glutathione is vital for enhanced immune function – it is the endogenous anti-oxidant that we mentioned earlier.
- Whey Protein has well-balanced levels of protein peptides that trigger a healthy immune response – lactoferrin and immunoglobulins.

- It has low levels of lactose (milk sugar – which can cause problems for people who are lactose intolerant)
- It has low levels of calories.
- It has low levels of fat.

THE MORE ACTIVE YOU ARE, THE MORE PROTEIN YOUR BODY NEEDS

Any form of "stress" on your body – including mental and emotional stress – that may occur should a severe phase 6 pandemic situation arise, will mean that your protein requirements will increase.

Studies show that optimal health demands that you have an optimal intake of amino acids, specifically, the branched-chained amino acids (BCAA's). Because a large portion of muscle tissue is made up of protein – of which amino acids are the building blocks – this greater requirement must come in the form of protein. Amino acids have many roles which include building cells and repairing tissues, forming antibodies to combat invading pathogens such as bacteria and viruses, they are part of our enzyme and hormonal systems, they build nucleoproteins (our genetic material – RNA and DNA), they carry oxygen throughout the body and participate in muscle activity.

When protein is broken down by the process of digestion, this results in the release of 22 known amino acids. Eight of these are "essential" (i.e. they cannot be manufactured by your body) the rest are "non-essential" (can be manufactured by your body if you have correct nutrition).

Whey Protein has very high concentrations of important amino acids including a large percentage (50%) of the BCAA's valine, leucine and isoleucine that are so vitally important for building and maintaining muscle tissue, giving our bodies the protein-rich nutrition they need to get and stay strong, and be optimally resistant to disease.

IMPROVED IMMUNE FUNCTION

Intense exercise, stress and vigorous physical activity can deplete our amino acid levels and this renders them less able to battle free-radicals, throughout our bodies. (See the chapter on Exercise). The amino acids in Whey Protein, L-glutamine and L-cysteine, help produce higher levels of Glutathione and ensure our immune systems are strong enough to fight infections and illness.

In one animal study, Whey Proteins were found to be protective against colon cancer [216,217,218,219,220] and there is even evidence to suggest Whey Protein may promote tumour regression (shrinkage) and normalisation.[221] Researchers have also conducted studies, whereupon a strain of human milk protein consisting of high levels of alpha-lactalbumin, a component of Whey Protein, was able to induce apoptosis (programmed cellular death) of cancer cells while leaving healthy cells intact. [222,223]

Furthermore, several clinical studies have determined that alpha-lactalbumin from Whey is highly effective at reducing stress. [224,225] The mechanism of action behind this extraordinary claim is that it raises brain serotonin (the "feel-good" chemical) activity while simultaneously reducing Cortisol (the "stress hormone") levels – which also means that there is good potential for alpha-lactalbumin to be used as a sleep aid.

Another protein-based component that figures prominently in the constitution of Whey Protein is lactoferrin. This is an iron-binding Whey Protein fraction that has been known to demonstrate an impressive anti-microbial capability of its own, among numerous other functions. These include controlling inflammation (which as we have seen, has relevance for protection against Swine Flu) and balancing cholesterol so that it is at optimum levels for health.

Scientists have identified lactoferrin's anti-inflammatory capabilities [226,227,228,229,230] which work through its stimulation of the anti-inflammatory cytokines (intracellular messengers) IL-4 and IL-10, and its simultaneous inhibition of the pro-inflammatory TNFα and IL-ß cytokines.

Research indicates that lactoferrin may act as a potent anti-inflammatory protein at local sites of inflammation including the respiratory[231] and gastrointestinal tracts.[232]

It is also important for Mucosal Immunity[233] which is of great relevance to protecting us from Swine Flu, since strong Mucosal Immunity helps us to be more resistant to viruses.

Lactoferrin's effects on cholesterol levels, on the other hand, seem to be based on its ability to reduce the oxidation of LDL ("bad") cholesterol.[234] This is important because oxidised LDL

The preferential attachment point for the hemagglutinin in the H5N1 virus is the α2,3 polymer of Sialic Acid. Tamiflu is an example of an anti-viral medicine that is based on trying to block the interaction between the Neuraminidase of influenza and the Sialic Acid receptor on the mucosal surface that the viral particle binds to. Sialic Acid binding SabA adhesion has been shown, in numerous studies, to be the binding site for various pathogenic organisms including H.pylori and various rotaviruses[236]. Research suggests that the Sialic Acid in Whey Protein may interfere with viral adherence capability [237,238,239,240].

Finally, there is a particularly innovative Whey Protein fraction called N-acetylneuraminic acid – commonly known as "Sialic Acid" – that has been receiving a great deal of attention in recent years. Sialic Acids are sugar molecules that are part of the glycomacropeptide content of Whey Protein.

In humans they are especially present in mucus and saliva and their biological role is to bind to invading pathogens for their subsequent excretion via the mucus membranes.

Whey Protein is of such great interest to scientists that the world's leading protein researchers and industry leaders have been gathering once a year over the last nine years in conferences to exchange information exclusively or primarily on the latest developments in Whey. In the conference held in Chicago, Illinois in September, 2005, Sialic Acids ranked among the most heavily-discussed topics of the entire conference.

There is also clinical evidence demonstrating that Sialic Acids may be responsible for the ability of glycoproteins (similar to the type found in Whey) to bind to E.coli and other types of bacteria, thus preventing their adhesion to the epithelial cell surface. This means that they can protect us from types of deadly bacteria such as E.coli, which can cause devastating gastro-intestinal problems, urinary tract infections, kidney infections etc.

The use of Whey Protein could then, possibly reduce the number of deaths and serious disablements that are related to E.coli food poisoning that we have often seen reported in the media.

Furthermore, while there has yet to be any research on this topic in regard to Swine Flu, there has been recent evidence showing that the Bird Flu virus (H5N1) has a propensity to attach itself to two particular types of polymers (tiny molecules strung in long repeating chains) that are themselves linked to Sialic Acid, thus opening the possibility of Sialic Acid's potential effectiveness against Bird Flu H5N1 – and possibly Swine Flu (H1N1).

It is not yet known whether Sialic Acid in Whey Protein will protect people from specific pandemic flu virus strains, however the science behind this proposition is as follows: many antiviral drugs – such as Tamiflu and Zanamivir were developed to inhibit the enzyme Neuraminidase (NA). This is a useful target for development of antiviral medication because of its essential role in the pathogenicity of many respiratory viruses.

As we read in our Chapter "What is a Virus", Neuraminidase removes Sialic Acid from the surface of infected cells and virus particles, which stops viruses from trying to re-enter an already infected cell, or even trying to "remix" its RNA, and this helps to promote the spread of the virus. Neuraminidase also plays a role in the initial penetration of the mucosal lining of the respiratory tract [241].

Interestingly, Neuramindase inhibitors such as Zanamivir were developed to be "analogues' of Sialic Acid [242]. So, hypothetically, at the moment, Sialic Acid could act as a Neuraminidase inhibitor for H1N1 although, of course, this hypothesis is yet to be tested.

There is a great deal of research in this area and the field is explosive in its literature output. As we learn more we will distribute this information via our CMA Monthly e-Newsletter Updates on The Complementary Medical Association's website (The-CMA.Org.UK).

OMEGA 3

Omega-3 Essential Fatty Acids are well-known inflammation fighters. Scientific trials clearly show that they fight inflammation and can often reduce the need, or even eliminate the requirement for, anti-inflammatory drugs which often have very harmful side effects. Aspirin and older non-steroidal anti-inflammatory drugs (NSAIDS), such as ibuprofen (e.g. Neurofen) carry warnings about the tendency of these drugs to cause stomach discomfort and even bleeding which can be, in some cases, severe enough to cause death.

Research demonstrates that 65% of people who take these drugs, long-term, will develop intestinal inflammation and 30% of long-term NSAID users will get gastroduodenal ulceration (stomach ulcers). In addition, drugs such as the "COX2 Inhibitors" Vioxx® (now banned) and Celebrex® have caused severe cardio-vascular events such as heart attack and stroke in people who took these drugs.

NSAIDS and COX 2 Inhibitors both work through their effects on a group of local, cellular hormones called eicosanoids. Eicosanoids are "messengers" that cells use to communicate with one another, thereby co-ordinating their activities. It is important to remember that inflammation is, in some cases, an important and useful response that your body produces to help us fight disease and to help us deal with injuries. However, to illustrate the action of eicosanoids and how these are moderated by Omega 3 Fatty Acids, we will call some eicosanoids "bad" if they promote undesirable inflammation, and call others "good" eicosanoids, if they have strong and powerful anti-inflammatory functions.

Your body's inflammatory response depends to a great degree on the balance of "good" and "bad" eicosanoids produced by your cells when they respond to your immune system's inflammatory call.

BAD EICOSANOIDS

"Bad" eicosanoids are made from the Omega-6 Fatty Acid called arachidonic acid – we've already discussed the effects of this in some detail. Most drug approaches to inflammation, from aspirin, NSAIDs, to the "COX-2 Inhibitor" drugs, like celecoxib [Celebrex®] and rofecoxib [Vioxx®] , work by inhibiting the formation of the series-2 Prostanoid Group of "bad" eicosanoids.

Prostanoids are formed from arachidonic acid by an enzyme called cyclooxygenase, or "COX". ("Prostanoid" is the term used to describe three types of eicosanoids: the prostaglandins, which are mediators of inflammation and anaphylaxis (the type of syndrome seen in severe allergic reactions), the thromboxanes which are mediators of vasoconstriction (constriction of blood vessels) and the prostacyclins, these are active in the resolution phase of inflammation.)

But while NSAIDS and COX2 Inhibitors certainly provide symptomatic relief of inflammatory symptoms such as pain and swelling in the short-term, COX-2 Inhibitors can actually accelerate the underlying inflammatory disease in the long-term.

They do this by diverting arachidonic acid into another, slower-acting and ultimately more destructive pathway; the lipoxygenase (LOX) enzyme pathway, which produces the damaging "series-4 leukotrienes".

Leukotrienes are the eicosanoids released by immune cells involved in your body's inflammatory responses and are more responsible for the long-term consequences of inflammation, which can result when a 'deranged' immune system attacks the very body that it was designed to defend.

What we have seen therefore, in the cases of people who have either died or been seriously injured as a result of taking COX2 Inhibitors, is that blocking the COX pathway alone results in an imbalance – an imbalance that ultimately trades short-term gain for long-term pain.

People who are experiencing generalised chronic inflammation – that's anyone who is following the "Western Diet" – and people who actually suffer from autoimmune disorders need a "dual pathway inhibitor"; a molecule which will shut down COX-2 and LOX alike, preventing the formation of all "bad" eicosanoids.

Giant pharmaceutical companies around the world are scrabbling to develop drugs that will achieve this dual pathway inhibitor – but Mother Nature has beaten them to it – with her Omega 3 Fatty Acids.

AN OMEGA 3 RECAP:

As we know, Omega 3 Fatty Acids are found in lean meat, oily fish, and in certain oils, such as walnut oil and flaxseed oil. They actually act on our DNA, activating, or inhibiting, transcription factors for NF-KappaB, the pro-inflammatory substance that is essential to and "kicks off" the process of inflammation.

Omega-3 fish oils are a rich source of Essential Fatty Acids (EFAs), such as docosahexanoic acid (DHA) and eicosapentaenoic acid (EPA). The levels of EFAs are typically three times greater in oils from the flesh of salmon, herrings, sardines, pilchards, and mackerel than in the oils that are extracted from cod liver.

There was a great deal of adverse publicity some years ago, regarding an overview of a number of trials on fish oils which showed that they were not of use in preventing cardio-vascular disease, and in fact may increase the death rate among people who were taking them. The research was based on trials that took place last century – before the dangers from toxic contaminants were really appreciated – so the oils used probably did contain high levels of toxic substances such as heavy metals including mercury.

Furthermore, this overview of the research produced a view that was diametrically opposed to the view taken by leading health advisory bodies including the USA's Food and Drug Administration – who, not long ago, actually prepared a statement that manufacturers of foods containing Omega 3's could use on their packaging to illustrate and promote the health benefits of the contents. Given the great concern over the levels of toxicity in fish oils, it is absolutely essential that you only take a fish oil that has been refined properly and is certified and guaranteed to be free of these harmful substances.

SUPEROXIDE DISMUTASE (SOD)

Considered to be the anti-ageing supplement - par excellence, Superoxide Dismutase, or 'SOD' for short, is found in and around every cell and plays a key antioxidant role. (In humans and other mammals, three forms of superoxide dismutase are present: SOD1 is located in the cytoplasm, SOD2 in the mitochondria and SOD3 is extracellular.) SOD is extremely important to heath and this is illustrated by the severe pathologies evident in mice genetically engineered to lack these enzymes. Mice lacking SOD2 die several days after birth, amidst massive oxidative stress. Mice lacking SOD1 develop a wide range of pathologies, including hepatocellular carcinoma (liver cancer), an acceleration of age-related muscle mass loss, an earlier incidence of cataracts and a reduced lifespan. Mice lacking SOD3 do not show any obvious defects and exhibit a normal lifespan, though they are more sensitive to hyperoxic injury.

Drosophila (fruit flies) lacking SOD1 have a dramatically shortened lifespan while flies lacking SOD2 die before birth.

Aside from its anti-ageing, antioxidant capabilities, SOD has many other health benefits. In fact, SOD has proven to be highly effective in the treatment of colonic inflammation in experimental colitis. Treatment with SOD decreases reactive oxygen species generation and oxidative stress and thus, inhibits endothelial activation and indicates that modulation of factors that govern adhesion molecule expression and leukocyte-endothelial interactions, such as antioxidants, may be important new tools for the treatment of inflammatory bowel disease.

SOD Research:
There have been numerous studies into the effects of SOD - however one in particular illustrates the anti-inflammatory effect of SOD - as derived from melon[143]. The study was undertaken to evaluate the antioxidant and anti-inflammatory effects of an extract of cantaloupe melon (Cucumis melo -

'CME') extract due to its high antioxidant activity. The study in mice evaluated the production of both pro and anti-inflammatory cytokines (TNFα and IL10 respectively) following exposure to CME. The trial results demonstrated that, in addition to its antioxidant properties, the anti-inflammatory properties of the CME extract were principally related to its capacity to induce the production of IL-10 by peritoneal macrophages (these are white blood cells found in the peritoneum in the abdominal cavity).

The problem with SOD is that it is very difficult to find forms that survive the journey through the intestinal tract and can be used by your body. One solution to this is linking the SOD to a wheat protein - gliadin (Triticum vulgare) - which enables the SOD to become bioavailable. In the trial mice were fed SOD - specially formulated with gliadin - and the results of the trial demonstrated that SOD - when prepared with gliadin - not only survives the journey through the intestinal tract, it is bioavailable - and produces a marked anti-inflammatory effect due to its ability to reduce the production of TNFα and increase the production of IL10. (IL10 - as with most cytokines has numerous functions - but of interest here is the fact that IL10 is capable of inhibiting synthesis of pro-inflammatory cytokines like IFN-γ, IL-2, IL-3, TNFα and GM-CSF made by cells such as macrophages and the Type 1 T helper cells.) Based upon this trial and other like it, we believe that SOD supplementation - when rendered bioavailable - is a useful adjunct to both the prevention and treatment of Swine Flu.

REFERENCES

1 Kasim-Karakas SE, Tsodikov A, Singh U, Jialal I. Responses of inflammatory markers to a low-fat, high-carbohydrate diet: effects of energy intake. Am J Clin Nutr. 2006 Apr;83(4):774-9.
2 Hennig B, Lei W, Arzuaga X, Ghosh DD, Saraswathi V, Toborek M. Linoleic acid induces proinflammatory events in vascular endothelial cells via activation of PI3K/Akt and ERK1/2 signaling. J Nutr Biochem. 2006 Mar 22; [Epub ahead of print]
3 De Caterina R, Zampolli A, Del Turco S, Madonna R, Massaro M. Nutritional mechanisms that influence cardiovascular disease. Am J Clin Nutr. 2006 Feb;83(2):421S-426S. Review.
4 De Souza CT, Araujo EP, Bordin S, Ashimine R, Zollner RL, Boschero AC, Saad MJ, Velloso LA. Consumption of a fat-rich diet activates a proinflammatory response and induces insulin resistance in the hypothalamus. Endocrinology. 2005 Oct;146(10):4192-9. Epub 2005 Jul 7.
5 Am J Clin Nutr. 2006 Mar;83(3):575-81. Mediterranean-inspired diet lowers the ratio of serum phospholipid n-6 to n-3 fatty acids, the number of leukocytes and platelets, and vascular endothelial growth factor in healthy subjects. Ambring A, Johansson M, Axelsen M, Gan L, Strandvik B, Friberg P. Department of Clinical Physiology, The Sahlgrenska Academy at Goteborg University, Goteborg, Sweden.
6 Seaman DR. The diet-induced proinflammatory state: a cause of chronic pain and other degenerative diseases? J Manipulative Physiol Ther. 2002 Mar-Apr;25(3):168-79. Review.
7 Aljada, A. American Journal of Clinical Nutrition, April 2004; vol 79: pp 682-690. News release, University of Buffalo.
8 Vasquez A. Chiropractic and Naturopathic Medicine for the Promotion of Optimal Health and Alleviation of Pain and Inflammation. http://optimalhealthresearch.com/major-monograph-05.
9 Mann NJ. Palaeolithic nutrition: what can we learn from the past? Asia Pac J Clin Nutr. 2004;13(Suppl):S17.
10 O'Keefe JH Jr, Cordain L. Cardiovascular disease resulting from a diet and lifestyle at odds with our Palaeolithic genome: how to become a 21st-century hunter-gatherer. Mayo Clin Proc. 2004 Jan;79(1):101-8.
11 Cordain L, Eaton SB, Miller JB, Mann N, Hill K. The paradoxical nature of hunter-gatherer diets: meat-based, yet non-atherogenic. Eur J Clin Nutr. 2002 Mar;56 Suppl 1:S42-52.
12 Eaton SB, Eaton SB 3rd. Palaeolithic vs. modern diets—selected pathophysiological implications. Eur J Nutr. 2000 Apr;39(2):67-70.
13 Simopoulos AP. Evolutionary aspects of omega-3 fatty acids in the food supply. Prostaglandins Leukot Essent Fatty Acids. 1999 May-Jun;60(5-6):421-9.
14 Vasquez A. Chiropractic and Naturopathic Medicine for the Promotion of Optimal Health and Alleviation of Pain and Inflammation. http://optimalhealthresearch.com/major-monograph-05.
15 Mann NJ. Palaeolithic nutrition: what can we learn from the past? Asia Pac J Clin Nutr. 2004;13(Suppl):S17.
16 O'Keefe JH Jr, Cordain L. Cardiovascular disease resulting from a diet and lifestyle at odds with our Palaeolithic genome: how to become a 21st-century hunter-gatherer. Mayo Clin Proc. 2004 Jan;79(1):101-8.
17 Cordain L, Eaton SB, Miller JB, Mann N, Hill K. The paradoxical nature of hunter-gatherer diets: meat-based, yet non-atherogenic. Eur J Clin Nutr. 2002 Mar;56 Suppl 1:S42-52.

18 Eaton SB, Eaton SB 3rd. Palaeolithic vs. modern diets—selected pathophysiological implications. Eur J Nutr. 2000 Apr;39(2):67-70.

19 Simopoulos AP. Evolutionary aspects of omega-3 fatty acids in the food supply. Prostaglandins Leukot Essent Fatty Acids. 1999 May-Jun;60(5-6):421-9.

20 Serra-Majem L, Roman B, Estruch R. Scientific evidence of interventions using the Mediterranean diet: a systematic review. Nutr Rev. 2006 Feb;64(2 Pt 2):S27-47.

21 Ambring A, Johansson M, Axelsen M, Gan L, Strandvik B, Friberg P. Mediterranean-inspired diet lowers the ratio of serum phospholipid n-6 to n-3 fatty acids, the number of leukocytes and platelets, and vascular endothelial growth factor in healthy subjects. Am J Clin Nutr. 2006 Mar;83(3):575-81.

22 Gerber M. Qualitative methods to evaluate Mediterranean diet in adults. Public Health Nutr. 2006 Feb;9(1A):147-51.

23 de Lorgeril M, Salen P. The Mediterranean-style diet for the prevention of cardiovascular diseases. Public Health Nutr. 2006 Feb;9(1A):118-23.

24 Alexandratos N. The Mediterranean diet in a world context. Public Health Nutr. 2006 Feb;9(1A):111-7.

25 Willett WC. The Mediterranean diet: science and practice. Public Health Nutr. 2006 Feb;9(1A):105-10.

26 Dernini S. Towards the advancement of the Mediterranean food cultures. Public Health Nutr. 2006 Feb;9(1A):103-4.

27 Serra-Majem L, Bach A, Roman B. Recognition of the Mediterranean diet: going a step further. Public Health Nutr. 2006 Feb;9(1A):101-2.

28 JAMA. 2004 Sep 22;292(12):1433-9. Comment in: JAMA. 2004 Sep 22;292(12):1490-2. JAMA. 2005 Feb 9;293(6):674; author reply 674-5. JAMA. 2005 Feb 9;293(6):674; author reply 674-5. Mediterranean diet, lifestyle factors, and 10-year mortality in elderly European men and women: the HALE project. Knoops KT, de Groot LC, Kromhout D, Perrin AE, Moreiras-Varela O, Menotti A, van Staveren WA. Division of Human Nutrition, Wageningen University, The Netherlands. Kim.Knoops@wur.nl

29 Mann NJ. Palaeolithic nutrition: what can we learn from the past? Asia Pac J Clin Nutr. 2004;13(Suppl):S17

30 O'Dea K. Westernisation, insulin resistance and diabetes in Australian aborigines. Med J Aust. 1991 Aug 19;155(4):258-64.

31 O'Dea K. Cardiovascular disease risk factors in Australian aborigines. Clin Exp Pharmacol Physiol. 1991 Feb;18(2):85-8.

32 O'Dea K. Westernization and non-insulin-dependent diabetes in Australian Aborigines. Ethn Dis. 1991 Spring;1(2):171-87.

33 Eyer J. Hypertension as a disease of modern society. Int J Health Serv. 1975;5(4):539-58.

34 Martinez-Gonzalez MA. The SUN cohort study (Seguimiento University of Navarra). Public Health Nutr. 2006 Feb;9(1A):127-31.

35 de Lorgeril M, Salen P. The Mediterranean-style diet for the prevention of cardiovascular diseases. Public Health Nutr. 2006 Feb;9(1A):118-23.

36 Willett WC. The Mediterranean diet: science and practice. Public Health Nutr. 2006 Feb;9(1A):105-10.

37 Bogani P, Galli C, Villa M, Visioli F. Postprandial anti-inflammatory and anti-oxidant effects of extra virgin olive oil. Atherosclerosis. 2006 Feb 17; [Epub ahead of print]

38 Rosenthal RL. Effectiveness of altering serum cholesterol levels without drugs. Proc (Bayl Univ Med Cent). 2000 Oct;13(4):351-5.

39 Gau GT. The hunt for the perfect heart health diet. Asia Pac J Clin Nutr. 2004;13(Suppl):S4.

40 De Lorgeril M. Nutritional trials for the prevention of coronary heart disease. Asia Pac J Clin Nutr. 2004;13(Suppl):S2.

41 Panagiotakos DB, Pitsavos C, Polychronopoulos E, Chrysohoou C, Zampelas A, Trichopoulou A. Can a Mediterranean diet moderate the development and clinical progression of coronary heart disease? A systematic review. Med Sci Monit. 2004 Aug;10(8):RA193-8. Epub 2004 Jul 23.

42 Panagiotakos DB, Pitsavos Ch, Chrysohoou Ch, Stefanadis Ch, Toutouzas P. The role of traditional mediterranean type of diet and lifestyle, in the development of acute coronary syndromes: preliminary results from CARDIO 2000 study. Cent Eur J Public Health. 2002 Jun;10(1-2):11-5.

43 Serra-Majem L, Roman B, Estruch R. Scientific evidence of interventions using the Mediterranean diet: a systematic review. Nutr Rev. 2006 Feb;64(2 Pt 2):S27-47.

44 Marin C, Perez-Jimenez F, Gomez P, Delgado J, Paniagua JA, Lozano A, Cortes B, Jimenez-Gomez Y, Gomez MJ, Lopez-Miranda J. The Ala54Thr polymorphism of the fatty acid-binding Protein 2 gene is associated with a change in insulin sensitivity after a change in the type of dietary fat. Am J Clin Nutr. 2005 Jul;82(1):196-200.

45 Urquiaga I, Guasch V, Marshall G, San Martin A, Castillo O, Rozowski J, Leighton F. Effect of Mediterranean and Occidental diets, and red wine, on plasma fatty acids in humans. An intervention study. Biol Res. 2004;37(2):253-61.

46 Biesalski HK. Diabetes preventive interventions in the Mediterranean diet. Eur J Nutr. 2004 Mar;43 Suppl 1:I/26-30.

47 Toobert DJ, Glasgow RE, Strycker LA, Barrera M Jr, Radcliffe JL, Wander RC, Bagdade JD. Biologic and quality-of-life outcomes from the Mediterranean Lifestyle Program: a randomized clinical trial. Diabetes Care. 2003 Aug;26(8):2288-93.

48 Perez-Jimenez F, Lopez-Miranda J, Pinillos MD, Gomez P, Paz-Rojas E, Montilla P, Marin C, Velasco MJ, Blanco-Molina A, Jimenez Pereperez JA, Ordovas JM. A Mediterranean and a high-carbohydrate diet improve glucose metabolism in healthy young persons. Diabetologia. 2001 Nov;44(11):2038-43.

49 Ryan M, McInerney D, Owens D, Collins P, Johnson A, Tomkin GH. Diabetes and the Mediterranean diet: a beneficial effect of oleic acid on insulin sensitivity, adipocyte glucose transport and endothelium-dependent vasoreactivity. QJM. 2000 Feb;93(2):85-91.

50 Colomer R, Menendez JA. Mediterranean diet, olive oil and cancer. Clin Transl Oncol. 2006 Jan;8(1):15-21.

51 Serra-Majem L, Roman B, Estruch R. Scientific evidence of interventions using the Mediterranean diet: a systematic review. Nutr Rev. 2006 Feb;64(2 Pt 2):S27-47

52 Menendez JA, Papadimitropoulou A, Vellon L, Colomer R, Lupu R. A genomic explanation connecting "Mediterranean diet", olive oil and cancer: Oleic acid, the main monounsaturated Fatty acid of olive oil, induces formation of inhibitory "PEA3 transcription factor-PEA3 DNA binding site" complexes at the Her-2/neu (erbB-2) oncogene promoter in breast, ovarian and stomach cancer cells. Eur J Cancer. 2006 Jan 4; [Epub ahead of print]

53 Lanzotti V. The analysis of onion and Garlic. J Chromatogr A. 2006 Apr 21;1112(1-2):3-22. Epub 2006 Jan 18.

54 Garcia Mediero JM, Ferruelo Alonso A, Paez Borda A, Lujan Galan M, Angulo Cuesta J, Chiva Robles V, Berenguer Sanchez A. [Effect of polyphenols from the Mediterranean diet on proliferation and mediators of in vitro invasiveness of the MB-49 murine bladder cancer cell line] Actas Urol Esp. 2005 Sep;29(8):743-9.
55 Hamdi HK, Castellon R. Oleuropein, a non-toxic olive iridoid, is an anti-tumor agent and cytoskeleton disruptor. Biochem Biophys Res Commun. 2005 Sep 2;334(3):769-78.
56 Gill CI, Boyd A, McDermott E, McCann M, Servili M, Selvaggini R, Taticchi A, Esposto S, Montedoro G, McGlynn H, Rowland I. Potential anti-cancer effects of virgin olive oil phenols on colorectal carcinogenesis models in vitro. Int J Cancer. 2005 Oct 20;117(1):1-7.
57 Wahle KW, Caruso D, Ochoa JJ, Quiles JL. Olive oil and modulation of cell signaling in disease prevention. Lipids. 2004 Dec;39(12):1223-31.
58 Cottet V, Bonithon-Kopp C, Kronborg O, Santos L, Andreatta R, Boutron-Ruault MC, Faivre J; European Cancer Prevention Organisation Study Group. Dietary patterns and the risk of colorectal adenoma recurrence in a European intervention trial. Eur J Cancer Prev. 2005 Feb;14(1):21-9.
59 Visioli F, Grande S, Bogani P, Galli C. The role of anti-oxidants in the mediterranean diets: focus on cancer. Eur J Cancer Prev. 2004 Aug;13(4):337-43.
60 Owen RW, Haubner R, Wurtele G, Hull E, Spiegelhalder B, Bartsch H. Olives and olive oil in cancer prevention. Eur J Cancer Prev. 2004 Aug;13(4):319-26. Review.
61 La Vecchia C. Mediterranean diet and cancer. Public Health Nutr. 2004 Oct;7(7):965-8. Review.
62 Simopoulos AP. The traditional diet of Greece and cancer. Eur J Cancer Prev. 2004 Jun;13(3):219-30. Review.
63 Gallus S, Bosetti C, La Vecchia C. Mediterranean diet and cancer risk. Eur J Cancer Prev. 2004 Oct;13(5):447-52.
64 Bosetti C, Gallus S, Trichopoulou A, Talamini R, Franceschi S, Negri E, La Vecchia C. Influence of the Mediterranean diet on the risk of cancers of the upper aerodigestive tract. Cancer Epidemiol Biomarkers Prev. 2003 Oct;12(10):1091-4.
65 Fortes C, Forastiere F, Farchi S, Mallone S, Trequattrinni T, Anatra F, Schmid G, Perucci CA. The protective effect of the Mediterranean diet on lung cancer. Nutr Cancer. 2003;46(1):30-7.
66 Hermann F, Spieker LE, Ruschitzka F, Sudano I, Hermann M, Binggeli C, Luscher TF, Riesen W, Noll G, Corti R. Dark chocolate improves endothelial and platelet function. Heart. 2006 Jan;92(1):119-20.
67 Grassi D, Necozione S, Lippi C, Croce G, Valeri L, Pasqualetti P, Desideri G, Blumberg JB, Ferri C. Cocoa reduces blood pressure and insulin resistance and improves endothelium-dependent vasodilation in hypertensives. Hypertension. 2005 Aug;46(2):398- 405. Epub 2005 Jul 18.
68 Vlachopoulos C, Aznaouridis K, Alexopoulos N, Economou E, Andreadou I, Stefanadis C. Effect of dark chocolate on arterial function in healthy individuals. Am J Hypertens. 2005 Jun;18(6):785-91.
69 Grassi D, Lippi C, Necozione S, Desideri G, Ferri C. Short-term administration of dark chocolate is followed by a significant increase in insulin sensitivity and a decrease in blood pressure in healthy persons. Am J Clin Nutr. 2005 Mar;81(3):611-4.
70 Mursu J, Voutilainen S, Nurmi T, Rissanen TH, Virtanen JK, Kaikkonen J, Nyyssonen K, Salonen JT. Dark chocolate consumption increases HDL cholesterol concentration and chocolate fatty acids may inhibit lipid peroxidation in healthy humans. Free Radic Biol Med. 2004 Nov 1;37(9):1351-9.
71 Engler MB, Engler MM, Chen CY, Malloy MJ, Browne A, Chiu EY, Kwak HK, Milbury P, Paul SM, Blumberg J, Mietus-Snyder ML. Flavonoid-rich dark chocolate improves endothelial function and increases plasma epicatechin concentrations in healthy adults. J Am Coll Nutr. 2004 Jun;23(3):197-204.
72 Innes AJ, Kennedy G, McLaren M, Bancroft AJ, Belch JJ. Dark chocolate inhibits platelet aggregation in healthy volunteers. Platelets. 2003 Aug;14(5):325-7.
73 Steinberg FM, Bearden MM, Keen CL. Cocoa and chocolate Flavonoids: implications for cardiovascular health. J Am Diet Assoc. 2003 Feb;103(2):215-23.
74 Mathur S, Devaraj S, Grundy SM, Jialal I. Cocoa products decrease low density lipoProtein oxidative susceptibility but do not affect biomarkers of inflammation in humans. J Nutr. 2002 Dec;132(12):3663-7.
75 Wan Y, Vinson JA, Etherton TD, Proch J, Lazarus SA, Kris-Etherton PM. Effects of cocoa powder and dark chocolate on LDL oxidative susceptibility and prostaglandin concentrations in humans. Am J Clin Nutr. 2001 Nov;74(5):596-602.
76 Curr Med Chem. 2006;13(9):989-96. Vascular dysfunction in aging: potential effects of resveratrol, an anti-inflammatory phytoestrogen. Labinskyy N, Csiszar A, Veress G, Stef G, Pacher P, Oroszi G, Wu J, Ungvari Z. Department of Physiology, New York Medical College, Valhalla, New York 10595, USA. zoltan_ungvari@nymc.edu.
77 Mol Interv. 2006 Feb;6(1):36-47. Resveratrol in cardioprotection: a therapeutic promise of alternative medicine. Das DK, Maulik N. Cardiovascular Research Center, University of Connecticut School of Medicine, Farmington, CT 06030-1110, USA.
78 Am J Clin Nutr. 2005 Feb;81(2):341-54. Comment in: Am J Clin Nutr. 2005 Aug;82(2):483; author reply 483-4. Origins and evolution of the Western diet: health implications for the 21st century. Cordain L, Eaton SB, Sebastian A, Mann N, Lindeberg S, Watkins BA, O'Keefe JH, Brand-Miller J. Department of Health and Exercise Science, Colorado State University, Fort Collins, CO 80523, USA. cordain@cahs.colostate.edu
79 Am J Clin Nutr. 2004 Feb;79(2):311-7. Fruit and vegetable intakes are an independent predictor of bone size in early pubertal children. Tylavsky FA, Holliday K, Danish R, Womack C, Norwood J, Carbone L. Health Science Center, University of Tennessee, Memphis, TN 38105, USA. ftylavsky@utmem.edu
80 MacLeay JM, Olson JD, Enns RM, Les CM, Toth CA, Wheeler DL, Turner AS. Dietary-induced metabolic acidosis decreases bone mineral density in mature ovariectomized ewes. Calcif Tissue Int. 2004 Nov;75(5):431-7. Epub 2004 Aug 12.
81 New SA. Intake of fruit and vegetables: implications for bone health. Proc Nutr Soc. 2003 Nov;62(4):889-99. Review. Erratum in: Proc Nutr Soc. 2004 Feb;63(1):187. 82 Macleay JM, Olson JD, Turner AS. Effect of dietary-induced metabolic acidosis and ovariectomy on bone mineral density and markers of bone turnover. J Bone Miner Metab. 2004;22(6):561-8.
83 Maurer M, Riesen W, Muser J, Hulter HN, Krapf R. Neutralization of Western diet inhibits bone resorption independently of K intake and

reduces cortisol secretion in humans. Am J Physiol Renal Physiol. 2003 Jan;284(1):F32-40. Epub 2002 Sep 24.

84 New SA. Nutrition Society Medal lecture. The role of the skeleton in acid-base homeostasis. Proc Nutr Soc. 2002 May;61(2):151-64.

85 Wiederkehr M, Krapf R. Metabolic and endocrine effects of metabolic acidosis in humans. Swiss Med Wkly. 2001 Mar 10;131(9-10):127-32. Review.

86 Am J Clin Nutr. 2002 Dec;76(6):1308-16. Comment in: Am J Clin Nutr. 2003 Oct;78(4):802-3; author reply 803-4. Estimation of the net acid load of the diet of ancestral preagricultural Homo sapiens and their hominid ancestors. Sebastian A, Frassetto LA, Sellmeyer DE, Merriam RL, Morris RC Jr. Department of Medicine and the General Clinical Research Center, University of California, San Francisco, California 94143, USA. anthony_sebastian@msn.com

87 Am J Clin Nutr. 2002 Dec;76(6):1308-16. Comment in: Am J Clin Nutr. 2003 Oct;78(4):802-3; author reply 803-4. Estimation of the net acid load of the diet of ancestral preagricultural Homo sapiens and their hominid ancestors. Sebastian A, Frassetto LA,Sellmeyer DE, Merriam RL, Morris RC Jr. Department of Medicine and the General Clinical Research Center, University of California, San Francisco, California 94143, USA. anthony_sebastian@msn.com

88 Wetz K. Attachment of neutralizing antibodies stabilizes the capsid of poliovirus against uncoating. Virology. 1993 Feb;192(2):465-72.

89 Warwicker J. Model for the differential stabilities of rhinovirus and poliovirus to mild acidic pH, based on electrostatics calculations. J Mol Biol. 1992 Jan 5;223(1):247-57.

90 Warwicker J. Model for the differential stabilities of rhinovirus and poliovirus to mild acidic pH, based on electrostatics calculations. J Mol Biol. 1992 Jan 5;223(1):247-57.

91 Wojtowicz H, Kloc K, Maliszewska I, Mlochowski J, Pietka M, Piasecki E. Azaanalogues of ebselen as antimicrobial and antiviral agents: synthesis and properties. Farmaco. 2004 Nov;59(11):863-8.

92 Cermelli C, Vinceti M, Scaltriti E, Bazzani E, Beretti F, Vivoli G, Portolani M. Selenite inhibition of Coxsackie virus B5 replication: implications on the etiology of Keshan disease. J Trace Elem Med Biol. 2002;16(1):41-6.

93 Chen Y, Maret W. Catalytic selenols couple the redox cycles of metallothionein and glutathione. Eur J Biochem. 2001 Jun;268(11):3346-53.

94 Proc Nutr Soc. 2006 May;65(2):169-81.Biofortification of UK food crops with selenium. Broadley MR, White PJ, Bryson RJ, Meacham MC, Bowen HC, Johnson SE, Hawkesford MJ, McGrath SP, Zhao FJ, Breward N, Harriman M, Tucker M. Warwick HRI, University of Warwick, Wellesbourne, Warwick CV35 9EF, UK.

95 Corradini E, Ferrara F, Pietrangelo A. Iron and the liver. Pediatr Endocrinol Rev. 2004 Dec;2 Suppl 2:245-8. Review.

96 Ramm GA, Ruddell RG. Hepatotoxicity of iron overload: mechanisms of iron-induced hepatic fibrogenesis. Semin Liver Dis. 2005 Nov;25(4):433-49. Review.

97 Glei M, Klenow S, Sauer J, Wegewitz U, Richter K, Pool-Zobel BL. Hemoglobin and hemin induce DNA damage in human colon tumor cells HT29 clone 19A and in primary human colonocytes. Mutat Res. 2006 Feb 22;594(1-2):162-71. Epub 2005 Oct 13.

98 Alkhenizan AH, Al-Omran MA. The role of Vitamin E in the prevention of coronary events and stroke. Meta-analysis of randomized controlled trials. Saudi Med J. 2004 Dec;25(12):1808-14.

99 Mazlan M, Sue Mian T, Mat Top G, Zurinah Wan Ngah W. Comparative effects of alpha-tocopherol and gamma-tocotrienol against hydrogen peroxide induced apoptosis on primary-cultured astrocytes. J Neurol Sci. 2006 Apr 15;243(1-2):5-12. Epub 2006 Jan 27.

100 Azlina MF, Nafeeza MI, Khalid BA. A comparison between tocopherol and tocotrienol effects on gastric parameters in rats exposed to stress. Asia Pac J Clin Nutr. 2005;14(4):358-65.

101 Ahmad NS, Khalid BA, Luke DA, Ima Nirwana S. Tocotrienol offers better protection than tocopherol from free-radical-induced damage of rat bone. Clin Exp Pharmacol Physiol. 2005 Sep;32(9):761-70. 102 Khanna S, Roy S, Slivka A, Craft TK, Chaki S,Rink C, Notestine MA, DeVries AC, Parinandi NL, Sen CK. Neuroprotective properties of the natural Vitamin E alpha-tocotrienol. Stroke. 2005 Oct;36(10):2258-64. Epub 2005 Sep 15.

103 Sen CK, Khanna S, Roy S. Tocotrienols: Vitamin E beyond tocopherols. Life Sci. 2006 Mar 27;78(18):2088-98. Epub 2006 Feb 3. Review.

104 Pertseva NG, Ananenko AA, Malinovskaia VV, Klembovskii AI, Burova VIa, Meshkova EN, Kleimenova NV. [The effect of reaferon and alpha-tocopherol on lipid peroxidation in experimental influenza] Vopr Virusol. 1995 Mar-Apr;40(2):59-62. Russian.

105 Gallop PM, Paz MA, Fluckiger R, Kagan HM. PQQ, the elusive coenzyme. Trends Biochem Sci. 1989 Aug;14(8):343-6.

106 Smidt CR, Steinberg FM, Rucker RB. Physiologic importance of pyrroloquinoline quinone. Proc Soc Exp Biol Med. 1991 May;197(1):19-26.

107 Killgore J, Smidt C, Duich L, Romero-Chapman N, Tinker D, Reiser K, Melko M, Hyde D, Rucker RB. Nutritional importance of pyrroloquinoline quinone. Science. 1989 Aug 25;245(4920):850-2.

108 Stites T, Storms D, Bauerly K, Mah J, Harris C, Fascetti A, Rogers Q, Tchaparian E, Satre M, Rucker RB. Pyrroloquinoline quinone modulates mitochondrial quantity and function in mice. J Nutr. 2006 Feb;136(2):390-6.

109 Steinberg F, Stites TE, Anderson P, Storms D, Chan I, Eghbali S, Rucker R. Pyrroloquinoline quinone improves growth and reproductive performance in mice fed chemically defined diets. Exp Biol Med (Maywood). 2003 Feb;228(2):160-6.

110 Stites TE, Mitchell AE, Rucker RB. Physiological importance of quinoenzymes and the O-quinone family of cofactors. J Nutr. 2000 Apr;130(4):719-27.

111 Zhang Y, Rosenberg PA. The essential nutrient pyrroloquinoline quinone may act as a neuroprotectant by suppressing peroxynitrite formation. Eur J Neurosci. 2002 Sep;16(6):1015-24.

112 He K, Nukada H, Urakami T, Murphy MP. Antioxidant and pro-oxidant properties of pyrroloquinoline quinone (PQQ): implications for its function in biological systems. Biochem Pharmacol. 2003 Jan 1;65(1):67-74.

113 Bishop A, Gallop PM, Karnovsky ML. Pyrroloquinoline quinone: a novel vitamin? Nutr Rev. 1998 Oct;56(10):287-93.

114 Yamaguchi K, Sasano A, Urakami T, Tsuji T, Kondo K. Stimulation of nerve growth factor production by pyrroloquinoline quinone and its derivatives in vitro and in vivo. Biosci Biotechnol Biochem. 1993 Jul;57(7):1231-3.

115 Kumazawa T, Sato K, Seno H, Ishii A, Suzuki O. Levels of pyrroloquinoline quinone in various foods. Biochem J. 1995 Apr 15;307 (Pt

2):331-3.

116 Utterback PL, Parsons CM, Yoon I, Butler J. Effect of supplementing selenium yeast in diets of laying hens on egg selenium content. Poult Sci. 2005 Dec;84(12):1900-1.

117 Barber SJ, Parker HM, McDaniel CD. Broiler breeder semen quality as affected by trace minerals in vitro. Poult Sci. 2005 Jan;84(1):100-5.

118 Choct M, Naylor AJ, Reinke N. Selenium supplementation affects broiler growth performance, meat yield and feather coverage. Br Poult Sci. 2004 Oct;45(5):677-83.

119 Trends Microbiol. 2004 Sep;12(9):417-23. Host nutritional status: the neglected virulence factor. Beck MA, Handy J, Levander OA. Department of Pediatrics and Nutrition, University of North Carolina at Chapel Hill, Chapel Hill, North Carolina, NC 27599, USA. melinda_beck@unc.edu

120 Int J Occup Med Environ Health. 2005;18(4):305-11. The role of selenium in cancer and viral infection prevention. Luty-Frackiewicz A. Department of Hygiene, Medical University of Wroclaw, Wroclaw, Poland. annalf@hyg.am.wroc.pl

121 Neill MG, Fleshner NE. An update on chemoprevention strategies in prostate cancer for 2006. Curr Opin Urol. 2006 May;16(3):132-7.

122 Lee SO, Yeon Chun J, Nadiminty N, Trump DL, Ip C, Dong Y, Gao AC. Monomethylated selenium inhibits growth of LNCaP human prostate cancer xenograft accompanied by a decrease in the expression of androgen receptor and prostate- specific antigen (PSA). Prostate. 2006 Apr 24; [Epub ahead of print]

123 Schrauzer GN. Interactive Effects of Selenium and Chromium on Mammary Tumor Development and Growth in MMTV-Infected Female Mice and Their Relevance to Human Cancer. Biol Trace Elem Res. 2006 Mar;109(3):281-92.

124 Goel A, Fuerst F, Hotchkiss E, Boland CR. Selenomethionine Induces p53 Mediated Cell Cycle Arrest and Apoptosis in Human Colon Cancer Cells. Cancer Biol Ther. 2006 May 5;5(5) [Epub ahead ofprint]

125 Luty-Frackiewicz A. The role of selenium in cancer and viral infection prevention. Int J Occup Med Environ Health. 2005;18(4):305-11.

126 Irons R, Carlson BA, Hatfield DL, Davis CD. Both selenoProteins and low molecular weight selenocompounds reduce colon cancer risk in mice with genetically impaired selenoProtein expression. J Nutr. 2006 May;136(5):1311-7.

127 Finley JW. Bioavailability of selenium from foods. Nutr Rev. 2006 Mar;64(3):146-51.

128 Prog Biophys Mol Biol. 2006 Feb 28; [Epub ahead of print] The challenge resulting from positive and negative effects of sunlight: How much solar UV exposure is appropriate to balance between risks of vitamin D deficiency and skin cancer? Reichrath J. Klinik fur Dermatologie, Venerologie und Allergologie, Universitatsklinikum des Saarlandes, 66421 Homburg/Saar, Germany.

129 Hawaii Med J. 2006 Jan;65(1):16-17, 20. Severe vitamin D deficiency in Hawai'i: a case report. Bornemann M. University of Hawaii, John A. Burns School of Medicine, Honolulu, HI 96813, USA.

130 Zittermann A. Vitamin D and disease prevention with special reference to cardiovascular disease. Prog Biophys Mol Biol. 2006 Feb 28; [Epub ahead of print]

131 Holick MF. High prevalence of vitamin D inadequacy and implications for health. Mayo Clin Proc. 2006 Mar;81(3):353-73.

132 Holick MF. Vitamin D: important for prevention of osteoporosis, cardiovascular heart disease, type 1 diabetes, autoimmune diseases, and some cancers. South Med J. 2005 Oct;98(10):1024-7.

133 Holick MF. Vitamin D: Its role in cancer prevention and treatment. Prog Biophys Mol Biol. 2006 Mar 10; [Epub ahead of print]

134 Holick MF. Sunlight and vitamin D for bone health and prevention of autoimmune diseases, cancers, and cardiovascular disease. Am J Clin Nutr. 2004 Dec;80(6 Suppl):1678S-88S.

135 Bertone-Johnson ER, Hankinson SE, Bendich A, Johnson SR, Willett WC, Manson JE. Calcium and vitamin D intake and risk of incident premenstrual syndrome. Arch Intern Med. 2005 Jun 13;165(11):1246-52.

136 Thys-Jacobs S. Micronutrients and the premenstrual syndrome: the case for calcium. J Am Coll Nutr. 2000 Apr;19(2):220-7.

137 Lips P. Vitamin D physiology. Prog Biophys Mol Biol. 2006 Feb 28; [Epub ahead of print]

138 Cantorna MT. Vitamin D and its role in immunology: Multiple sclerosis, and inflammatory bowel disease. Prog Biophys Mol Biol. 2006 Feb 28; [Epub ahead of print]

139 Matsuzaki J, Tsuji T, Zhang Y, Wakita D, Imazeki I, Sakai T, Ikeda H, Nishimura T. 1alpha,25- Dihydroxyvitamin D3 downmodulates the functional differentiation of Th1 cytokine-conditioned bone marrow-derived dendritic cells beneficial for cytotoxic T lymphocyte generation. Cancer Sci. 2006 Feb;97(2):139-47.

140 Lips P. Vitamin D physiology. Prog Biophys Mol Biol. 2006 Feb 28; [Epub ahead of print

141 Grant WB. Epidemiology of disease risks in relation to vitamin D insufficiency. Prog Biophys Mol Biol. 2006 Feb 28; [Epub ahead of print]

142 Pozzilli P, Manfrini S, Crino A, Picardi A, Leomanni C, Cherubini V, Valente L, Khazrai M, Visalli N; IMDIAB group. Low levels of 25- hydroxyvitamin D3 and 1,25-dihydroxyvitamin D3 in patients with newly diagnosed type 1 diabetes.Horm Metab Res. 2005 Nov;37(11):680-3.

143 Vouldoukis I, Lacan D, Kamate C, Coste P, Calenda A, Mazier D, Conti M, Dugas B. Antioxidant and anti-inflammatory properties of a Cucumis melo LC. extract rich in superoxide dismutase activity. J Ethnopharmacol. 2004 Sep;94(1):67-75. PubMed PMID: 15261965.

CHAPTER 22

HOMEOPATHY

WHAT IS HOMEOPATHY?

The term 'homeopathy' is derived from the Greek homoios (same) and pathos (suffering). Homeopathy is a non-toxic, holistic medical system, based on the principle of "like treats like" (Law of Similars). What does this mean? At its basic level it means that a substance that causes specific symptoms of illness in a healthy person can be used, successfully, to treat those same symptoms in someone who is ill.

For example, "Belladonna" – otherwise known as "deadly nightshade" – is used to treat an illness like scarlet fever, due to the fact that the symptoms of Belladonna poisoning are very similar to those of scarlet fever. So, in a case of scarlet fever, the patient will exhibit symptoms including a high fever, redness and glassy eyes. Belladonna poisoning shows the same set of symptoms – therefore there is a "match".

Another good example of "like treats like" is the use of "Allium cepa", or common onion, to treat a cold. When one has a fairly normal "head cold", there are a number of symptoms that we all tend to produce – these include things like watery eyes, scratchy throat, sneezing and so on. All these symptoms are similar to those that you might get if you cut up a raw onion. However, homeopaths very rarely prescribe a "raw" substance.

DILUTION

Substances that homeopaths use are subjected to a process of repeated dilution and a special kind of percussive shaking (known as sucussion), to make a remedy that is safe to use. Homeopaths believe sufficient "likeness" remains between the remedy and the symptoms of the illness to stimulate the body's self-healing abilities. The process of dilution and sucussion is just one of the reasons for friction between some members of the Conventional scientific establishment and those who support homeopathy. Critics of homeopathy say of this dilution process:

"It can't work because there's nothing there".

However, homeopaths believe (and experience shows) that this process of repeated dilution and sucussion, known as "potentisation", has the effect of making the remedy more powerful in terms of its healing capacity.

THE VITAL FORCE

Another key principle of homeopathy is the idea that the body is regulated by a "vital force". This vital force is dynamic and in a constant state of flux, dealing with all the stimuli that could disturb your healthy equilibrium, otherwise known as "homeostasis" – keeping your body balanced, and keeping you healthy. Thus, if your vital force is below par, your healthy balance can be disrupted, homeostasis can be disturbed and then illness can occur.

Symptoms of disease are seen by homeopaths as signs that your vital force is fighting something that has disturbed your body's natural healthy balance, this could be a pathogen, such as a bacterium, or a virus, for example. In the wider scheme of things, the vital force can also be disrupted by anything that disturbs the equilibrium - such as stress, shock, malnutrition etc. So, homeopaths view symptoms that our bodies produce as guiding signs as to what exactly has been disrupted.

When you take the time to think about the homeopathic understanding of symptoms, you can see that it is quite logical. For example, if we get a bacterial infection - such as food poisoning - the symptoms that we produce can include vomiting and diarrhoea. These symptoms are your body's way of protecting you by getting the bacteria out of your body as quickly as possible. Rather than suppress these symptoms, homeopaths administer remedies that assist this self-healing process. And, it is this homeopathic assistance – or stimulation – of our self-healing process that often enables us to get better, faster and with fewer complications than with some Conventional Medicine.

This is different to the way that Conventional Medicine views symptoms: Conventional Medicine generally views symptoms as "undesirable" things that "must be suppressed". In our example of food poisoning above, if you were to take a drug that suppressed your vomiting and diarrhoea, it may well lead to other far more serious problems, as the bacterium that is making you ill has no way out of your body. So, a doctor will then need to prescribe antibiotics to kill the bacteria. Of course, the antibiotics will also kill off all our "good" bacteria and then we are exposed to other potentially more serious illnesses. These will require more medication, and so it goes on. The over-prescription of antibiotics has worsened the current MRSA and TB epidemics, as bacteria that cause these diseases have become resistant to antibiotics.

Homeopaths do not "throw the baby out with the bathwater" however and recognise that there are very definite situations where it is absolutely sensible to utilise Conventional Medical approaches, and examples of these include life saving surgery and drugs e.g. the justifiable use of appropriately prescribed antibiotics in critical situations, such as bacterial meningitis, but only if the infective pathogen has been proven to respond to antibiotic treatment.

THE LAW OF CURES

The "Law of Cures" concept is also of paramount importance in homeopathy. According to this system, the healing process adheres to the three basic laws of cure: That symptoms move down from the top of the body; outward from the inside of the body; and from the most important organs to the least important, with long standing complaints taking longer to disappear than those that developed more recently.

This Law was devised by Dr Constantine Hering in 1835. Hering was a gifted Allopathic (Conventional) doctor who was a "healthy sceptic", and was set the task of disproving homeopathy. At some point during his research into homeopathy, Hering was treated successfully for a septic cut and this caused him to reconsider whether homeopathy may have some value. He then began various experiments which demonstrated to him that there was indeed value in the approach.

Hering's Law of Cures helps homeopaths and their patients to have a fuller understanding of how treatment is progressing. The homeopath will always encourage the patient to be actively involved in observing changes in symptoms after treatment – where possible – and accurately reporting these changes, so that progress towards health can be properly monitored. This involvement of the patient as part of the treatment is another way that homeopathy differs from Conventional Medicine. In Conventional Medicine, patients are expected to passively receive treatment and are not necessarily encouraged to interact with the doctor to any great degree.

WHAT ARE HOMEOPATHIC REMEDIES MADE OF?

The remedies are made from plant, mineral and animal materials, which are chopped, soaked in a mixture of 90% alcohol:10% water, for up to a month and then strained. The retained liquid is known as the "mother tincture", of which one drop is diluted in 99 drops of alcohol and then rapidly shaken (sucussion). This process of dilution and sucussion is continued, until the required potency is achieved. In the final stage, a few drops of the liquid are added to a jar of plain tablets. It is these pills that will be given to you by the homeopath.

CASE TAKING

The type of remedy given to a patient depends upon their particular constitutional make-up and symptom picture. In order to ascertain which of the 2,000 or so remedies should be given to the patient, and at which potency, the homeopath "takes the patient's case". This case-taking process involves a great deal of questioning of the patient, by the homeopath and acute and careful observation of the patient too. In addition to talking about the symptoms that the patient currently has, he or she will also be asked about their likes and dislikes of foods, drinks, temperatures, weather and so on. As well as listening to, and noting down, all of the patient's current symptoms, the homeopath will delve deep into their patient's past life history and will also ask about family history too.

All of this observation and questioning helps the homeopath to build up a really accurate picture of the patient – as an individual. The homeopath is attempting to understand the "underlying" reasons why a person would manifest the particular symptoms that they are experiencing. The homeopathic remedy addresses these underlying symptoms, which then helps the person to return to a state of health.

By painstaking case-taking, the homeopath can prescribe a carefully selected remedy that exactly matches the patient's symptoms – using the basis of the Law of Similars – or "like treats like" as described above.

It is this extremely careful and totally individualised approach to prescribing that again differentiates homeopathy from Conventional Medicine. In Conventional Medicine, all patients with a generalised diagnosis – such as high blood pressure receive much the same medication – even though doctors know that high blood pressure can occur for many different underlying reasons. Homeopaths view this approach as a "sticking-plaster" tactic, one that is designed to keep the patient's symptoms under control but doesn't address the real reasons that are causing the problem.

The absolutely individualised approach that homeopathy takes and the fact that homeopaths treat the underlying reasons for a person's illness, mean that homeopathy has an excellent track record in successfully treating those chronic (long term) illnesses that Conventional Medicine cannot cure but can merely suppress. A good example of this would be the Conventional Medical suppression of eczema with steroids – the use of which is certainly not curative and, as soon as the patient stops using the steroids, the eczema comes back.

Of course, there are other issues with using drugs – such as steroids - to suppress symptoms and many of these lead to other side-effect problems later on for the patient. Homeopathy however, treats the underlying symptoms and assists the body in curing itself, gently and permanently.

EXAMPLES OF HOMEOPATHIC PRESCRIBING

To illustrate how homeopaths differentiate between the thousands of remedies we can look at the following simplified example. A patient presents to the homeopath complaining of constipation. There are many remedies that can have constipation as part of the "remedy picture" and the homeopath's job is to differentiate between these.

LET'S LOOK AT TWO VERY DIFFERENT REMEDIES

Nux vomica is typically suited to people who are impatient, competitive and highly strung. They often have digestive problems and constipation in particular.

Calc. carb is seen as a potential remedy for quiet, cautious, slightly obsessive patients who are often overweight and tend to suffer from joint pain. People needing Calc. carb can also suffer from constipation.

So, by careful analysis of the patient's case – taking into account all of his or her symptoms, (mental, emotional, physical etc.) the homeopath can decide which is the correct remedy.

HOW DO WE KNOW HOW HOMEOPATHIC REMEDIES WORK?

Over the last 200 years since homeopathy has been in existence, there have been thousands of "provings" of homeopathic remedies to find out what types of symptoms they can be used to treat.

A "proving" is similar to a placebo (inactive substance) controlled drug trial – where two sets of people are given a drug, or a dummy pill, and not told which group is taking the active substance.

The main difference here, between homeopathy and Conventional Medicine, is that homeopathic remedies are trialled on people, not animals. This is a sensible approach as animals react very differently to humans. Their physiology is very dissimilar indeed. Also, the people involved in a proving are healthy subjects when they begin to take the remedy (or placebo – they don't know which they are getting). Any symptoms that they produce as a result of taking the pills are carefully noted by the people running the experiment. It is this information that is used to formulate a very deep understanding of exactly what a homeopathic remedy will do. Then – according to the Law of Similars (or "like treats like"), this remedy can be prescribed to people who are ill in order to match the same symptom picture.

DO ALL HOMEOPATHS WORK IN THE SAME WAY?

There are two main approaches to homeopathic prescribing: the "Classical" approach and the "Complex".

The Classical School tends to look for a single remedy that matches the patient's "Constitutional Type", or symptom picture, perfectly, treating them with single doses of that one remedy. This was the system devised by Hahnemann – the inventor of homeopathy. The latter approach –

Homeopathy

Complex Prescribing – developed in the late nineteenth century by a British homeopath, Richard Hughes, focuses on organ imbalances rather than the person's "Constitutional Type" and tends to use low-potency remedies, often incorporating herbal extracts. Often many remedies are prescribed at a time. This is known as "poly-pharmacy" and this approach is used extensively in Europe by homeopaths and also by Conventional Medical doctors for whom homeopathic medicines are considered to be just another medical tool.

Worldwide, many practitioners, however, combine both systems. Indeed, every homeopath works in an individual way and may subscribe to slightly different theories from those referred to here, with regard to how their practice is carried out. Homeopathy can treat a wide variety of ailments and it is particularly suitable for home use to treat common conditions. Basic, low-potency homeopathic remedies are available at health shops, as well as most chemists and supermarkets. Homeopathic remedies are safe and effective to use at home – as long as the person using the remedies has a proper understanding of the principles of "like treats like" so that they can make sure that they have selected the correct remedy, in the correct potency, in order to match the patient's symptoms.

Homeopaths are keen for their patients to keep a small homeopathic first aid kit at home as many remedies can be easily and simply used to alleviate all sorts of common ailments such as colds, cuts and bruises, "normal" influenza, period pains, toothaches, abscesses, sore throats and so on. Obviously any chronic or more complex condition should be treated by a properly qualified homeopath. A listing of qualified practitioners is available on The Complementary Medical Association's website (The-CMA.Org.UK), you'll also find homeoapths registered with a number of other organisations including; the Alliance of Registered Homeopaths, the Society of Homeopaths, the British Homeopathic Association and the Homeopathic Medical Association.

WHY ARE SOME CONVENTIONAL DOCTORS AND 'SCIENTISTS' SO OPPOSED TO HOMEOPATHY?

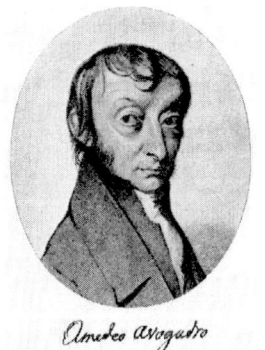

Amadeo Avogadro

First of all, not all doctors are opposed to homeopathy – in fact there are hundreds of medical doctors in the UK who also practice homeopathy, these doctors will tend to be registered with the British Homeopathic Association. In addition, there are also a number of NHS homeopathic hospitals in the UK.

Historically though, many scientists and doctors have, in the past, been vehemently opposed to homeopathy and have said that it cannot work. This is because they believed that due to the process of dilution and sucussion – "potentisation" – that the remedies undergo – there would not be enough of the original substance left in the remedy to make any difference to a person. This is a very difficult problem and certainly one that homeopaths have no absolutely proven explanation for – as yet.

Certainly in the higher potencies such as those that are diluted and sucussed over 23 times – "Avogadro's Number" – there will be no original molecule to be found – it is a mathematical improbability. The brilliant Italian scientist, Avogadro, born in 1776, made many discoveries, and those that have contributed most to science that we use today concern his "Principle":

> "Equal volumes of all gases at the same temperature and pressure contain the same number of molecules."

Avogadro's work later led scientists to discover the theory of "moles": a molecular weight in grams (mole) of any substance contains the same number of molecules, therefore according to Avogadro's Principle, the molar volumes of all gases should be the same. So, the number of molecules in one mole is now called "Avogadro's Number".

Avogadro's Number is very large, and currently scientists put this at 6.0221367×10^{23}. The size of such a number is enormously difficult to comprehend.

Here are a few examples of illustrations that help us to visualise this number:

- An Avogadro's Number of standard soft drink cans e.g. cans of cola, would cover the surface of the earth to a depth of over 200 miles.
- If you had Avogadro's Number of peas and spread them across the United States of America, the country would be covered in peas to a depth of over 9 miles.
- If you could count atoms at the rate of 10 million per second, it would take you about 2 billion years to count the atoms in one mole.

So, given the vastness of Avogadro's Number and the fact that homeopathic remedies often exceed this dilution, 24c (c = centesimal i.e. a dilution of 1:100), just one dilution step above Avogadro's Number, is considered by homeopaths to be a low potency. They will frequently prescribe remedies at 30c, 200c or even up to 1,000c or 10,000c. So how could homeopathy possibly work?

CLUSTERED/ STRUCTURED WATER

Well, as with many inventions and discoveries, a scientist working on a totally different project stumbled upon a strange phenomenon that explains how homeothapic remedies might work – in spite of their enormous dilutions. Dr Shui Yin Lo – a former Visiting Associate Professor in the Chemistry Department at California Institute of Technology who went on to hold the post of Director of Research and Development at American Technologies Group – was performing experiments on how to improve car engine efficiency when he made a startling discovery.

Dr Lo found that water molecules, which are completely random in their normal state, begin to form clusters when a substance is added to water and the water is vigorously shaken. This is the exact process homeopaths use to create their medicine. Dr Lo's research shows that every substance exerts its own unique influence on the water, so each cluster shape and configuration is unique to the substance added[1].

With each dilution and shaking, the clusters in the water grow bigger and stronger. (This might explain why homeopaths find that remedies exert a more intense influence on the body, the higher the homeopathic potency levels.) This water, which homeopaths call "potentised," is considered by scientists to be "Structured Water," because the water molecules have taken on a shape influenced by the original substance. Interestingly, the clusters start to assume a shape that resembles the structure of the original substance itself. So, in spite of the fact that the chemical can no longer be detected, its "image" is there, taken on by the water molecules.

This would mean that the presence – or not – of the original material that the remedy is made from is irrelevant – it seems that the water is actually reflecting the shape of the original molecules – almost like a fractal which is a mathematically generated pattern that looks the same when seen at any magnification or reduction. Homeopaths have been aware of the theory of clustered water for some time, but this is the first time that this phenomenon has actually been proven.

Robust scientific research such as this is helping doctors and scientists to understand that there is a "plausible mechanism of action" at play in the creation of homeopathic medicines[2,3,4,5,6,7,8,9,10,11]. In fact, over 1,500 studies which explore water clusters and their effects appear on PubMed. However, of course not all doctors and scientists are actually familiar with this research – yet.

To read more about the fascinating subjects of water clusters and the structure of water, visit one of the best websites on this area of research; lsbu.ac.uk/water/. This has been written by Professor Martin Chaplin, who is Professor of Applied Science, Water and Aqueous Systems Research and Head of the Food Research Centre at London South Bank University.

RESONANCE AND SYSTEMIC MEMORY

Even if Dr Lo's discovery does provide the answers to what actually happens during the dilution and sucussion process, we still have no idea how the remedies actually work in your body although hypotheses are emerging. These point to "Resonance" and "Systemic Memory" as possible mechanisms of action.

Researchers in the Department of Medicine at the University of Arizona[12] explain that a mechanism of action may be elucidated when modern dynamical systems analysis is applied to high-dilution therapies. Furthermore, they propose the hypothesis that complex patterns of emergent information and energy are stored, to various degrees, in physical, chemical and biological systems. This is supported by the idea of the logic of "recurrent feedback loops", which applies to all dynamical network systems.

When you add the concept of "Resonance", which is a dynamic pattern-recognition process into the equation, many of the classic observations using high-dilution therapies can be explained. The researchers conclude by pointing out that the "Systemic Memory Resonance" hypothesis may provide a plausible biophysical mechanism for explaining how high-dilution therapies contribute to healing. Most interestingly, they also make the connection that this may, but by extension, explain how information and energy in low-dilution and chemical drugs contribute to healing as well.

ULTRA-HIGH DILUTIONS

There is currently hot scientific debate as to whether Ultra High Dilutions (UHDs) (homeopathic remedies come into this category) can have any biological, systemic or other effect. Many scientists believe that, in fact, they do. As one researcher at the Royal Free Hospital School of Medicine in London put it:

> *"Given that the existence of UHD effects would revolutionise science and medicine and given the considerable empirical evidence of them, the philosophies of science tell us that possible UHD effects warrant serious investigation by Conventional scientists and serious attention by scientific journals."* [13]

In 2007 a meta-analysis (a form of research that looks at the overall results of a number of studies) of trials into UHDs in-vitro showed that 75% of the experiments included in the analysis had positive results[14].

The fact remains that we still do not – at this time – have a real understanding of what is actually going on in our body when we take a homeopathic remedy. However, this should not upset doctors and scientists too much, as according to the British Medical Association's "Clinical Evidence" website, the physical effects of over 85% of the medicines and procedures used by doctors in Conventional Medicine are not entirely understood either. Both the homeopathic and the Conventional Medical sectors require more research.

MORE REASONS FOR CONVENTIONAL SCIENCE'S OPPOSITION TO HOMEOPATHY

- Historically, there has been strong opposition from the Medical Associations in the UK and the USA. For example, the American Medical Association was actually formed in the late 1800's with the original mission to eradicate the competitive medical practices of the times: Homeopathy and osteopathy[16]. This was because by 1900, there were 22 homeopathic medical schools, more than 100 homeopathic hospitals and 10% of American physicians were homeopathic doctors. The major reason for homeopathy's popularity at that time stemmed from its success in treating the many various epidemic diseases that occurred during the 1800's. Death rates in homeopathic hospitals were anywhere from 1/8 to 1/2 of those in orthodox Conventional Medical hospitals. So, Conventional doctors were losing money but homeopaths were well off.

- Advances in modern medical pharmacology (antibiotics, anti-inflammatories, steroids, etc.) The pharmaceutical companies have actively and covertly campaigned against homeopathy. But isn't that just a little paranoid? Surely the pharmaceutical industry is there to help us?

No, – this is not necessarily the case. The pharmaceutical companies can't make substantial profits on homeopathic medicines and the single (i.e. not specific "complex") remedies cannot be patented, so this is not in the interest of their shareholders. Pharmaceutical companies are first and foremost, big businesses.

For a pharmaceutical company to perform profitably it needs to keep people "just ill enough" for them to continue to use their drugs. There is a conflict of interest as it is clearly not sensible for any drug company to actually "cure" a particular disease.

For example – Gilead and Roche – the companies who respectively invented and currently manufacture Tamiflu, have made billions of dollars from both the Swine Flu and Bird Flu outbreaks. There is huge money to be made from selling drugs and very little to be made from homeopathic medicine and furthermore, as homeopathic medicines do actually make people better, this means that there would be no requirement for repeat prescriptions of the pharmaceutical company's drug.

- Homeopathy performs reasonably but not outstandingly well in standard Random Controlled Trials (RCTs). This is because homeopathy – in order for it to "be" homeopathy, requires that remedies are prescribed according to each individual's own particular symptoms. In RCTs it is not possible to mimic this individualised approach as, for these tests to be valid and have any significant statistical meaning, the same medicine must be given to one group – regardless of each individual's symptoms. So, essentially, the wrong "tool" is being used to test homeopathy. It's a bit like trying to test gravity with a thermometer!

Homeopathy performs very well however, when it is given a chance to be examined properly – in the conditions and circumstances that it is actually prescribed in – that of individualisation. There are many examples of excellent, robust scientific trials[15] that have taken this individualised approach and the positive outcomes of these demonstrate that patients treated homeopathically

Samuel Hahnemann

experience an average of more than 78% improvement in symptoms.

SCIENTIFIC RESEARCH IN HOMEOPATHY

The 2008 conference of this title covered all the Scientific Research that has been done to date on homeopathy – including work from the emerging medical field of Homotoxicology. To watch the full Conference see the "Scientific Research in Homeopathy" DVD (from The-CMA.Org. UK).

HISTORY (IN BRIEF)

Hippocrates, the Greek "Father of Medicine", advocated the virtues of the *"like cures like"* theory in the 5th century B.C. The genius German doctor, Samuel Hahnemann, rekindled this principle in the late eighteenth century. Dr Hahnemann was an immensely gifted doctor who became disillusioned with the medicine of the day. While many medicines in common usage were undoubtedly effective, many patients died from their side effects.

This was not surprising when many of the commonly used medicines contained heavy metals such as mercury and lead – and even arsenic was frequently used. **Hahnemann wanted to take a more scientific approach.** So, in the spirit of true empiricism, Hahnemann took regular doses of quinine, an extract of cinchona bark used to treat malaria, and soon developed malaria-like symptoms.

By using himself as a guinea pig, Hahnemann was able to prove that small doses of a substance that stimulated the symptoms of an illness in a healthy person could be used to combat that illness in someone who was sick.

He continued to conduct numerous trials - known as "provings" - following the methods outlined above, with much success. Interestingly, Hahnemann conducted what we now recognise to be Placebo Controlled Trials and his contribution to science undoubtedly deserves greater recognition. Hahnemann went on to write up the basis, theory and philosophy of this "New Medicine" in his encyclopaedic series of classic works, "The Organon of Medicine".

Hahnemann enjoyed enormous success in treating thousands of cases homoeopathically. One of the earliest tests of his homeopathic system was in the treatment of an epidemic in 1813 when Typhus Fever (carried by lice) came through Leipzig and spread among the population as a result of Napoleonic troops retreating from the Russian front. Hahnemann treated 180 cases of Typhus Fever and lost just two people – at a time when the typical death rate among those Conventionally treated was over 30%.

Dr. Constantine Hering and Dr. James Tyler Kent developed Hahnemann's ideas further, introducing the "Law of Cure" and "Constitutional Type" concepts respectively. The American Institute of Homeopathy was founded in 1844 and enjoyed enormous success in the Spanish Flu pandemic of 1918, but by the 1930's its practice in the States was virtually non-existent due to severe opposition from the then burgeoning pharmaceutical industry.

In fact, as we have said, the American Medical Association was actually formed "to stamp out the scourge of homeopathy," as stated in its charter. Homeopathy in the USA went into a steep decline until its resurgence in America began in the 1970's.

However, in Britain, this holistic medicine has proved to be consistently popular with patients, so much so that it was included as part of the National Health Service when it was founded in 1948. There are currently five NHS homeopathic hospitals in the UK. Most homeopaths however, operate in private practice.

In Europe, homeopathic medicine is considered to be a completely normal therapeutic approach, for example in the Netherlands 40% of doctors practice homeopathy. Throughout Europe many doctors will opt to take extra training in homeopathy after they finish their basic medical training.

HOMEOPATHY AND SWINE FLU (H1N1)

Homeopathy was used to great effect all over the world in the Spanish Flu (H1N1) pandemic of 1918.

In fact, although homeopathy is often relegated to the sidelines of medicine, usually because critics say that it lacks a plausible mechanism of action in today's scientific framework, homeopathy was used to treat enormous numbers of people – successfully.

One of the most compelling reports comes from The Journal of the American Institute for Homeopathy in 1921. This long report was verified by a number of highly reliable sources and contributors – who were all well respected Conventional Medical doctors in their day.

One of these, Dr Dean W A Pearson of Philadelphia, reported that 24,000 cases of flu were treated allopathically (Conventionally) and had a death rate of 28.2% and another group of people, 26,795 cases, were treated homoeopathically and had a mortality rate of just 1.05%.

In 1920, respected doctor, Dr W A Dewey, wrote an article for the Journal of the American Institute of Homeopathy titled; "Homeopathy In Influenza - A Chorus of Fifty In Harmony" which demonstrates that homeopathy was successfully used in the Spanish Flu epidemic of 1918.

Homeopathy

Dewey wrote to a number of doctor homeopaths across the USA and these are some of the responses he received:

- **"Dr Dean W. A. Pearson** *of Philadelphia collected 26,795 cases of influenza treated by homeopathic physicians with a mortality of 1.05%, while the average old school (Conventional Medicine) mortality is close to 30%".*

- *"Thirty physicians in Connecticut responded to my request for data. They reported 6,602 cases with 55 deaths, which is less than 1%".*

- Dr. H. A. Roberts was a physician on a troop ship at the time. He provided two stories to Dewey:

"In the transport service I had 81 cases on the way over. All recovered and were landed. Every man received homeopathic treatment. One ship lost 31 on the way."
H. A. Roberts, MD, Derby, Connecticut.

- Dr Roberts second report:
(Another boat pulled alongside Dr Roberts' boat to get any spare coffins – its mortality rate was so high. On his return to port, the commander asked Roberts);

"Used all your coffins?" To which Roberts, who had been treating his ship's men with homeopathy, replied; *"Yes, and lost not one man!"*

- *"In a plant of 8,000 workers we had only one death. The patients were not drugged to death. Gelsemium was practically the only remedy used. We used no aspirin and no vaccines".*
Frank Wieland, MD, Chicago.

- *"I did not lose a single case of influenza; my death rate in the pneumonias was 2.1%. The salycilates, including aspirin and quinine, were almost the sole standbys of the old school (Conventional Medicine) and it was a common thing to hear them speaking of losing 60% of their pneumonias"*
Dudley A. Williams, MD, Providence, Rhode Island.

- *"Fifteen hundred cases were reported at the Homeopathic Medical Society of the District of Columbia with but fifteen deaths. Recoveries in the National Homeopathic Hospital were 100%".*
E. F. Sappington, M. D., Philadelphia.

- *"I have treated 1,000 cases of influenza. I have the records to show my work. I*

have no losses. Please give all credit to homeopathy and none to the Scotch-Irish-American!"
T. A. McCann, MD, Dayton, Ohio.

• One physician in a Pittsburgh hospital asked a nurse if she knew anything better than what he was doing, because he was losing many cases.

"Yes, doctor, stop aspirin and go down to a homeopathic pharmacy, and get homeopathic remedies."

The doctor replied: *"But that is homeopathy."*

"I know it, but the homeopathic doctors for whom I have nursed have not lost a single case."
W. F. Edmundson, MD, Pittsburgh.

• *"There is one drug which directly or indirectly was the cause of the loss of more lives than was influenza itself. You all know that drug. It claims to be salicylic acid. Aspirin's history has been printed. Today you don't know what the sedative action of salicylic acid is. It did harm in two ways. Its indirect action came through the fact that aspirin was taken until prostration resulted and the patient developed pneumonia"*
Frank L. Newton, MD, Somerville, Massachusetts.

• *"Aspirin and other coal tar products are condemned as causing great numbers of unnecessary deaths. The omnipresent aspirin is the most pernicious drug of all. It beguiles by its quick action of relief of pain, a relief which is meretricious. In several cases aspirin weakened the heart, depressed the vital forces, increased the mortality in mild cases and made convalescence slower. In all cases it masks the symptoms and renders immeasurably more difficult the selection of the curative remedy. Apparently aspirin bears no curative relation to any disease and it ought to be prohibited".*
Guy Beckly Stearns, MD, New York.

• *"Three hundred and fifty cases and lost one, a neglected pneumonia that came to me after she had taken one hundred grains of aspirin in twenty-four hours".*
Cora Smith King, MD, Washington, DC.

• *"I had a package handed to me containing 1,000 aspirin tablets, which was 994 too many. I think I gave about half a dozen. I could find no place for it. My remedies were few. I almost invariably gave Gelsemium and Bryonia. I hardly ever lost a*

case if I got there first, unless the patient had been sent to a drug store and bought aspirin, in which event I was likely to have a case of pneumonia on my hands".
J.P.Huff, MD, Olive Branch, Kentucky.

HAS HOMEOPATHY HAD ANY OTHER SUCCESS IN TREATING OTHER EPIDEMICS APART FROM THE 1918 SPANISH FLU?

There are many more compelling examples of homeopathy being used successfully in various epidemics and pandemics around the world since Hahnemann's time. Furthermore, the evidence stands up to scrutiny and is highly reliable. Nowadays there are numerous well-conducted trials that demonstrate that homeopathy does indeed work very effectively and most doctors do acknowledge its efficacy:

THE TYPHUS EPIDEMIC 1813

The background to this typhus epidemic was telling: Having marched through Germany and on to Russia, Napoleon began his calamitous retreat from Moscow. By August, 1813, he was back in Saxony with a new army; he defeated the Allies at Dresden and then moved north-west to Leipzig, where he encamped outside the city accompanied by his unreliable ally, the King of Saxony.

On the 18th October Napoleon fought a major battle against the Allies, who were commanded by Prince Karl Schwarzenberg. On the next day Napoleon's Saxon allies turned against him; he was defeated and had to leave Germany, never to return. Leipzig celebrated the defeat of the French but the city was full of wounded men. Hahnemann took part in treating the casualties and the victims of the epidemic that broke out in the city. When the epidemic hit Leipzig,

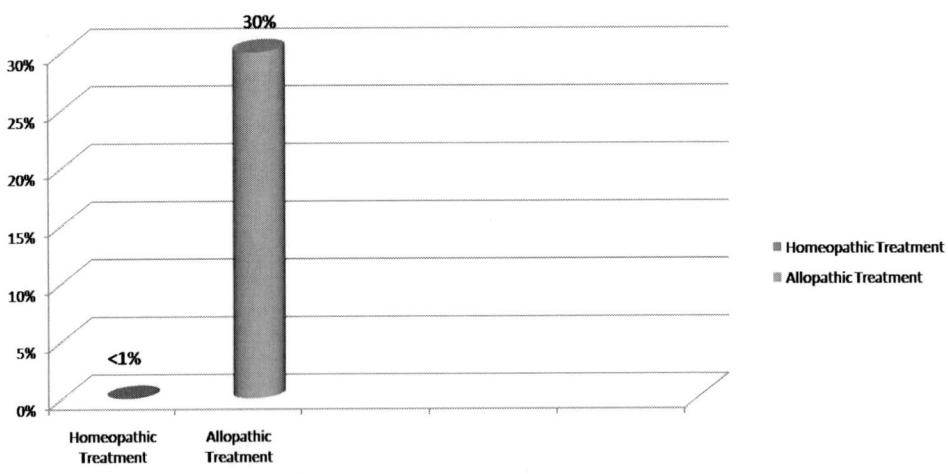

Mortality Rate in Typhus Fever Epidemic 1813

Hahnemann treated 180 people and lost only 2 (less than 1%) – Allopathic mortality rates were >30% It should be noted that in modern times, prompt treatment of the disease with antibiotics reduces the mortality rate to approximately 1%. When untreated, typhoid fever usually lasts for three weeks to a month. Death occurs in between 10% and 30% of untreated cases.

THE CHOLERA EPIDEMIC OF 1831

When Cholera finally reached Europe in 1831, the mortality rate for those treated with the Conventional Medicines of the time (Allopathy), was between 40% (Imperial Council of Russia) to 80% (Osler's Practice of Medicine).

Out of five people who contracted Cholera, two to four of them died under Conventional (allopathic) treatment.

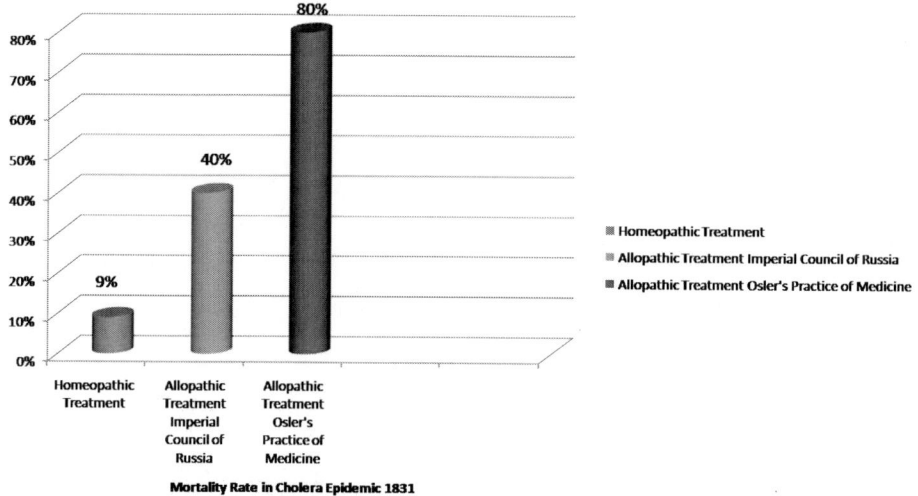

Respected doctors of the day reported the following:

•   The excellent physician Dr. Quin, based in London, reported the mortality in the ten homeopathic hospitals in the UK in 1831-32 as 9%;
•   Dr. Roth, personal doctor to the King of Bavaria, reported that under homeopathic care the mortality was 7%;
•   Admiral Mordoinow of the Imperial Russian Council reported 10% mortality under homeopathy.

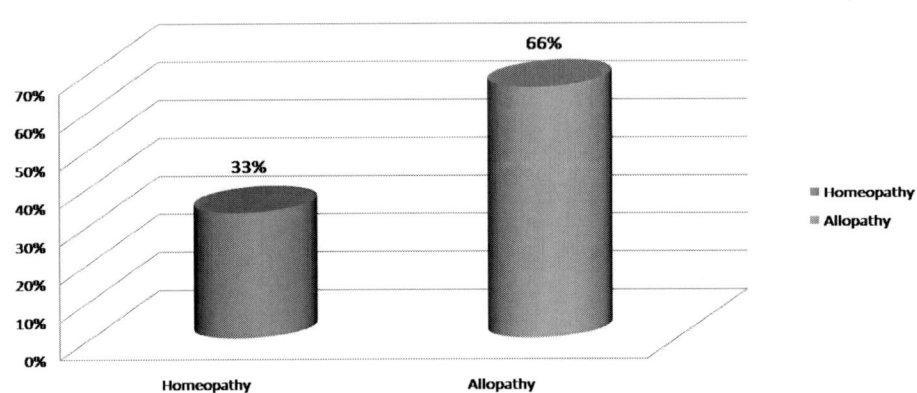

Furthermore, Dr. Wild, Allopathic editor of Dublin Quarterly Journal, reported in Austria in 1831 (see graph above), the Allopathic mortality was 66% and the homeopathic mortality was 33% *"and on account of this extraordinary result, the law interdicting the practice of Homeopathy in Austria was repealed."*

JOSEPH PULTE AND THE CHOLERA EPIDEMIC, CINCINNATI – 1849

The homeopathic historian Julian Winston retold this anecdote on his website, which elegantly illustrates the manner in which people initially rejected homeopathy and then thoroughly embraced it, when it was demonstrated to be highly effective:

"There is a story told about Joseph Pulte, one of the earliest homeopaths in Cincinnati. When he began his practice, many people were so angered by a homeopath being in town that they pelted the house with eggs. He was becoming discouraged

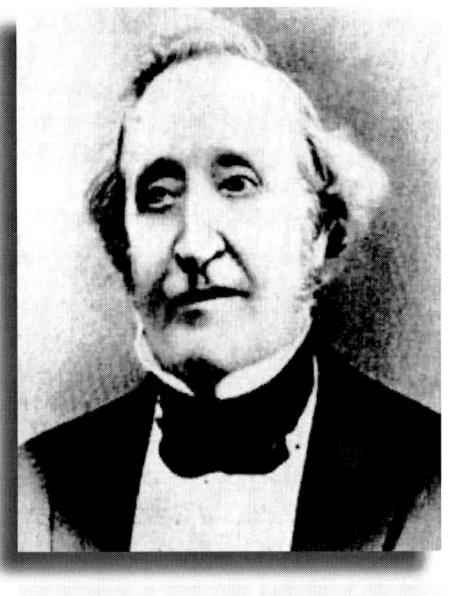

Joseph Pulte

enough to think of leaving. His wife said, "Joseph, do you believe in the truth of homeopathy?" He replied in the affirmative. "Then," she said, "you will stay in Cincinnati."

Shortly after, when the Cholera epidemic swept through, Pulte was able to boast of not having lost a single patient - and he was accepted into the community. In the Epidemic of 1849, people crowded to his door and stood in the street because the waiting room was full."

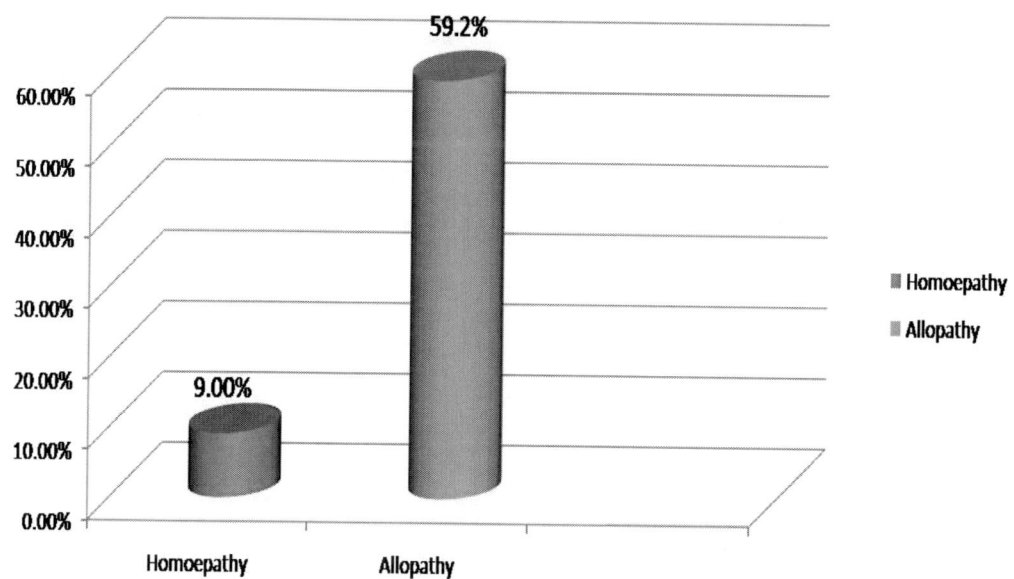

MORTALITY RATE IN THE CHOLERA EPIDEMIC 1854

THE CHOLERA EPIDEMIC OF 1854

In 1854 a Cholera Epidemic struck London and homeopathy continued to be effective in its treatment. A medical breakthrough was made during this epidemic as it was the first time the medical community (Dr John Snow, to be precise) was able to trace the outbreak of a disease to a source - in this case - a public water pump. When the pump was closed, the epidemic soon ceased. All in all 10,738 people died.

The House of Commons requested a report regarding the various methods of treating the epidemic. When the report was issued, no homeopathic figures were included. The House of Lords requested an explanation, and it was admitted that if the homeopathic figures were to be included in the report, it would "skew the results' so it was suppressed.

Upon examination, the buried report revealed that under allopathic care the mortality was 59.2% while under homeopathic care mortality was only 9%.

Homeopathy

CHOLERA EPIDEMIC IN RIO DE JANEIRO 1855

388 cases of cholera were treated with homeopathy with a 2% death rate, while the allopathic infirmary had a 40-60% death rate.

In 1878, Saturnino de Meirelles and others re-created the old Instituto Homeopatico do Brasil and in 1880, they changed the name to Instituto Hahnemanniano do Brazil, which still exists. Homeopathy appears to be thriving in Brazil and is still an important part of national health care initiatives.

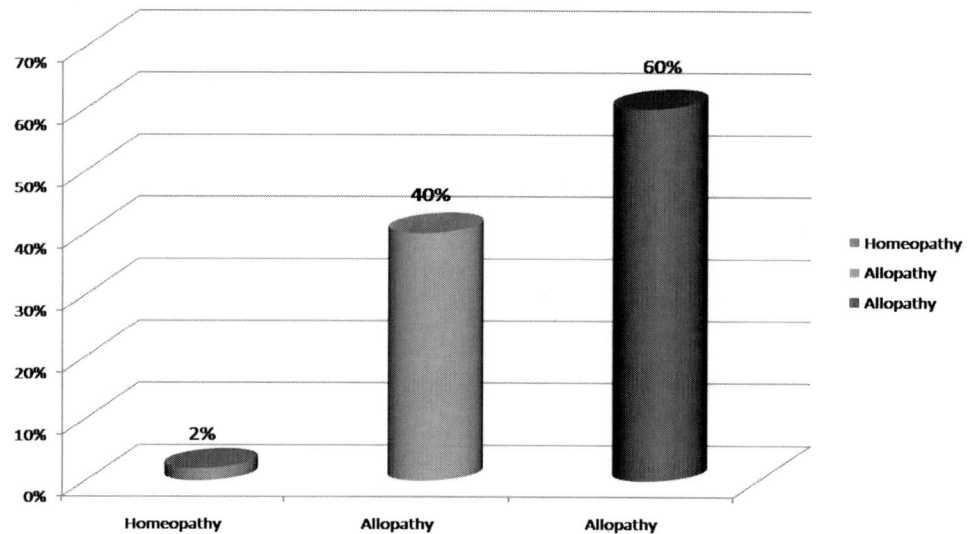

Cholera Epidemic Rio 1855

Hand bill from the New York City Board of Health, 1832. The outdated public health advice demonstrates the lack of understanding of the disease and its actual causative factors.

The Survivor's Guide to Swine Flu

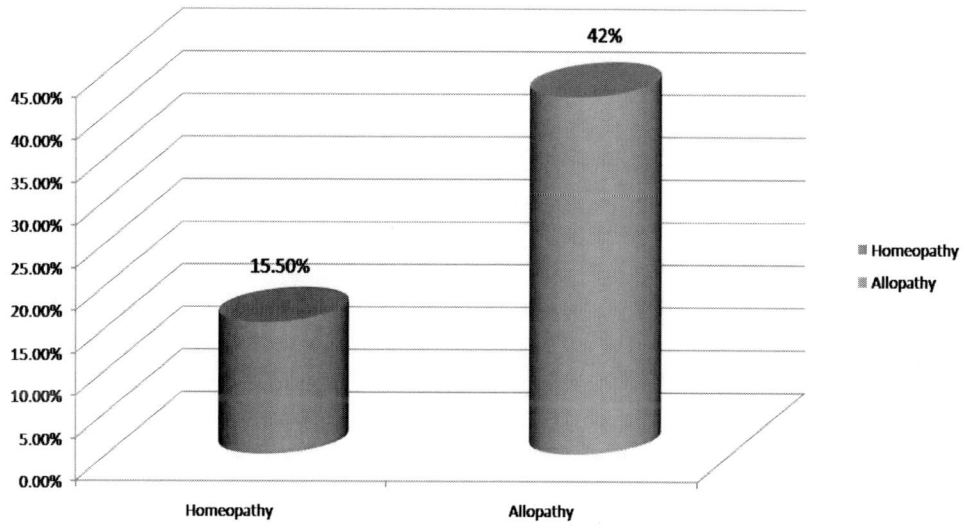

Cholera Epidemic 1892 Hamburg

HAMBURG 1892:

In the Hamburg cholera epidemic of 1892, allopathic mortality was 42%, homeopathic mortality was 15.5% In all, about 8,600 people died.

Although the city government knew about Dr John Snow's discovery linking the spread of cholera to the public water supply, they made no attempt to make any policy changes that could have prevented these deaths. The government was largely held responsible for this calamity and eventually revised their strategies for dealing with epidemics. This was the last serious European cholera outbreak.

Cholera is still a real health threat and is one of the most rapidly fatal illnesses known. A healthy person may become hypotensive within an hour of the onset of symptoms; in a particularly virulent outbreak, infected patients can die within three hours if treatment is not provided.

Usually, the disease progresses from the first liquid stool to shock in 4 to 12 hours, and death can occur in 18 hours to several days without oral rehydration therapy.

(Interestingly, Type O blood groups are most susceptible and Type AB least so)

Homeopathy

YELLOW FEVER IN THE SOUTHERN STATES OF THE USA: 1850'S

Yellow fever broke out in the southern states of the USA during the 1850s. Eventually it was discovered that the disease was borne by mosquitoes. The allopathic mortality from Yellow Fever among people treated with the Conventional Medicine of the time was between 15-85% depending upon location.

Homeopaths such as the respected doctors Holcome, and Davis based in Natchez, reported mortality rates of 6.43% and 5.73%, respectively.

In 1878, the mortality in New Orleans was 50% under allopathic care, and 5.6% with homeopathic care. Infection figures were in 1,945 cases in the same epidemic, so this represents a good sample size.

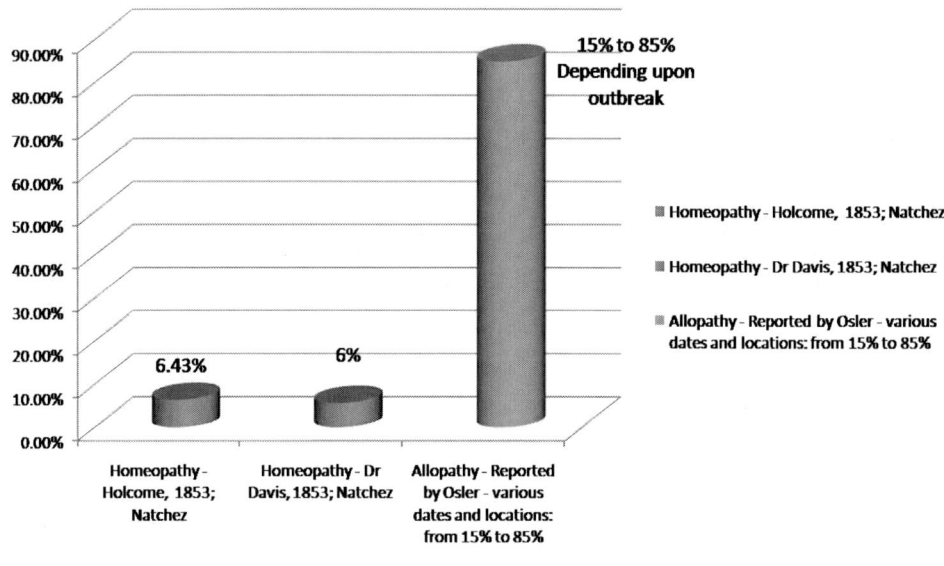

Yellow Fever 1850

To further illustrate the successes of homeopathic intervention in yellow fever, the following information is drawn from a "President's Address" given by Dr. A. L. Monroe of Louisville, Kentucky, given 8pm Friday evening, December 10, 1886, at the 3rd Annual Meeting of the Southern Homeopathic Medical Association:

> *"Yellow fever statistics showing average proportion of death losses during yellow fever epidemic of 1878 in Southern United States. These statistics represent the mean average of losses as calculated by a commission of yellow fever experts visiting*

the infected districts immediately after the epidemic: Allopathic, 15.50 per cent; homeopathic, 6 per cent.

Here we have a mass of statistics compiled by careful, conscientious workers, representing in the aggregate of at least 1,000,000 prescriptions given to 500,000 patients, and the work extending over a term of years of practice of at least 1000 physicians of each school."

Speaking at the same conference, Dr. A. L. Monroe also stated:

AND ON SMALLPOX:

"The first set [see chart below] I desire to present to your notice was compiled by a reputable life insurance company [my emphasis] in 1874, from the death reports of the cities of Boston for 1870, 1871 and 1872; Philadelphia for 1872, the year of the great epidemic of small-pox there; Newark for 1872 and 1873. The table presents the average death loss to number of patients treated during that time by the representatives of the two great schools of medicine."

By "*the two great schools of medicine*", Dr Monroe referred to both homeopathy and Allopathy.

Smallpox

	Allopathic Av. Loss	Homeopathic Av. Loss
Boston, 1870, '71 and '72	1735	885
New York, 1870 and '71	1576	848
Philadelphia,'70, '71	1903	1287
New York '72, '73	2046	1124
Brooklyn '72, '73	2280	1028
General average	1908	1034

DIPHTHERIA

Another epidemic disease which was greatly feared by many as it was so dangerous was diphtheria – however this was again treated successfully with homeopathy. Since the advent of widespread vaccination, it is a disease not often seen in our modern world.

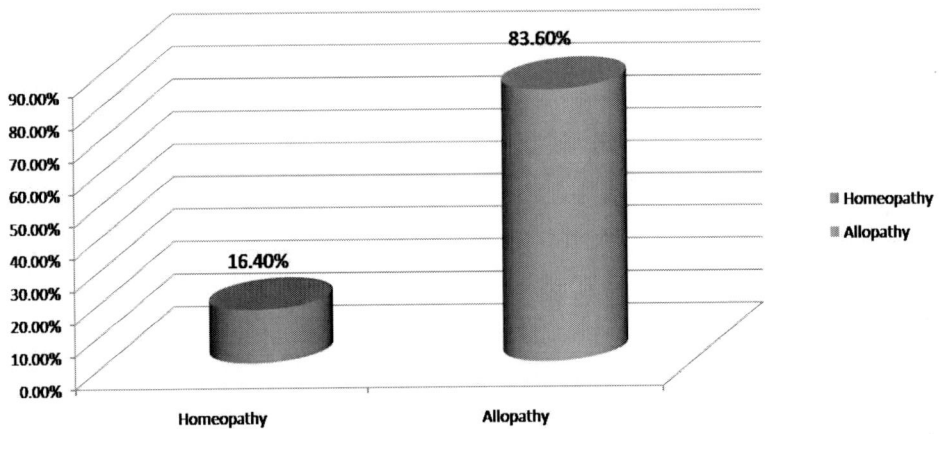

Diptheria 1862-1864

Diphtheria appeared periodically but rarely manifested the same types of symptoms and so was a very difficult disease to treat. This means that each practitioner had to really individualise his or her homeopathic prescription to match the patient's symptoms exactly.

A remedy which had been effective in treating it one year might not be the same remedy needed the next year.

Records of three years of diphtheria in Broome County, New York from 1862 to 1864, show that there was a report of an 83.6% mortality rate among the Conventional doctors (allopaths) and a 16.4% mortality rate among the homeopaths. (Bradford)

An aside . . . Regarding diphtheria, some evidence has been collected during controlled studies in the lab which support the idea of using a nosode (a remedy made from the disease e.g. in this case, sputum from a person with diptheria) as a prophylactic: In 1932, Chavanon published that 45 children had changed from Schick test positive to Schick test negative (demonstrating antibody to diphtheria) after being treated with Diptherinum. Patterson and Boyd repeated this test in 1941, and 20 out of 33 children treated converted to Schick test negative. Roux again repeated the study in 1946 with similar results.

RESULTS FROM MORE RECENT EPIDEMICS ARE AS FOLLOWS:

MENINGITIS EPIDEMIC IN BUENOS AIRES 1974

In 1974, during an epidemic of meningitis, 18,640 children were treated homoeoprophylactically (i.e. treated homeopathically to prevent them from getting the disease) and 6,340 were not. In the treated group four cases of meningitis were reported, in the untreated group, 32 cases were reported. Thus, the homeopathically treated group had an infection rate of 0.021% and the untreated group had an infection rate of 0.5%[16].

MENINGITIS IN 1998 IN BLUMENAU, BRAZIL

On the basis of the success of homeopathic prophylaxis in Buenos Aires, a large-scale investigation of the use of homeoprophylaxis was undertaken in persons up to 20 years of age. In the first six months of administration, the following results were obtained: of the 65,826 protected homeopathically, one case was reported and of the 23,532 not protected, 7 cases were reported. (The homeopathically treated group had an infection rate of 0.0015% and the infection rate in the untreated group was 0.02%)

A 12-month follow-up reported 3 cases in the protected group and 13 cases in the unprotected group. Statistical analysis demonstrated a 95% protection in children under six months and 91% protection in children over 12 months[17]

LEPTOSPIROSIS IN OCTOBER 2007 IN CUBA

In a Cuban Medical Conference in December 2008, Dr. Concepción Campa, Dr. Luis E. Varela, Dr. Esperanza Gilling, MCs. Rolando Fernández, Tec. Bárbara Ordaz, Dr. Gustavo Bracho, Dr. Luis García, Dr. Jorge Menéndez, Lic. Natalia Marzoa and Dr. Rubén Martínez presented a paper based upon their experiences in preventing the outbreak of Leptospirosis (Weil's Disease) – a deadly water-born disease that is rapidly fatal.

[NB: The results of this initiative were so astounding that I have translated the original abstract of the paper from Spanish, as the implications, for medicine as a whole, are extraordinary]:

Background: The Finlay Institute is a science institute based in Cuba that specialises in the production of vaccines. The situation medically in Cuba is rather different from the rest of the world in that, as Cuba is a Communist country, their medical system is more open and driven by the needs of people – and their drug-producing organisations are not 'simply in it for the profit' as they are here in the West. This means that there is a huge emphasis on producing medicines that are effective – and very importantly – inexpensive! There is no profit motive at all. Furthermore, medical training in Cuba is outstanding – some of the world's best doctors are trained in Cuba.

THE PRESENTATION:

The Finlay Institute is a centre dedicated to the development and production of vaccines. We also make our WHO-qualified facilities available for all homeopaths and homeopathic medicine.

The Finlay Institute acts as a supporting institution for research, production and development of high quality homeopathic products. However, in accordance with the social objective of addressing the prevention of infectious diseases, we are focused on homeo-prophylaxis as a viable strategy to attenuate the impact of preventable diseases on the developing world, the ones that need it the most.

Thus, development and evaluation of nosodes (homeopathically prepared remedies based upon pathological susbstances related to the disease, e.g. a remedy made from sputum could be made to treat a cough), is our main approach to make up the shortfall of current Conventional strategies based on vaccination.

As with vaccination interventions, the massive application of prophylactic nosodes gives rise to a greater impact on population health, compared with individualised therapies.

In addition, due to the easy administration and low economic resources needed, homeopathic prophylaxis becomes extremely suitable and accessible for developing countries and probably the best option for emergency situations comprising epidemic outbreaks and natural disasters.

The Cuban experiences of massively administrated nosodes supports the use of homeopathic prophylaxis as a promising solution to confront dangerous epidemiological situations.

During the October-November period of 2007, three provinces of the eastern region of Cuba were affected by strong rainfalls, causing flooding over vast areas, with severe damage to sanitary and health systems.

The risk of leptospirosis infection was raised to extremely dangerous levels with about 2 million people exposed to potentially contaminated water.

Considering this situation, the Finlay Institute prepared a leptospira nosode 200 C, using 4 circulating strains and following international quality standards.

A multidisciplinary team travelled to the affected regions to conduct the massive administration

of the nosode. Co-ordinated action with public health system infrastructures allowed the administration of a preventive treatment consisting of two doses (7-9 days apart) of the nosode to about 2.4 million of people (4.8 million doses).
Up to 95% percent of total population in the three provinces at risk were treated.

The epidemiology surveillance after the intervention showed a dramatic decrease of morbidity two weeks after and a reduction to zero mortality of hospitalised patients. The number of confirmed leptospirosis cases remains at low levels and below the levels that we would normally expect to see according to the seasonal trends and rainfall levels.

A reinforcing dose of the remedy was given after the hit of the hurricane IKE, but using the same nosode diluted up to 10 MC. Strict epidemiologic surveillance continues to be carried out on these provinces.

The results supported the design of new strategies for leptospirosis control. This experience could be extended to other diseases and other countries. The Finlay Institute is offering our facilities and specialists to spread this alternative approach to all regions needing emergent alternatives for epidemic control and prevention.

It will be clear from the information outlined above that, exactly as we have seen in historic outbreaks of Swine Flu, 1918-1919, and as we state throughout this book, homeopathy is a potentially enormously useful tool in treating epidemics and pandemics, including this recent outbreak of H1N1.

Although we have data about the effectiveness of homeopathic remedies in the case of H1N1 back in 1918, we have no data about whether or not homeopathy will work for H1N1 if it mutates to become more lethal, however we can confidently state the following:

> Based upon media reports and, in the case of H1N1 previous outbreaks, we now have a very clear symptom picture of how H1N1 presents itself. In fact, because H1N1 in its serious form produces an aggressive illness, it is a fairly straightforward matter for homeopaths to be able to identify a small group of homeopathic remedies that will "fit the picture" presented by anyone who contracts this disease. By using this particular symptom picture we have devised a homeopathic protocol that we believe, given our huge amounts of research in this area, will be helpful.

In dealing with any type of pandemic flu, whether it is Swine Flu, Bird Flu, or another type, there are three approaches that a homeopath will need to take:

Homeopathy

1. PREVENTION

The first is prevention (prophylaxis) i.e. "setting people up" so that they are optimally-resistant to the disease.

2. TREATMENT

The second is treatment (acute prescribing). Treating the presenting symptoms during an attack of H1N1 and also dealing with opportunistic infections that may set in after the acute phase of H1N1. This will involve treatment for the symptoms of the initial infection of H1N1. Serious cases of H1N1 have shown that after the first few days, the disease tends to develop into Acute Respiratory Distress Syndrome (ARDS) and this too will need to be treated.

3. RECOVERY/CONSTITUTIONAL PRESCRIBING

The third approach is "constitutional prescribing" – to "mop up the mess" left by a devastating infection – in order to help the person return to health as quickly as possible and to avoid as much post-viral complication as possible.

1. MORE ABOUT PREVENTION

It is possible to utilise particular homeopathic remedies that have a good track record of preventing flu. These include the remedies Influenzinum and Thymuline. (It should be pointed out that homeopathic prophylaxis is still controversial - in spite of the evidence from Brazil and Cuba. Critics of homeopathy point out that there have been no studies in humans that confirm that homeopathic prophylaxis is guaranteed to prevent you from contracting the disease, but then again, there is no Conventional Medicine that can do this either. The information here is based upon observation and historical data and is included here so that you can make up your own mind as to whether to try homeopathic proplylaxis.

HOW IT WORKS

Each year, the drug companies distribute a new flu vaccine, and each year, homeopathic pharmacies uses this vaccine to prepare the homeopathic remedy - Influenzinum.

The problem that we see in this approach – with specific regard to the current Swine Flu, or potential future Bird Flu, or indeed other pandemic flu outbreaks – is that the vaccine for this virus has not yet been produced and one will not be able to be made until scientists have seen exactly how the particular virus (H1N1, H5N1, etc.) is mutating.

Thymuline is a homeopathic remedy that is designed to stimulate your immune system and up-regulate the activity of the thymus gland which is responsible for producing your immune system's T cells.

We believe that it may be useful to take Thymuline as a prophylactic remedy but we would NOT advise taking it if you have actually caught Swine Flu, or Bird Flu as it may theoretically, stimulate a Cytokine Storm.

PROPHYLAXIS IS NOT REALLY 'HOMEOPATHY':

These two remedies are not prescribed "homeopathically", as for a prescription to be "homeopathic" it must be prescribed to exactly match the symptoms that the person is displaying. However, as we have seen above, there are many examples throughout the history of homeopathy where certain remedies have been used to confer immunity upon people when under threat from various epidemics.

HOMEOPATHIC PREVENTION AND CONVENTIONAL VACCINES – AN OVERVIEW

As discussed in an earlier chapter, Conventional flu vaccinations carry a small but real risk of causing life-threatening diseases such as Guillain-Barré Syndrome (a devastating viral disorder involving the spinal cord and nerves).

As we have discussed, flu vaccinations are also likely to contain undesirable additives such as adjuvants and preservatives which can have harmful effects. In addition, should governments choose to launch a new type of vaccine – some have talked of an RNA vaccine - this will have been untested to any great degree and may have intrinsic problems. (AZT, to choose but one example, was rushed onto the market to fight what was supposed to be another "plague" – AIDS - and caused devastating effects.)

Last, but by no means least, it is unlikely that a specific vaccine for a manifestation of H1N1 that would have mutated to become as lethal as it was in 1918, could be developed in time and in sufficient quantity to immunise the entire population.

There is extreme suspicion even from the medical community that anti-viral drugs such as Tamiflu, or Relenza will be of no real use at all, and a study in the Lancet – the journal of the British Medical Association (BMA), was very critical of these drugs and.....

> *"Could find no credible evidence of the effects of neuraminidase inhibitors on the avian influenza".*

Furthermore, the paper went on to comment that the authors were *"concerned about side effects of these drugs"*. (Lancet, February 2006).

Since then, the WHO has admitted that most (99%) of the seasonal H1N1 strains are resistant to Tamiflu.

2. MORE ABOUT TREATMENT

As we have seen, homeopathic treatment of epidemic and pandemic influenza has a long and successful history. According to homeopathic principles, remedies should be prescribed according to the exact presentation of symptoms when they appear.

A detailed list of the remedies that we believe will be most frequently required follows.

The decision to recommend these particular remedies is based upon what we do know about the way that H1N1 has manifested itself so far – in humans. We have carefully examined the symptoms and the remedies that we discuss are the ones that most closely match the symptoms that people have actually suffered from.

In addition, we have looked at pandemics throughout history and examined the particular symptoms that these produced. We are also bearing in mind the very successful use of particular homeopathic remedies in 1918 for which we have good historical medical evidence for their success.

3. MORE ABOUT RECOVERY/CONSTITUTIONAL PRESCRIBING

Homeopathic constitutional prescribing will be valuable in helping people to return to health after they have survived a flu infection, as that is the time when a devastated immune system will need all the help it can get.

The types of conditions that we would expect to see after a pandemic include Post Traumatic Stress Disorder, Post Viral Syndrome and may other generalised ailments which will be nigh-on impossible to diagnose in Conventional Medical terms as whole new syndromes are likely to emerge. (For example, the relatively "new" disease Chronic Fatigue Syndrome is thought to be causatively linked in many cases to viral infections. There are over 400 research studies on PubMed which allude to or confirm this relationship). This is where the true individualised nature of case-taking and prescribing based upon an individual's own particular symptoms really comes into its own.

(See your CMA Registered homeopath to receive an individualised prescription that will be based upon your own particular symptom picture. In the UK you can find a qualified, registered homeopath, or other Complementary Medical practitioners, on the CMA's website (The-CMA.

Org.UK), or in the USA at the National Center for Homeopathy's website (Homeopathy.Org).

"CAN I TAKE HOMEOPATHIC REMEDIES WITH ANTI-VIRAL DRUGS LIKE TAMIFLU?"

YES YOU CAN. IF YOU CAN GET TAMIFLU.

You can take homeopathic medicines alongside any other medication. In fact, homeopathic medicines work in a completely different way to Conventional Medicines. Homeopathic medicines are "energetic substances" that work on your body's "vital force", in order to help you to return to a state of healthy balance. Conventional Medicines are physical chemicals that work directly on your body's molecules and cells.

One important point to note though is that some Conventional drugs, such as steroids, are thought to antidote homeopathic medicines as they disrupt your body's function to such a degree that the homeopathic remedy doesn't stand a chance of working – it is as if the Conventional drug is fighting against your body's attempts to return to health because the aim of many Conventional drugs is to suppress – not cure symptoms. This is the opposite to homeopathy – which aims to help your body return, gently and permanently to a state of good health.

REFERENCES

1 Med Hypotheses. 2000 Jun;54(6):948-53. Water clusters in life. Lo SY, Li WC, Huang SH.
R & D Department, American Technologies Group, Inc., Monrovia, CA, USA.
2 A.K.Vallance,Can Biological Activity be Maintained at Ultra-high Dilution? An Overview of Homeopathy, Evidence and Bayesian Philosophy, The Journal of Alternative and Complementary Medicine 1998 4:1;49-76
3 Teschke O, de Souza EF. Water molecule clusters measured at water/air interfaces using atomic force microscopy. Phys Chem Chem Phys. 2005 Nov 21;7(22):3856-65. Epub 2005 Sep 20.
4 Dougherty RC, Howard LN. Analysis of excess Gibbs energy of electrolyte solutions: a new model for aqueous solutions. Biophys Chem. 2003 Sep;105(2-3):269-78.
5 Watterson JG. A role for water in cell structure. Biochem J. 1987 Dec 1;248(2):615-7.
6 Watterson JG. The role of water in cell architecture. Mol Cell Biochem. 1988 Feb;79(2):101-5.
7 Ludwig R. Water: From Clusters to the Bulk. Angew Chem Int Ed Engl. 2001 May 8;40(10):1808-1827.
8 Ju SP, Yang SH, Liao ML. Study of molecular behavior in a water nanocluster: size and temperature effect. J Phys Chem B Condens Matter Mater Surf Interfaces Biophys. 2006 May 11;110(18):9286-90.
9 Singh NJ, Park M, Min SK, Suh SB, Kim KS. Magic and Antimagic Protonated Water Clusters: Exotic Structures with Unusual Dynamic Effects. Angew Chem Int Ed Engl. 2006 May 3; [Epub ahead of print]
10 Ackland GJ, Guerin JA. Structure of an amphiphilic lattice gas, and its relationship to
microclustering of methanol in water. Phys Rev E Stat Nonlin Soft Matter Phys. 2006 Feb;73(2 Pt 1):021504. Epub 2006 Feb 7.
11 E. Tiezzi, NMR evidence of a supramolecular structure of water, Annali di Chimica 93 (2003) 471-476.
12 Med Hypotheses, 2000 Apr; 54 (4): 634-7. Plausibility of homeopathy and Conventional chemical therapy: the systemic memory resonance hypothesis. Schwartz GE, Russek LG, Bell IR, Riley D. Department of Medicine, University of Arizona, Tucson 85721 – 0068, USA.
13 J Altern Med. 1998 Spring; 4(1): 49-76. Comment in : J Altern Complement Med. 1998 Summer: 4(2): 132-5. Can biological activity be maintained at ultra-high dilution? An overview of homeopathy, evidence and Bayesian philosophy. Vallance AK,Medical School Registry, Royal Free Hospital School of Medicine, London, UK.
14 Witt CM, Bluth M, Albrecht H, et al. The in vitro evidence for an effect of high homeopathic potencies – a systematic review of the literature. Complementary Therapies in Medicine, 2007; 15: 128–138.
15 For a discussion of recent reports of a meta-analysis of homeopathic trials in The Lancet please visit the website of The Faculty of Homeopaths, which is the organisation that represents medical doctors who also properly qualified to practice homeopathy. http://www.trusthomeopathy.org/research/
16 Coulter, H. [1982, 2nd edition] Divided Legacy: The Conflict between Homoeopathy and the American Medical Association, pp.298-302.
17 Mroninski C, Adriano E & Mattos G (1998/99) Menigococcinum: Its protective effect against meningococcal disease, Homoeopathic Links,

18 Much historical data has been collated by the late (loved and missed) homeopath and historian Julian Winston. His website can be found at http://www.julianwinston.com/

CHAPTER 23

HOMEOPATHIC TREATMENT OF SWINE FLU (H1N1)

The information that follows is a selection of homeopathic remedies that have been shown, historically, to be useful in treating severe Swine Flu (H1N1) symptoms.

As with all serious, life-threatening diseases – there is a possibility that despite the treatments given, a person may still die. If Swine Flu strikes, you need to decide which treatments you are going to use. As you know – current Government advice recommends that you should seek medical advice immediately, if you suspect that you may have been exposed to the Swine Flu virus.

You may be offered Tamiflu – if it is available. This needs to be taken within the first 48 hours of exposure and may lessen the duration of the flu. (Current estimates state that Tamiflu may shorten the duration of a Swine Flu attack by one day.) In addition, as discussed previously, there is now significant evidence to indicate that many strains of H1N1 are actually now Tamiflu resistant.[1,2,3,4,5,6,7,8]

If you are considering using a Complementary Medical approach to treat yourself - and incorporating homeopathic medicines, please read on.

There are several historical precedents in recommending these particular remedies (out of over 2,000 possible homeopathic remedies). They have been proven to work well, time and again, and to save countless lives. As you have seen, we have excellent data from the Spanish Flu pandemic (and other epidemics), as to which remedies were most often indicated, and as the doctors at that time kept such meticulous notes, we do know that homeopathic treatment achieved far superior results compared to the conventional treatment of the time.

HOW DO WE KNOW WHAT THESE REMEDIES DO? A RECAP

When you read the brief remedy "pictures" below you will notice some very quirky symptoms that seem quite strange to anyone unfamiliar with the way that homeopathy works.

As you know, homeopathic research has been ongoing for the last two hundred years. The remedies are tested on healthy people, to see what symptoms they produce from taking a particular remedy and homeopathy works on the principle that "like treats like" or as Hahnemann put it *"Similar Similibus Curentur"*. So, the remedies that produce symptoms in a healthy person will cure those same symptoms in a sick person.

Remember, unlike most Conventional Medicine, homeopathic remedies are tested on people – not on animals and therefore, people undergoing the tests or "provings" as they are known, have been able to describe their symptoms in great detail.

It is interesting to consider that on the occasions that Conventional Medicine tests its medicines on people, they often tend to be sick people, which is a slightly about-face way of undertaking research, as each person who experiences a disease is a unique individual and will express the disease in their own unique way, so there would inevitably be a lot of "noise" in research results and inconsistencies.

In fact, a quote from Dr Alan Roses, the World-Wide Vice-President of Genetics at GlaxoSmithKline in December 2003 revealed that;

> *"The vast majority of drugs – more than 90% – only work in 30-50 % of the people".*

THE REMEDIES MOST LIKELY TO BE REQUIRED, TO TREAT SWINE FLU (H1N1)

FIRST, AN EXPLANATORY NOTE:

Homeopaths often refer to illnesses by using the name of the remedy that best matches the symptoms. So, they may speak of a "Gelsemium Flu", or an "Aconite Flu" etc. This doesn't mean that the flu has been caused by these remedies, merely that this remedy is the one that should be used for a patient who is experiencing that particular set of symptoms.

HOW TO TAKE A HOMEOPATHIC REMEDY

Remedies are energetic substances and are easily antidoted, so it is important not to handle them. Observe the following important guidelines:

- Do not take a remedy 20 minutes before, or after, eating, drinking or smoking

- Remove the cap from the top of the vial.

- Shake the tablet out of its container into the cap.

- Drop the tablet under your tongue and let it dissolve. After about 5 minutes, if the tablet has not completely dissolved, you can crunch it and swallow it.

- Avoid mint, coffee and camphor as these can antidote remedies. (Camphor is found in some lip salves, mothballs, some decongestant nasal sprays and in some chest-rubs such as Vicks.)

GELSEMIUM: (GELS)

Historically, Gelsemium has been the most effective remedy for flu. It was used extensively in 1918 and people who were fortunate enough to receive this form of treatment had a phenomenal reported survival rate of over 99% as compared to less than 70% among those who were treated with the conventional medicine of that time – aspirin etc.

KEY CHARACTERISTICS:
Flu with chills and paralytic weakness.

"Gelsemium Flu" symptoms come on slowly and will often occur as a result of exposure to infection. In general, Gelsemuim symptoms may also develop due to the stresses caused by worry or even "anticipatory anxiety" such as having to speak in public and so on. (Anticipatory fear of contracting H1N1? Stress from the economic downturn we are going through?)

One of the main characteristics of the Gelsemuim state is that there is a generalised weakness and shakiness, with great fatigue. The person just wants to lie in bed and may complain of wobbly legs.

An odd characteristic of a Gelsemium flu is that the patient may have a splitting headache which is better after urinating.

Chills run up and down the back and the patient may have a very sore throat. The head feels heavy and eyelids are droopy and there may even be visual disturbance such as double vision.

Another odd Gelsemium characteristic is that pain is felt "in the bones".

The face is hot and flushed. There is a putrid taste in the patient's mouth and the mouth may tremble. There may be a sensation of a lump in the throat and possibly a pain from the throat to the ear.

The person may have diarrhoea and much, frequent urination. (This profuse urination makes them feel better.)

The patient is thirstless in spite of the fact that they may indeed have a fever – and this can contribute to dehydration. However the Gelsemium patient does not perspire.

Symptoms are better for breathing and being in fresh air, moving around and bending forward.

The patient feels worse in damp weather or before a thunderstorm and if exposed to tobacco smoke and they are also worse in the early part of the morning (around 10am).

BRYONIA: (BRY)

After Gelsemium, Bryonia was a frequently used homeopathic remedy used for treating patients in the 1918 Spanish Flu.

KEY CHARACTERISTICS:

Bryonia Flu produces a severe, splitting headache and the patient just wants to be left alone.

The onset of a Bryonia Flu is slow.

The patient is achy all over and may complain of a violent headache, which is worsened by any movement at all e.g. coughing or even moving the eyes.

The Bryonia headache can be ameliorated by firm pressure and sleep.

The Bryonia patient is thirsty and dehydration is a risk.

They must drink large quantities of water.

They may vomit immediately after eating or drinking.

Mentally, they are irritable – they may talk anxiously about business and they just want to be alone.

They feel better from rest, cold things, pressure on painful parts.

Pains are described as stitching or tearing.

Symptoms in the Bryonia patient are worsened by noise, excitement, touch, bright lights, eating, warmth or movement.

They feel worse after eating and coughing and symptoms are at their peak at 3am and 9pm.

ACONITE: (ACON)

Aconite is described as "the first remedy for inflammatory fevers" in the homeopathic literature. Also conditions with "acute, sudden and violent invasion, with fever call for it".

KEY CHARACTERISTICS:
Symptoms come on very suddenly, often after exposure to cold, or from a fright, shock or other stressful event. Symptoms may begin at night.

A person with Aconite Flu shows great restlessness and anxiety, even great fear, particularly fear of death. They may even predict the time of their death, so convinced are they that they will die.

Physically, there is a high fever, sore throat and the patient feels better in fresh air. They may need the window to be opened.

Respiratory symptoms include the following – constant pressure in the left side of the chest, oppressed breathing on the least motion.

The cough is hoarse, hacking, dry and croupy and breathing is loud and laboured.

The patient is very sensitive to inspired (breathed in) air, there will be shortness of breath.

Hot feeling in lungs and blood comes up with when coughing up phlegm.

They feel worse in a warm room, in the evening or at night, when exposed to tobacco smoke, lying on the affected side or hearing music.

The face is red, hot and flushed which becomes deathly pale on rising.

An important point to note about the use of Aconite, is that it is to be used only in the early stages of disease – at the point where the symptoms are strong e.g. high fever – it should not be used after pathological change sets in – other remedies will be indicated at that stage.

Aconite should not be used for low fevers.

Note that vinegar can antidote Aconite and acid fruits, coffee and lemonade can modify its action so these are all best avoided.

Aconite works fast and must be repeated frequently in severe states such as might be seen in Swine Flu.

ARNICA: (ARN)

KEY CHARACTERISTICS:
The bruising remedy – par excellence. This "bruising" can be experienced mentally and emotionally as well as physically. Often in the case of flu one can feel bruised all over and Arnica will address this sensation.

An Arnica Flu will present with a feeling of soreness, as if bruised internally and externally.

The paradoxical thing about the Arnica state is that the patient will insist that they are well even when they are obviously not.

They may complain that the bed feels too hard (from the bruised sensation), they are also fearful of someone touching them – their body feels so bruised that this would be unbearable.

Their head is hot and body cold.

A patient requiring Arnica may desire vinegary things, like pickles for example.

Arnica is strongly indicated in influenza (with a low fever as opposed to Aconite – which is prescribed for high fever) and is also an excellent remedy for haemorrhage – seen to a great degree in 1918.

One odd symptom in the Arnica picture is the tendency for skin to turn black and blue – this was often seen in 1918 Spanish Flu.

The Arnica cough is violent and spasmodic – it is painful and historical reports tell us that children will cry before coughing due to anticipating the pain.

In homeopathy text books there is a strong indication that Arnica is useful in treating pleurodynia, which is usually a rare complication of coxsackievirus B infection and is defined as the sudden occurrence of lancinating (stabbing) chest pain attacks, commonly associated with fever, malaise, and headaches – co-incidentally these symptoms all appear as part of the Arnica symptom picture.

Aconite is a complementary remedy to Arnica so it is useful to know that it could be used after Aconite – which is often used at the very beginning of an illness where there is marked violence and rapidity of onset.

Arnica is antidoted by Camphor – which as mentioned above - is an ingredient in things like Vicks Vaporub and its ilk and some lip balms.

ARSENICUM ALBUM: (ARS ALB)

KEY CHARACTERISTICS:

An Arsenicum Flu presents with great restlessness and anxiety. Often this anxiety is "anticipatory" (like Gels. and Arg. Nit.) and the person is fearful of events that they anticipate rather than those events that are actually happening in the present moment.

Vomiting and/or diarrhoea are extremely common Arsenicum symptoms, as are burning pains which could be described as being like hot needles, which are improved by hot applications (e.g. a hot water bottle).

The patient feels chilly, restless and they feel great anxiety and fear of death – they look very worried.

They want to be alone – but not totally alone – they will want the security of knowing that there is someone in the next room for example.

Arsenicum patients are thirsty but can only take small sips.

Their face is swollen, pale, looks almost yellow, cold but covered with sweat.

There is an intense photophobia, or aversion to bright light.

The Arsenicum fever is intermittent, with a very high temperature.

The patient may be delirious.

All symptoms are generally worse between 1 and 2am.

They are better from hot drinks, heat and keeping the head elevated.

And lastly, a point worth noting is that Arsenicum, when given in very high potencies can, according to homeopathic literature, "give quiet and ease to the last moments of life".

BAPTISIA: (BAPT)

Baptisia was another of the main remedies used in 1918.

KEY CHARACTERISTICS:

Bluish skin discolouration – this could be similar to the heliotrope cyanosis seen in 1918 Spanish Flu.

Flu with high fever and a feeling of being bruised all over.

The onset of a Baptisia Flu is sudden and the patient complains of feeling sore all over and bruised.

They may complain of a sensation of "feeling scattered", or may talk about being "in bits".

Dehydration in a Baptisia Flu case is a big risk as there is profuse sweating with a high fever and the patient is extremely thirsty.

As there is also a risk of "gastric flu-like symptoms" with vomiting (as soon as the person has drunk or eaten) and diarrhoea, this exacerbates the dehydration problems. This vomiting and severe diarrhoea has been seen in people who have contracted H1N1.

The person needing Baptisia will look sluggish and dazed and their face may be a dull red colour.

The Baptisia fever is characterised by chills with soreness all over the body. (Chills can worsen at around 11am.)

The patient is worse for humid heat and in foggy conditions.

Baptisia is a rather short acting remedy and may need to be frequently repeated.

Bryonia and Arsenicum both follow Baptisia well and may be needed after Baptisia has done its work.

BELLADONNA: (BELL)

KEY CHARACTERISTICS:

A Belladonna Flu is characterised by a high fever, face is red and pupils dilated, with a "staring" quality. (In Conventional Medicine, Atropine, a constituent of Belladonna is used to dilate the pupils and paralyse pupil accommodation so that examination of the internal area of the eye may be undertaken.)

When a very high fever comes on rapidly after exposure to infection or from the head getting cold, wet, or overheated e.g. sunstroke or exposure to other high temperatures, Belladonna is indicated.

Mentally, the patient may be confused or be prone to delirium and have a very high temperature. A throbbing headache is typical of Belladonna.

The patient's face is bluish-red and looks flushed.

They may have a sore throat and their tongue may resemble a strawberry.

In Belladonna cases, the symptoms tend to be quite marked and strong. People who are normally quite vital and strong will tend to produce symptoms that respond to Belladonna as symptoms are aggressive and require a strong vital force to manifest symptoms of such intensity.

The patient feels better when they stand or sit upright and are better in a warm room.

Symptoms are worsened by any noises, bright light or movement.

They are worse from lying down and symptoms are often exacerbated at night.

One Belladonna "oddity" is that symptoms tend to affect the right side of the body – so for example, if the patient has a sore throat, this will be worse on the right side.

The patient will be thirsty for cold water but will have a dread of drinking.

The patient may cough up blood and the cough may be tickling, short and dry – worse at night.

Belladonna is antidoted by Camphor, Coffee and Aconite.

Belladonna is a fast acting remedy and will need to be frequently repeated.

EUPATORIUM PERFOLIATUM: (EUP PER)

KEY CHARACTERISTICS:

A traditional remedy for Dengue fever also known as "breakbone fever", the Eupatorium Flu produces symptoms that make the person feel that their bones are broken.

Eupatorium symptoms are truly terrible and are present in the most severe flus, with patients actually feeling that their bones really are broken.

In addition, there will be soreness and a generalised bruised feeling all over and extreme muscle aches.

The patient will moan and groan with pain.

The action of Eupatorium as a remedy is very fast and it relieves pains very rapidly.

Any movement worsens the patient and they will have what can be described as a "bursting headache", which is made worse by coughing.

They may sneeze a great deal, the chest is sore and the nose is runny.

The patient is thirsty for iced water and this brings on chills in the small of the back.

The patient feels better for perspiration but this is not copious and it doesn't improve the headache symptoms.

The patient benefits from conversation and feels better for talking.

MERCURIUS SOLUBILIS: (MERC SOL)

KEY CHARACTERISTICS:

The Mercury Flu produces a high fever with excessive salivation, bad breath and copious offensive perspiration that brings no relief.

Patients are very thirsty and their temperature goes up and down like a barometer.

Mercury is a very destructive remedy and people requiring it may produce mouth ulcers (apthous ulcers) and may also have swollen glands.

In a Mercury Flu, there is much sneezing and the nostrils are raw and ulcerated – the discharge is corrosive. The nose may bleed.

The face looks pale, puffy and dirty-looking.

The tongue may have a furrow in it, lengthwise and the tongue feels heavy, thick and has a moist coating with indentations of teeth marks.

The throat is bluish-red and swollen and the patient has a constant desire to swallow with pain worse on the right side.

There is an intense thirst for cold drinks and continuous hunger.

Stools can be greenish, bloody and slimy.

There is a general tendency to perspiration but this does not bring relief.
The fever is worse in the evening and into the night.

The patient feels worse at night in wet, damp weather, lying on their side, perspiring and in a warm room/bed.

NUX VOMICA: (NUX VOM)

KEY CHARACTERISTICS:

Nux Vomica Flus are characterised by oversensitivity. This means that the sufferer is over-reactive to stimuli and is also irritable.

They are very chilly and they may be impatient, irritable, even angry and may take offence at the slightest thing.

The oversensitivity of this state means that the patient is very sensitive to light, noise and odours.

They may have digestive problems and will frequently be constipated.

They may feel that they have a nail being driven into the top of the head, sometimes a frontal headache with the desire to press the head against something.

There is marked photophobia (sensitivity to light).

Loud noises are very irritating to the patient and may anger him or her.

The nose is stuffy and may bleed. In addition, they may have bloody saliva.

They feel nauseous in the morning and feel worse after eating.

The Nux Vomica patient has shallow, oppressed breathing and a tight hacking cough with bleeding – a symptom seen in some people with H1N1. The cough brings on a bursting headache.

The body feels burning hot – especially the face and the patient feels chilly but does not want to be covered.

Nux produces a dry heat of the body and it does not feel sweaty.

Nux is antidoted by Coffee and it is said to act best if given in the evening.

RHUS TOXICODENDRON: (RHUS TOX)

KEY CHARACTERISTICS:

The Rhus Tox Flu will often come on after exposure to cold and damp and the patient feels stiff and painful.

The keynote is that there will be initial pain on moving which will wear off if movement is continued and will return again if movement is continued beyond the individual's point of tolerance.

The patient is restless and always moving around – they can't get comfortable.

The person is worried and anxious, weepy, and often worse at night.

An odd characteristic of Rhus Tox is that the patient may have a red triangular tip on their tongue.

They may have swollen glands, with a "sticking" pain on swallowing.

The Rhus Tox patient has a bitter taste in their mouth and a desire to drink milk.

They are very thirsty in general and may feel drowsy after eating.

Any cough that they may have can be characterised as dry and "teasing", which runs from midnight to the morning, during a chill or when putting the hands out of the bed.

They may cough up blood if they over-exert themselves and as they are restless this is a strong likelihood.

Rhus Tox patients feel as if their chest is "oppressed" and they can't get their breath properly.

Limbs feel stiff and paralysed.

The fever in a Rhus Tox case is intermittent, restless and chilly, followed by heat.

The patient feels better for warm applications (e.g. hot water bottle) on any parts affected.

HOW DO I CHOOSE WHICH HOMEOPATHIC REMEDY TO USE?

First of all, it is always best to consult a qualified homeopath who will be able to prescribe a Constitutional Remedy for you which will be designed to make you as optimally healthy as possible by clearing up any ailments that you may be suffering from at the moment.

However, it is also wise to carry a selection of all the eleven homeopathic remedies featured above, remedies that have been shown to have been effective in 1918. Also, learn the symptoms of each of the 'remedy pictures' in this Chapter. Generally, when a homeopathic remedy is needed for flu, you'll need to prescribe quickly - rather than having to spend time differentiating between various remedies.

HOW DO I KNOW WHICH DOSE TO TAKE?

Remedies are available in various potencies, however when treating an acute condition like flu it is best to stick to the lower potencies of 6c or 30c. When chosen well, the correct homeopathic remedy will work very quickly - you'll usually notice a marked difference in symptoms within half an hour. This is why it is essential to make sure that you are taking the right remedy - the wrong rememdy will do nothing.

By contrast, a constitutional remedy - prescribed by a homeopath to address your case as a whole and to treat ongoing chronic conditions may well be prescribed in much higher potencies.

HOW OFTEN SHOULD I TAKE THE REMEDIES FOR FLU?

You can take low-potency remedies for acute conditions like flu every hour. What tends to happen in practice is that as soon as people start to feel better they tend to forget to take the remedy. This is fine. There is no need to continue taking the remedy once you begin to feel better - as opposed to anti-biotics for example where if you have to take them it is absolutely necessary to finish the entire course.

REFERENCES

1: Hauge SH, Blix HS, Borgen K, Hungnes O, Dudman SG, Aavitsland P. Sales of oseltamivir in Norway prior to the emergence of oseltamivir resistant influenza A(H1N1) viruses in 2007-08. Virol J. 2009 May 12;6:54. PubMed PMID: 19435505; PubMed Central PMCID: PMC2685787.

2: Eshaghi A, Bolotin S, Burton L, Low DE, Mazzulli T, Drews SJ. Genetic microheterogeneity of emerging H275Y influenza virus A (H1N1) in Toronto, Ontario, Canada from the 2007-2008 respiratory season. J Clin Virol. 2009 Jun;45(2):142-5. Epub 2009 May 17. PubMed PMID: 19451021.

3: Vicente D, Cilla G, Montes M, Mendiola J, Pérez-Trallero E. Rapid spread of drug-resistant influenza A viruses in the Basque Country, northern Spain, 2000-1 to 2008-9. Euro Surveill. 2009 May 21;14(20). pii: 19215. PubMed PMID: 19460286.

4: Rungrotmongkol T, Intharathep P, Malaisree M, Nunthaboot N, Kaiyawet N, Sompornpisut P, Payungporn S, Poovorawan Y, Hannongbua S. Susceptibility of antiviral drugs against 2009 influenza A (H1N1) virus. Biochem Biophys Res Commun. 2009 Jul 31;385(3):390-4. Epub 2009 May 20. PubMed PMID: 19463784.

5: García J, Sovero M, Torres AL, Gomez J, Douce R, Barrantes M, Sanchez F, Jimenez M, Comach G, de Rivera I, Agudo R, Kochel T. Antiviral resistance in influenza viruses circulating in Central and South America based on the detection of established genetic markers. Influenza Other Respi Viruses. 2009 Mar;3(2):69-74. PubMed PMID: 19496844.

6: Hurt AC, Ernest J, Deng YM, Iannello P, Besselaar TG, Birch C, Buchy P, Chittaganpitch M, Chiu SC, Dwyer D, Guigon A, Harrower B, Kei IP, Kok T, Lin C, McPhie K, Mohd A, Olveda R, Panayotou T, Rawlinson W, Scott L, Smith D, D'Souza H, Komadina N, Shaw R, Kelso A, Barr IG. Emergence and spread of oseltamivir-resistant A(H1N1) influenza viruses in Oceania, South East Asia and South Africa. Antiviral Res. 2009 Jul;83(1):90-3. Epub 2009 Mar 24. PubMed PMID: 19501261.

7: Cheng PK, Leung TW, Ho EC, Leung PC, Ng AY, Lai MY, Lim WW. Oseltamivir- and amantadine-resistant influenza viruses A (H1N1). Emerg Infect Dis. 2009 Jun;15(6):966-8. PubMed PMID: 19523305.

8: Wang SQ, Du QS, Huang RB, Zhang DW, Chou KC. Insights from investigating the interaction of oseltamivir (Tamiflu) with neuraminidase of the 2009 H1N1 swine flu virus. Biochem Biophys Res Commun. 2009 Aug 28;386(3):432-6. Epub 2009 Jun 10. PubMed PMID: 19523442.

CHAPTER 24

OTHER COMPLEMENTARY MEDICAL APPROACHES THAT MAY BE USEFUL IN THE FIGHT AGAINST SWINE FLU (VIRAL INFECTION)

There are a number of highly promising approaches that should be considered when looking at ways of both preparing yourself to be as optimally healthy as possible and also to treat Swine Flu, should you be unfortunate enough to catch it. It is important to point out at this stage that none of the approaches discussed below have been used in trials to combat H1N1 specifically and while they may have anti-viral properties and be effective against other viruses, their effectiveness against H1N1 is, as yet, unknown.

SILVER

Silver has been used over the centuries in a number of medical applications and is the subject of much current medical research.[1,2,3,4,5,6,7,8] What is of immediate interest to us as we face the prospect of Swine Flu is the more recent use of silver against viruses.

There is growing evidence that a particular form of silver called "Colloidal Silver" is an effective antimicrobial treatment. A colloid is a suspension of a substance in a liquid. In the case of Colloidal Silver, extremely tiny particles of silver are suspended in water. They measure 0.01 to 0.001 microns in diameter and to put this into some perspective, one micron is one millionth of a metre or 4/100,000 of an inch.

Other Complementary Medical Approaches

The particles are so tiny and consist of only between 5 to 20 silver atoms and they have a positive electrical charge. They bounce off each other and this causes them to defy gravity.

This means that they remain suspended in water for months or years – if stored correctly – away from extremes of heat and light.

A BRIEF OUTLINE OF JUST A FEW OF THE CONDITIONS SILVER HAS BEEN USED TO TREAT

Silver has been used for centuries to speed wound healing, treat infections and purify water. The ancient Macedonians covered wounds with silver plates to speed healing. Historically, silver was used in its normal metallic state that we are all familiar with. Nowadays, various forms of silver are used in conventional medical settings – i.e. for the prevention of infection in burns victims and silver is also used in sticking plasters (band-aids) as an antimicrobial agent.

Silver was used extensively right from the turn of the 19th Century and into the 1940s when the advent of antibiotics meant that silver was no longer popular. Silver – in various forms - was used to treat many different ailments, just a few examples include pneumonia, tuberculosis and pleurisy,[9] sexually transmitted diseases e.g. gonorrhea and syphillis, cuts, wounds, leg ulcers, pustular eczema, impetigo and boils, acute meningitis and epidemic cerebro-spinal meningitis, infectious diseases such as Mediterranean fever, erysipelas, cystitis, typhus, typhoid fever, and tonsillitis[10]; eye disorders such as dacryocystitis, corneal ulcers, conjunctivitis and blepharitis[11]; and various forms of septicemia, including puerperal fever, peritonitis and post-abortion septicaemia[12].

Several trials have demonstrated that Colloidal Silver can kill viruses.

The main area of research is in the field of HIV and certainly colloidal silver seems to be performing well. Researchers at Temple University of Philadelphia USA, Brigham Young University USA, and the University Medical Centre in Geneva, Switzerland all report the antiviral activity of Colloidal Silver and the main mechanism of action seems to be that silver has been shown to be a potent inhibitor of HIV protease. Of course, it is far too early to tell whether colloidal silver will be active against H1N1 until trials on this particular virus are undertaken.

One concern that we have is that there are reports of a condition called Argyria – where the skin of a person using silver in various forms turns a bluish grey. Argyria is not treatable or reversible. The reports of Argyria seem to relate to people who have used silver nitrate or other silver salts. At present, there is only controversial evidence that this condition has been caused by the use of colloidal silver.

However, we are continuing our research in this area to ascertain the safety of Colloidal Ssilver and will report on our findings in our CMA Monthly e-Newsletter Updates that you can access via The Complementary Medical Association's website (The-CMA.Org.UK). We will continue to look for more evidence that Colloidal Silver may be useful in the battle against Swine Flu and will report our findings as soon as possible.

REFERENCES

1: Spratt DA, Pratten J, Wilson M, Gulabivala K. An in vitro evaluation of the antimicrobial efficacy of irrigants on biofilms of root canal isolates. Int Endod J. 2001 Jun;34(4):300-7. PubMed PMID: 11482142.

2: van Hasselt P, Gashe BA, Ahmad J. Colloidal silver as an antimicrobial agent: fact or fiction? J Wound Care. 2004 Apr;13(4):154-5. PubMed PMID: 15114827.

3: Araujo Castillo R, Pinto Valdivia JL, Ramírez D, Cok García J, Bussalleu Rivera A. [New ultrashort scheme for helicobacter pylori infection eradication using tetracycline, furazolidone and colloidal bismuth subcitrate in dyspeptic patients with or without peptic ulceration in the National Hospital Cayetano Heredia]. Rev Gastroenterol Peru. 2005 Jan-Mar;25(1):23-41. Spanish. PubMed PMID: 15818420.

4: Lansdown AB. Silver in health care: antimicrobial effects and safety in use. Curr Probl Dermatol. 2006;33:17-34. Review. PubMed PMID: 16766878.

5: Tien DC, Tseng KH, Liao CY, Tsung TT. Colloidal silver fabrication using the spark discharge system and its antimicrobial effect on Staphylococcus aureus. Med Eng Phys. 2008 Oct;30(8):948-52. Epub 2008 Feb 20. PubMed PMID: 18069039.

6: Zhang Y, Peng H, Huang W, Zhou Y, Yan D. Facile preparation and characterization of highly antimicrobial colloid Ag or Au nanoparticles. J Colloid Interface Sci. 2008 Sep 15;325(2):371-6. Epub 2008 Jun 5. PubMed PMID: 18572178.

7: Benn TM, Westerhoff P. Nanoparticle silver released into water from commercially available sock fabrics. Environ Sci Technol. 2008 Jun 1;42(11):4133-9. Erratum in: Environ Sci Technol. 2008 Sep 15;42(18):7025-6. PubMed PMID: 18589977.

8: Zhu C, Xue J, He J. Controlled in-situ synthesis of silver nanoparticles in natural cellulose fibers toward highly efficient antimicrobial materials. J Nanosci Nanotechnol. 2009 May;9(5):3067-74. PubMed PMID: 19452971.

9 B. Duhamel (1912) "Electric Metal Colloids and Their Therapeutical Applications" Lancet, Jan. 13.

10 A. Searle, The Use of Colloids in Health and Disease, London: Constable & Co., 1920, pp67-111.

11 A. Legge Roe (1915) "Collosol Argentum and its Opthalmis Uses" Br. Med. J., Jan.16, 104.

12 G. van Amber Brown (1916) "Colloidal Silver in Sepsis" Am.J.Obstetrics, Jan- June, 136-141.

FUNGI

Medicinal Fungi show enormous potential to combat many diseases. They have been thoroughly researched and our knowledge of Medicinal Fungi is enriched because they have been used for thousands of years in Traditional Chinese Medicine. There are five species of Fungi that show the greatest healing potential: Trametes, Maitake, Shiitake, Cordyceps and Reishi. Just a handful of studies have shown that these Fungi:

- Boost heart health[1]
- Lower the risk of cancer [2]
- Act as Potent Antiviral Agents [3,4,5,6,7]
- Act as Anti-Fungal, Anti-Bacterial and Anti-Parasitic agents [8,9,10,11,12,13,14,15,16,17]
- Reduce inflammation[18]
- Balance blood sugar levels [19,20,21,22]
- Lower cholesterol [23,24,25]

Maitake, Shiitake, Cordyceps and Reishi mushrooms have many similar properties. They all boost your body's immune function; all support cardiovascular health and all have demonstrated qualities which would make them very useful in the prevention of, and treatment of, certain forms of cancer. Additionally, each medicinal mushroom also has very specific effects.

- **Maitake** is specifically recommended for balancing blood sugar levels
- **Shiitake** treats nutritional deficiencies, impotence, candida, high blood pressure and high LDL cholesterol
- **Reishi** promotes respiratory health, eases stress and is a cardio-vascular tonic
- **Cordyceps** is an excellent stamina and libido enhancer, kidney tonic and anti-oxidant
- **Trametes** of all the medicinal mushrooms, is perhaps one of the most researched and is currently prescribed by health professionals across the globe to assist in the recovery and prevention of some potentially lethal conditions. Trametes is a wood-rotting polypore that grows on the side of felled oak logs and other dead or dying hardwoods. It has a very strong mycelium, which is able to penetrate the log in a short amount of time. Its voracious attitude is echoed in its powerful medicinal actions. As mentioned, this mushroom shows a varied array of health-enhancing properties, however it is primarily used in cancer treatments as a preventative and as a curative. Extracts of this mushroom account for 16% of Japan's national expenditure on cancer treatments.

Trametes components are thought to enhance T-cell proliferation and are used as an immune-stimulant, antibiotic, anti-viral and a treatment for hepatitis and infections of the lungs, digestive and urinary systems. The most well known studies of this remarkably curative Fungus have been carried out in Japan.[26,27,28,29]. Trametes contains some of the most potent anti-viral agents found in the mushroom kingdom. Two of these, PSP and PSK have been shown to be highly effective at inhibiting the replication of Herpes simplex 1, HIV, Hepatitis B and other debilitating viruses.

Anti-viral agents from other mushrooms have also been identified, such as lentinan from Shiitake (Lentinula edodes), and Ganaderiol-F, Ganoderic acid and Lucidumol from Reishi.

OF PARTICULAR RELEVANCE TO SWINE FLU

It is possible that some of the fungi discussed above may be extremely useful in preparing your immune system to be as resistant to viral infection as possible – and of course they are strongly antiviral. However, we are concerned that certain fungi – an example of which is Trametes – are highly potent immune stimulators – which would be of concern if used as a treatment for H1N1. It appears that Trametes does in fact, stimulate TNFα and a number of other inflammatory cytokines that are implicated in the Cytokine Storm phenomenon.

At this point in time we do not recommend their use to treat Swine Flu, but we will continue to research the importance of fungi in relation to Swine Flu and will report our findings and recommendations in our Monthly Updates via The Complementary Medical Association's website The-CMA.Org.UK

REFERENCES

1 Tao & Feng, 1990; Gau et al. 1990
2 Ikekawa, 1969, 1989, 2001; Ooi and Liu, 1999,2000
3 Suzuki et al., 1990
4 Eo et al. 2000
5 Kim et al. 1999
6 Brandt & Piriano, 2000
7 Zhou et al., 1990
8 Anke, 1989
9 Okamato et al., 1993
10 Ng et al., 1996
11 Sudirman, 1999
12 Thomas et al., 1999
13 Hirasawa et al., 1999
14 Hatvani, 2001
15 Trutneva et al., 2001
16 Suay et al.,2000
17 Stamets, 2002
18 Stavinoha et al., 1990,1996; Stavinoha, 1997;
19 Tomoda et al., 1986
20 Horio et al., 2001
21 Ohtsuru et al., 2001
22 Kubo et al., 1994
23 Li et al. 2001
24 Tao & Feng, 1990
25 Gau et al., 1990

26 Ebin & Murata, 1994

CHAPTER 25

SUMMARY OF RECOMMENDATIONS - AN OVERVIEW OF THE GUIDELINES AND ADVICE IN THIS BOOK

Should Swine Flu continue to spread rapidly and prove to be as virulent as when it started in Mexico and you, or someone close to you, are unfortunate enough to catch it, we've made sure that you know what your Conventional and Complementary Medical options are. Should you wish follow our advice, or not, the choice is yours and you will be able to make informed decisions and take responsibility for your well-being and that of your loved ones.

As well as the treatments that Conventional Medicine has to offer, you now know that there are a series of homeopathic remedies that Complementary Medical practitioners have used successfully against major pandemics and various outbreaks of influenza over the years.

These remedies are, in the eyes of professional, qualified Complementary Medical practitioners, tried and tested. Some have hisorically been successfully used to treat many thousands of people with an H1N1 infection and they are the remedies that homeopaths in particular rely on when treating cases like this. Whether you choose to take advantage of them, or not, is your decision.

And, even if Swine Flu continues to spread and become more virulent, our advice is:

> *"Don't panic, plan carefully and ensure that you are as optimally healthy as you can be".*

Summary of Recommendations

How can we make sure we really are 'as healthy as we can be'?

Our recommendations, supported by vast amounts of scientific research, consist of getting you into the best shape possible, given your current state of health. At the heart of this advice is the need to adopt an anti-inflammatory diet and lifestyle and learn how to use the supplements, herbs and remedies in this book in order to give yourself the best chance possible.

Should the best happen and you don't contract Swine Flu, you haven't wasted your time following our recommendations, you'll be fitter, healthier and less predisposed to developing a whole range of chronic diseases such as heart disease, arthritis, Type 2 diabetes and even certain cancers. You'll even look better, feel more energetic and experience better moods as our recommendations carry a whole host of anti-ageing benefits too!

DETAILED SUMMARY OF RECOMMENDATIONS

There are really four stages that you need to plan for:

1. Preparing yourself prior to a truly virulent, highly toxic Phase 6 pandemic

2. What to do should H1N1 mutate to be more virulent and a severe pandemic occurs

3. What to do if you catch Swine Flu

4. Dealing with the after effects

STAGE ONE: PREPARE YOURSELF PRIOR TO A TRULY VIRULENT, HIGHLY TOXIC PANDEMIC

Preparedness for a more extreme pandemic includes psychological preparation, by which we mean that you should read and implement the ideas and tips outlined in our Psychology of Survival section. This could mean the difference between life and death. It is vital to ensure that you make preparations so that know that you know you have safe shelter, plentiful food supplies and clean water in the event of a serious pandemic, and that you are able to implement correct sanitation measures that will help to keep you healthy.

REMEMBER THE 6 'P's

Prior Preparation Prevents P*** Poor Performance

Begin now to stockpile water, food and other essential items outlined in this book. Remember to rotate your stocks. Remember that Governments in the UK and the USA are telling us that services and supplies of foods, utilities and water may be disrupted for a period of three months, if a serious pandemic hits, so make sure you know how, and where, you can store your supplies.

- Avoid foods and drinks that will compromise your immune system.
- It is important to exercise to stay healthy – but only in moderation.
- Get into healthy habits such as correct hand washing and nose blowing – habits only become ingrained by practicing them.

In order to optimise your immune system you need correct nutrition, supplements and herbs to create the best health possible and to be optimally resistant to viruses.

Follow the Palæo-Mediterranean Diet. This is ideally a permanent lifestyle change, given that this diet is designed to make you as healthy as possible, reduce your predisposition to inflammation and help you to be resistant to degenerative diseases, as well as acute illnesses such as viruses.

Every day, you need to take a balanced mixture of high quality, bioavailable Multi-vitamin/ Mineral supplements, that include anti-oxidant nutrients. These should ideally be taken in one balanced supplement that contains all of the vitamins and minerals outlined below.

We realise it may well be difficult to find supplements that contain these extremely specialised ingredients, and we are currently advising a number of companies in order to help them to formulate supplements to these specifications. We will provide information about this on The CMA website (The-CMA.Org.UK).

You need to take a high quality Omega 3 fish oil, as well as the anti-inflammatory, anti-oxidant, anti-viral, anti-bacterial herbs mentioned below that contain standardised extracts of herbs and you will also need to take a superior Whey Protein supplement.

THE SUPPLEMENTS YOU TAKE EVERY DAY SHOULD CONTAIN THE FOLLOWING:

VITAMINS (THESE MUST BE NON-SYNTHETIC AND BIOAVAILABLE AND IDEALLY IN THE FORMS BELOW)

- Vitamin A Complex: (Such as retinol palmitate) with natural-source, mixed carotenoids (that should include alpha-carotene, beta-carotene, cryptoxanthin, lutein, lycopene, zeaxanthin)
- Vitamin B Complex: B1 (thiamin), B2 (riboflavin), B3 (niacin, this should be as inositol hexanicotinate), B5 (d-Ca pantothenate), B6 (pyridoxine), B12 (cyanocobalamin), folic

acid, biotin, choline bitartrate, inositol (ideally from inositol hexanicotinate), and if possible include the "new" Vitamin B – phylloquinone (PQQ)
- Vitamin C Complex: Vitamin C (Magnesium Ascorbate, plus mixed citrus bioflavonoids, quercetin dihydrate)
- Vitamin D3 (Cholecalciferol)
- Vitamin E Complex: **Tocopherols**: alpha-tocopherol, beta-tocopherol, gamma-tocopherol, delta-tocopherol, **Tocotrienols**: alpha-tocotrienol, beta-tocotrienol, gamma-tocotrienol, delta-tocotrienol

MINERALS (NON-SYNTHETIC, BIOAVAILABLE AND IDEALLY IN THE FORMS BELOW)

- Boron (Citrate)
- Calcium (Citrate-Malate)
- Chromium (Picolinate)
- Copper (Citrate)
- Iodine (Potassium Iodide)
- Magnesium (Citrate, Ascorbate)
- Manganese (Glycinate)
- Molybdenum (Na Molybdate)
- Selenium (Se-Methylselenocysteine)
- Silicon (Na Metasilicate)
- SOD (Superoxide Dismutase - with Gliadin)
- Vanadium (Citrate)
- Zinc (Citrate)

OMEGA 3 ESSENTIAL FATTY ACIDS

These must be guaranteed to be highly purified. Ideally, they should contain high levels of Eicosapentaenoic Acid (EPA), and lower levels of Docosahexaenoic Acid (DHA)

HERBS

All of which MUST contain biologically relevant, confirmed, standardised amounts of the necessary active substances:

- Turmeric (Curcumin)
- Resveratrol (Trans-Resveratrol – not Cis-Resveratrol)
- Ginger
- Rosemary
- Olive Leaf Extract

WHEY PROTEIN

This should be an advanced Whey Protein formulation, which is high in alpha-lactalbumin and bioactive peptide subfractions such as lactoferrin and ideally it should also ideally incorporate Sialic Acid.

STAGE TWO: WHAT TO DO SHOULD H1N1 MUTATE TO BE MORE VIRULENT AND A SEVERE PANDEMIC OCCURS

- Put your survival plans into place.
- Continue with the Paleo-Mediterranean Diet; (fresh, organic products wherever possible).
- Continue to take the herbs, vitamins, minerals and supplements, recommended above.
- Make sure that you are properly hydrated.
- Care for your immune system by avoiding sugars, "bad fats" and alcohol and making sure you exercise only in moderation.

Obviously if a more deadly version of Swine Flu hits, you will be doing everything that you can to avoid catching it. However, it is vital to take care not to get ill from dangerous opportunistic infections other than Swine Flu.

One example of this is diarrhoea that can occur if you are drinking water that is not as clean as it should be. This can rapidly lead to severe problems and needs to be taken seriously. If you do get a bout of diarrhoea remember to take your ORS and also take any of the following:

HERBS

- Psyllium husks/seeds
- Carob
- Chamomile

SUPPLEMENTS

- Acidophilus
- Sb
- MultiVitamins
- Charcoal tablets
- Garlic
- Kelp
- Potassium

Summary of Recommendations

- Omega 3

HOMEOPATHY

- Arsenicum
- Croton Tig
- Gratiola
- Colocynthus
- China

STAGE THREE: WHAT TO DO IF YOU CATCH SWINE FLU

COMPLEMENTARY MEDICAL APPROACHES:

Depending on type of flu, take one of these homeopathic remedies every 2 hours, or as frequently as needed. You will be able to judge the frequency that you need by carefully noticing whether symptoms are changing. If symptoms improve, reduce the frequency of dosage – if they worsen, increase the frequency - or consider changing the remedy.

- Gelsemium
- Bryonia
- Aconite
- Arnica
- Arsenicum Album
- Baptisia
- Belladonna
- Eupatorium Perfoliatum
- Mercurius Solubilis
- Nux Vomica
- Rhus Toxicodendron

Carry on taking the Multi-Vitamin/Mineral, Herbs, Omega 3 and Whey Protein as in your preparation phase. Consider too the other anti-inflammatory supplements that we cover in this book.

If you can, try to follow the Palæo-Mediterranean Diet as much as possible.

CONVENTIONAL MEDICINE

If you do choose to use Conventional Medical anti-viral drugs such as Tamiflu – and you can get them, you need to make sure that you take these within 48 hours of the onset of Swine Flu for them to stand a chance of being effective. Before giving Tamiflu to children under twelve, please check current medical guidelines - as undesireable side effects have occured in young children and some more vulnerable adults.

STAGE FOUR: AFTER EFFECTS OF A SERIOUS PANDEMIC

You should continue to take the Multi-Vitamin/Minerals, Herbs, Omega 3 and Whey Protein as outlined above, make sure you are properly hydrated and in addition the following suggestions may have some benefit:

ADAPTOGENS

Adaptogens such as the following may be of use after an H1N1 infection, however there is much research still to be done to ascertain if this is indeed the case. We will report our findings in our CMA Monthly e-Newsletter Updates available via The Complementary Medical Association's website (The-CMA.Org.UK). Effective adaptogens include:

- Ginseng
- Rhodiola Rosea
- Liquorice
- Ashwagandha
- Sutherlandia
- Immune boosting Fungi such as Trametes

OTHER IMMUNE BOOSTING HERBS

As mentioned, you must continue to take the anti-inflammatory, anti-viral, anti-bacterial herbs that we recommend for general use.

In addition, if you are recovering from a bout of Swine Flu, it is possible that at this stage Echinacea and Black Elderberry may well come into their own. These herbs boost your immune system and they may well protect you from any opportunistic infections that might occur after H1N1 infection.

A post viral opportunistic infection (bacterial pneumonia) was a pattern seen in the Spanish Flu of 1918 and killed many people. It is vital to remember that **these herbs should not be taken to treat Swine Flu** as research indicates that they can increase levels of the cytokines that are thought to be responsible for the Cytokine Storm phenomenon.

In order to find a qualified homeopath, naturopath, nutritionist, herbalist or any other professional, fully qualified practitioner, please visit The Complementary Medical Association's website (The-CMA.Org.UK). Over the next few months, The CMA will be expanding their databases to include the names of homeopaths and other qualified practitioners country by country.

(If you are a qualified practitioner and feel that you should be included in this database please email The CMA; Info@The-CMA.Org.UK

APPENDIX

THE SIX PHASES OF A PANDEMIC

Experts at the World Health Organisation (WHO) have been preparing for a worldwide influenza pandemic in recent years. They were responding to the effects of Bird Flu and what could happen if this started to spread easily amongst the human population. Now, with the virulent spread of Swine Flu the world is now officially in the middle of a pandemic caused by influenza.

In the last century there were three major pandemics and it has been almost 40 years since the last one in 1968.

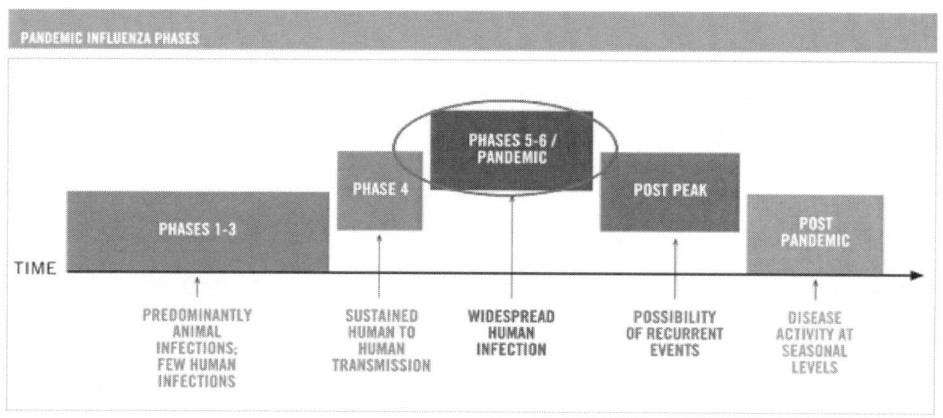

http://www.who.int/csr/disease/avian_influenza/phase/en/

The WHO has a grading system to monitor the progression of a pandemic and they list six separate phases, from 1 to 6, with 6 being the most dangerous level. This six-level alert system acts as a method of informing the world of the importance of the threat. It also helps countries, Governments, industry and even individuals to be aware of the need to take increasingly more intense preparedness activities.

OFFICIAL WHO DEFINITIONS

Phase 1 In nature, influenza viruses circulate continuously among animals, especially birds. Even though such viruses might theoretically develop into pandemic viruses, in Phase 1 no viruses circulating among animals have been reported to cause infections in humans.

In Phase 2 an animal influenza virus circulating among domesticated or wild animals is known to have caused infection in humans, and is therefore considered a potential pandemic threat.

In Phase 3, an animal or human-animal influenza reassortment virus has caused sporadic cases or small clusters of disease in people, but has not resulted in human-to-human transmission sufficient to sustain community-level outbreaks. Limited human-to-human transmission may occur under some circumstances, for example, when there is close contact between an infected person and an unprotected caregiver. However, limited transmission under such restricted circumstances does not indicate that the virus has gained the level of transmissibility among humans necessary to cause a pandemic.

Phase 4 is characterized by verified human-to-human transmission of an animal or human-animal influenza reassortant virus able to cause "community-level outbreaks." The ability to cause sustained disease outbreaks in a community marks a significant upwards shift in the risk for a pandemic. Any country that suspects or has verified such an event should urgently consult with WHO so that the situation can be jointly assessed and a decision made by the affected country if implementation of a rapid pandemic containment operation is warranted. Phase 4 indicates a significant increase in risk of a pandemic but does not necessarily mean that a pandemic is a foregone conclusion.

Phase 5 is characterized by human-to-human spread of the virus into at least two countries in one WHO region. While most countries will not be affected at this stage, the declaration of Phase 5 is a strong signal that a pandemic is imminent and that the time to finalize the organization, communication, and implementation of the planned mitigation measures is short.

Phase 6, the pandemic phase, is characterized by community level outbreaks in at least one other country in a different WHO region in addition to the criteria defined in Phase 5. Designation of this phase will indicate that a global pandemic is under way.

During the post-peak period, pandemic disease levels in most countries with adequate surveillance will have dropped below peak observed levels. The post-peak period signifies that pandemic activity appears to be decreasing; however, it is uncertain if additional waves will occur and countries will need to be prepared for a second wave.

Previous pandemics have been characterized by waves of activity spread over months. Once the level of disease activity drops, a critical communications task will be to balance this information with the possibility of another wave. Pandemic waves can be separated by months and an immediate "at-ease" signal may be premature.

In the **post-pandemic period**, influenza disease activity will have returned to levels normally seen for seasonal influenza. It is expected that the pandemic virus will behave as a seasonal influenza A virus. At this stage, it is important to maintain surveillance and update pandemic preparedness and response plans accordingly. An intensive phase of recovery and evaluation may be required.

Source: WHO; http://www.who.int/csr/disease/avian_influenza/phase/en/

Changes from one phase to another are triggered by several factors, which include the epidemiological behaviour of the disease and the characteristics of circulating viruses. The Director-General of WHO decides the level of the phase and also makes decisions on when to move from one phase to another.

On April 27th 2009, the WHO upgraded the current Swine Flu outbreak to a Level 4.

Two days later on April 29th it raised its Pandemic Alert status to Level 5.

On June 11th the WHO announced that the criteria for a pandemic have been met and moves to Level 6. (http://www.searo.who.int/LinkFiles/Influenza_A(H1N1)_Chronology_of_Influenza_A(H1N1).pdf)

During this Pandemic stage little public unrest has occurred as Swine Flu continues to spread, and the call on public health resources around the world has been manageable. There have been no shortages of health treatments.

If the Swine Flu virus does mutate to cause higher lethality, civil unrest might occur, similar to, but on a much larger scale than the problems seen with Hurricane Katrina.

The Survivor's Guide to Swine Flu

IN THE EVENT THAT YOU DO BECOME ILL, USE THE FOLLOWING FORM TO MAKE A NOTE OF ANY CONDITIONS THAT YOU AND YOUR FAMILY MEMBERS MAY HAVE – IN THE EVENT THAT YOU ARE UNABLE TO REPORT THESE TO MEDICAL STAFF.

Name

Any Existing Medical Conditions

Allergies/Sensitivities

Blood Type

Current Medications/Dosages

Current Symptoms

The Survivor's Guide to Swine Flu

USE THIS FORM TO MAKE A NOTE OF ANY EMERGENCY CONTACTS THAT MIGHT BE IMPORTANT. CARRY THIS LIST WITH YOU AND MAKE SURE YOUR FAMILY DOES TOO. IF YOU ARE TRAVELLING ABROAD DO MAKE SURE THAT TELEPHONE NUMBERS ARE IN THE INTERNATIONAL DIALLING CODE FORMAT FOR ACCESS TO YOUR COUNTRY.

Contacts Name/Phone Number

Next of Kin/Emergency Contact

Hospitals near: Work   School   Home

General Practitioner/Family Doctor

Pharmacy

Employer contact and emergency information

School contact and emergency information

Religious/spiritual organisation – if appropriate

Qualified Homeopath

Qualified Herbalist

Qualified Nutritionist

Other Complementary Medical Practitioner

Remember to put an 'In Case of Emergency' (ICE) number into your mobile phone - this should be the contact number for your next of kin - or someone that you would want to be contacted in an emergency situation. Emergency service personnel are trained to scroll though a mobile phone's address book to try to find an ICE number. You might want to save various contact numbers such as ICE Mum, ICE Brother, and so on.